OXFORD MEDICAL PUBLICATIONS

Echocardiography

Published and forthcoming Oxford Specialist Handbooks

General Oxford Specialist Handbooks
A Resuscitation Room Guide (Banerjee and Hargreaves)

Oxford Specialist Handbooks in End of Life
Cardiology: From advanced disease to bereavement (Beattie, Connelly, and Watson)
Nephrology: From advanced disease to bereavement (Brown, Chambers, and Eggeling)

Oxford Specialist Handbooks in Anaesthesia
Cardiac Anaesthesia (Barnard and Martin eds.)
Neuroanaesthesia (Nathanson and Moppett eds.)
Obstetric Anaesthesia (Clyburn, Collis, Harries, and Davies eds.)
Paediatric Anaesthesia (Doyle ed.)

Oxford Specialist Handbooks in Cardiology
Cardiac Catheterisation and Coronary Intervention. (Mitchell, West, Leeson, Banning)
Pacemakers and ICDs (Timperley, Leeson, Mitchell and Betts eds.)
Echocardiography (Leeson, Mitchell, and Becher eds.)
Heart Failure (Gardner, McDonagh and Walker)
Nuclear Cardiology (Kelion, Loong, and Sabharwal)

Oxford Specialist Handbooks in Neurology
Epilepsy (Alarcon, Nashaf, Cross, and Nightingale)
Parkinson's Disease and Other Movement Disorders (Edwards, Bhatia, Quinn, and Swinn)

Oxford Specialist Handbooks in Paediatrics
Paediatric Gastroenterology, Hepatology, and Nutrition (Beattie, Dhawan, and Puntis eds.)
Paediatric Nephrology (Rees, Webb, and Brogan)
Paediatric Neurology (Forsyth and Newton eds.)
Paediatric Oncology and Haematology (Bailey and Skinner eds.)
Paediatric Radiology (Johnson, Williams, and Foster)

Oxford Specialist Handbooks in Surgery
Hand Surgery (Warwick)
Neurosurgery (Samandouras)
Otolaryngology and Head and Neck Surgery (Corbridge and Warner)
Renal Transplantation (Talbot)
Urology (Reynard, Sullivan, Turner, Feneley, Armenakas, and Mark eds.)
Vascular Surgery (Hands, Murphy, Sharp, and Ray-Chauduri)

Oxford Specialist Handbooks in
Cardiology

Echocardiography

Edited by

Paul Leeson
Honorary Consultant Cardiologist,
John Radcliffe Hospital, and
BHF Clinical Science Fellow,
University of Oxford,
Oxford, UK

Andrew R.J. Mitchell
Consultant Cardiologist,
Jersey General Hospital,
Jersey, Channel Islands, and
Honorary Consultant Cardiologist,
John Radcliffe Hospital,
Oxford, UK

and

Harald Becher
Consultant Cardiologist,
John Radcliffe Hospital, and
Professor of Cardiac Ultrasound,
University of Oxford,
Oxford, UK

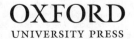

OXFORD
UNIVERSITY PRESS

OXFORD
UNIVERSITY PRESS

Great Clarendon Street, Oxford OX2 6DP

Oxford University Press is a department of the University of Oxford.
It furthers the University's objective of excellence in research, scholarship,
and education by publishing worldwide in

Oxford New York

Auckland Cape Town Dar es Salaam Hong Kong Karachi
Kuala Lumpur Madrid Melbourne Mexico City Nairobi
New Delhi Shanghai Taipei Toronto

With offices in

Argentina Austria Brazil Chile Czech Republic France Greece
Guatemala Hungary Italy Japan Poland Portugal Singapore
South Korea Switzerland Thailand Turkey Ukraine Vietnam

Oxford is a registered trade mark of Oxford University Press
in the UK and in certain other countries

Published in the United States
by Oxford University Press Inc., New York

© Oxford University Press, 2007

British Library Cataloguing in Publication Data

Data available

Library of Congress Cataloging in Publication Data

Data available

Typeset by Newgen Imaging Systems (P) Ltd., Chennai, India
Printed in China
on acid-free paper
through Asia Pacific Offset.

ISBN 978–0–19–921575–1 (flexicover: alk.paper)

10 9 8 7 6 5 4 3 2

Foreword

> 'A picture is worth ten thousand words'—Chinese proverb.
> 'Mutum est pictura poema' (A picture is a mute poem.)—Latin proverb.
> 'What is the use of a book,' thought Alice, 'without pictures or
> conversations?'—Lewis Carroll.

What, after all, is echocardiography but pictures of the heart? Do we need another book on echocardiography—about pictures of the heart? After reading this fine volume I can answer unequivocally yes. I have been an echocardiographer for over thirty-five years, beginning with my intro-duction to echocardiography as a Fellow at Stanford University Medical Center in the late 1960s and continuing through many years directing the Echocardiography laboratory at the University of Iowa. I was, as a former American Secretary of State put it, 'Present at the creation', participating in the founding of the American Society of Echocardiography and later serving as its President. I watched the field develop through the 'ice pick' days of M-mode echocardiography, to the introduction of two-dimensional echo—initially as crude parallel linear echos, then moving on to the fami-liar sector format. Along came Doppler flow velocity, tissue Doppler, three and four-dimensional echo, transesophageal echo, and intracardiac echo.

Each of these advances has been accompanied by fine volumes, written by names that continue to resonate in our field: Feigenbaum, Weyman, Nanda, Seward, Tajik, Otto, and far too many others to list. Why, then, another book?

As Dr. Johnson said, 'Painting can illustrate but cannot inform'. This manual of echocardiography is special because it goes past the simply illustrative. The book informs by extensive use of tables and graphs, as well as text. Look, for example, at Chapter 6 on Stress Echocardio-graphy. Besides excellent illustrations, this chapter includes detailed technical points on patient preparation, instrument set up and perform-ance, avoiding artifacts, exercise and pharmacologic protocols, pre-op assessment; even sample consent documents and reporting schemes are provided.

This volume is constructed to be maximally useful to both novices and experienced personnel, echocardiographers, and sonographers. Emerging from one of the leading academic centers in the United Kingdom, it is a major achievement, both as a technical manual and an authoritative source. Clinical practice will be reinforced by this volume, while neo-phytes will find it an invaluable reference. A major diagnostic technology in cardiovascular disease deserves and is well served by this important contribution. Use it and enjoy it.

Richard E. Kerber, MD, FASE, FAHA, FACC
Past President, American Society of Echocardiography
Professor of Medicine and Emergency Medicine
University of Iowa, USA

Preface

Echocardiography remains the most important non-invasive cardiac investigation. During the last decade, exciting new technologies have become available—transoesophageal echocardiography, complex Doppler, and stress echocardiography studies are now routinely performed in a large number of hospitals.

This handbook originates from the demands of our trainees and sonographers for practical guidelines that describe how to apply current imaging technology to address the common key issues in adult echocardiography. The book follows the natural workflow of echocardiography, detailing what to record and how to analyse and report studies. The British and American Society of Echocardiography and the European Association of Echocardiography have also started to provide guidelines for specific questions. Therefore this handbook incorporates all the current guidelines relevant to clinical practice.

The book was designed as a comprehensive compendium of focused approaches for specific clinical questions. We hope it will be used both as a means to learn how to perform echocardiography and as a trusted, easily accessible reference for those who are already proficient.

PL
ARJM
HB

Acknowledgements

We would like to express our sincere thanks to the many individuals who read the text during its preparation and gave advice on its development.

Contents

Contributors

We would like to express our sincere thanks to the following people for their expert contributions and advice that were used as the basis for the following sections (in alphabetical order):

John Chambers
Consultant Cardiologist,
Cardiothoracic Centre,
Guy's and St. Thomas'
Hospital, London, UK
Chapter 3: Aortic stenosis

Jonathan Goldman
Consultant Cardiologist,
VA Hospital, San Francisco,
CA, USA.
*Chapter 3: Left ventricular and
left atrial measures*

Andreas Haggendorf
Professor of Cardiac Medicine,
University of Leipzig, Germany
*Chapter 2: Echocardiography
views*

Lucy Hudsmith
SpR in Cardiology, John Radcliffe
Hospital, Oxford, UK.
*Chapter 3: Tricuspid and
pulmonary valves*

Xu Yu Jin
Consultant Surgical Echocardiolo-
gist, John Radcliffe Hosptial,
Oxford, UK.
*Chapter 5: Intraoperative tran-
soesophageal echocardiography*

Graham Leech
Honorary Consultant
Clinical Scientist, St George's
Hospital, London, UK
Chapter 1: Ultrasound

Tom Marwick
Professor of Medicine,
University of Queensland,
and Director of Echocardiography,
Princess Alexandra Hospital
Brisbane, Australia.
*Chapter 3: Left ventricular
function*

Michael Stewart
Consultant Cardiologist, The James
Cook University Hospital,
Middlesbrough, UK.
Chapters 3 and 5: Aorta

Jonathan Timperley
SpR in Cardiology, John Radcliffe
Hospital, Oxford, UK.
Chapters 3 and 5: Mitral stenosis

All other sections were written by Paul Leeson and Harald Becher.
The text was illustrated by Paul Leeson.
Paul Leeson, Andrew Mitchell, and Harald Becher edited the book.

Symbols and abbreviations

↓	decreased
↑	increased
↔	normal
2D	two-dimensional
3D	three-dimensional
A	A-wave velocity
Ao	aorta
AR	aortic regurgitation
AS	aortic stenosis
ASD	atrial septal defect
AV	aortic valve
CFM	colour flow mapping
CO	cardiac output
CT	computerized tomography
CW	continuous wave (Doppler)
d	diastole
DET	deceleration time
E	E-wave velocity
ECG	electrocardiogram
ed	end diastole
EROA	effective regurgitant orifice area
es	end systole
ETT	exercise tolerance test
FS	fractional shortening
Hep. V	hepatic veins
IV	intravenous
IVC	inferior vena cava
IVRT	isovolumetric relaxation time
IVS	interventricular septum
IVSd	interventricular septum diastolic diameter
IVSs	interventricular septum systolic diameter
JVP	jugular venous pressure
LA	left atrium
LAA	left atrial appendage
LAs	left atrial systolic diameter
LCC	left coronary cusp
LLPV	left lower pulmonary vein

LUPV	left upper pulmonary vein
LV	left ventricle
LVDd	left ventricular diastolic diameter
LVDs	left ventricular systolic diameter
LVID	left ventricular internal diameter
LVOT	left ventricular outflow tract
LVPW	left ventricular posterior wall
LVPWd	left ventricular posterior wall diastolic thickness
LVPWs	left ventricular posterior wall systolic thickness
MI	mechanical index
MR	mitral regurgitation
MS	mitral stenosis
MV	mitral valve
MVA	mitral valve area
NCC	non-coronary cusp
NYHA	New York Heart Association
P1/2 time	pressure half time
Pmax	peak pressure
Pmean	mean pressure
PA	pulmonary artery
PDA	patent ductus arteriosus
PFO	patent foramen ovale
PHT	pressure half time
PISA	proximal isovelocity surface area
PR	pulmonary regurgitation
PS	pulmonary stenosis
PV	pulmonary valve
PW	pulsed wave (Doppler) *or* posterior wall
RA	right atrium
RAA	right atrial appendage
RCC	right coronary cusp
RLPV	right lower pulmonary vein
RUPV	right upper pulmonary vein
RV	right ventricle
RVd	right ventricular diastolic diameter
RVOT	right ventricular outflow tract
s	systole
SAX	short axis
SV	stroke volume
SVC	superior vena cava
TDI	tissue Doppler imaging
TOE	tranoesophageal echocardiography

TOE	tranoesophageal echocardiography
TR	tricuspid regurgitation
TV	tricuspid valve
Vmax	peak velocity
Vmean	mean velocity
vti	velocity time integral
VSD	ventricular septal defect

References

Reference textbooks

Feigenbaum, H. *Echocardiography*, 6th edition. Lippincott, Williams, & Wilkins 2004.

Otto CM. *Textbook of clinical echocardiography*, 3rd edition. WB Saunders and Co Ltd 2004.

Perrino AC, Reeves ST. *A practical approach to transesophageal echocardiography*. Lippincott Williams, & Wilkins 2003.

Rimmington H, Chambers J. *Echocardiography: guidelines for reporting—a practical handbook*. Taylor and Francis. 1998.

Sidebotham D, Merry A, Legget M, Bashein G. *Practical perioperative transoesophageal echocardiography*. Butterworth–Heinemann Ltd 2003.

Websites

American Society of Echocardiography: http://www.asecho.org
British Society of Echocardiography: http://www.bsecho.org
European Association of Echocardiography:
http://www.escardio.org/bodies/associations/EAE
American Heart Association: http://www.americanheart.org/
British Cardiovascular Society: http://www.bcs.com/
European Society of Cardiology: http://www.escardio.org/
British Heart Foundation: http://www.bhf.org.uk/

Papers and guidelines

Recommendations for Evaluation of the Severity of Native Valvular Regurgitation with Two-dimensional and Doppler Echocardiography. A report from the American Society of Echocardiography's Nomenclature and Standards Committee and The Task Force on Valvular Regurgitation, developed in conjunction with the American College of Cardiology Echocardiography Committee, The Cardiac Imaging Committee Council on Clinical Cardiology, the American Heart Association, and the European Society of Cardiology Working Group on Echocardiography. *J Am Soc Echocardiogr* 2003; **16**: 777–802.

Recommendations for Chamber Quantification: A Report of the American Society of Echocardiography Guidelines and Standards Committee and the Chamber Quantification Writing Group, Developed in Conjunction with the European Association of Echocardiography. *J Am Soc Echocardiogr* 2005; **18**: 1440–1463.

Waggoner AD, Ehler D, Adams D, Moos S, Resenbloom J, Gresser C, Perez JE, Douglas PS. Guidelines for the Cardiac Sonographer in the Performance of Contrast Echocardiography: Recommendations of the American Society of Echocardiography. *J Am Soc Echocardiogr* 2001; **14**: 417–420.

Chambers J, Masani N, Hancock J, Graham J, Wharton G, Ionescu A. A Minimum Dataset for a Standard Adult Transthoracic Echocardiogram. From the British Society of Echocardiography Education Committee.

Masani N, Chambers J, Hancock J, Graham J, Wharton G. BSE Echocardiogram Report: Recommendations for Standard Adult Transthoracic Echocardiography. From the British Society of Echocardiography Education Committee.

Becher H, Chambers J, Fox K, Jones R, Leech GJ, Masani N, Monaghan M, More R, Nihoyannopoulos P, Rimington H, Senior R, Warton G; British Society of Echocardiography Policy Committee. BSE procedure guidelines for the clinical application of stress echocardiography, recommendations for performance and interpretation of stress echocardiography: a report of the British Society of Echocardiography Policy Committee. *Heart* 2004 Dec; **90** Suppl 6: vi 23–30.

The following tables and figure are adapted from *J Am Soc Echocardiography* 2003 and 2005 with permission from the American Society of Echocardiography: Tables 3.2, 3.5, 3.7, 3.9, 3.11, 3.12, 3.17, 3.18, 3.19, 5.1, 5.4, 5.5, 5.6, 5.8, 5.9, 5.10, 7.1, 7.2, 7.3, 7.4, 7.6, and 7.8, and Fig. 7.1.

The minimal dataset in Chapter 2 and reporting descriptive terms in Chapter 7 have been adapted with permission from the British Society of Echocardiography guidelines.

Detailed contents

Ultrasound

Introduction

Modern cardiac ultrasound scanners are very sophisticated. They generate real-time moving images of the heart, together with quantitative data on blood flow and tissue motion displayed either as 2D tomographic ('slice') images or, more recently, rendered 3D 'volume' images.

It is not necessary for a user to know how a computer processes data, so it is reasonable to ask why clinical users need to know how echo machines work. The justification for including this chapter is that some knowledge of the principles of ultrasound imaging is fundamental to understanding clinical applications. Limitations both of fundamental physics and current technology can result in image distortion and artefacts that might result in misdiagnoses. Also, an understanding of the concepts behind how images are generated helps the operator to optimize, interpret, and analyse images.

Echocardiography employs high frequency sound waves to generate images of the heart and to detect blood flow within the cardiac chambers and blood vessels. It was originally developed from marine sonar and there are many similarities between the ways in which information from echocardiography and that from a depth-sounder are gathered and displayed. The physical principles underlying imaging of the heart's structure and studying blood flow are fundamentally different, and will be considered separately, but in practice images and blood flow data are usually displayed and recorded superimposed or concurrently.

The echo machine derives a great deal of information from echoes generated from the ultrasound beam it transmits into the body. These include: specular echoes from which real-time 2D/3D images and M-mode traces are formed to study cardiac structures and their motion patterns; and Doppler signals backscattered from blood and tissues that can be processed to provide spectral displays and colour flow maps. Additional processing produces derived data such as strain rate and power mode imaging. It can be likened to a toolkit, all powered by a single source, the ultrasound beam. Each tool has its own particular applications; to use it optimally requires appreciation of its features, strengths, and weaknesses. Together they form a powerful, non-invasive diagnostic armoury, which has revolutionized cardiac diagnosis in almost every area of clinical activity from primary care to the operating room.

Basic concepts

Vibrations are transmitted through a solid, liquid, or gaseous medium as pressure fluctuations—waves of alternating compression and rarefaction. In soft body tissues pressure waves travel at about 1500m/sec (compared with 300m/sec in air).

Velocity, frequency, and wavelength

- There is a fundamental relationship between propagation velocity, the frequency (pitch) of the waves, and their wavelength (the distance between two successive maxima or minima in the train of pressure cycles). This states that:

    propagation velocity = frequency × wavelength

- Thus, in soft body tissues, at a frequency of 1000Hz (= Hertz, or cycles per second), the wavelength is 1.5m. Common sense dictates that this wavelength is too great to image the heart, which is only about 15cm across and which contains structures less than 1mm thick. To achieve a wavelength of 1mm, the frequency has to be 1,500,000Hz, or 1.5MHz.
- The human ear responds only to frequencies from about 30Hz to 15,000Hz, and, since the word *sound* implies a sensation generated in the brain, the term *ultrasound* is used to describe the frequencies used in echocardiography.

Reflection, refraction, diffraction

Pressure waves and light waves share many properties.
- When a beam of light passes from one medium to another, part of the energy is reflected and the path of the transmitted portion is deviated by refraction. In the same way, when pressure waves encounter an interface between two different body tissues, blood and muscle, for example, some of the incident energy is reflected. Such echoes are called 'specular' (mirror-like).
- Another characteristic shared by light and pressure waves is diffraction, whereby the path of the waves 'bends' around the edge of an obstacle. The degree to which this is apparent depends on the relative sizes of the wavelength and the obstacle. Thus sound waves, whose wavelength in air is of the order of 1m, appear to bend around a given obstacle much more than light waves, having a wavelength of 0.000,001m. Ultrasound used for medical imaging typically has a wavelength of the order of 0.001m (1mm), almost exactly half-way between that of sound and light. Ultrasound can therefore be thought of as being similar to a rather poorly focused flashlight; it can be aimed at regions of the heart of interest, but is far from an infinitely fine 'laser' probe.

Compression waves

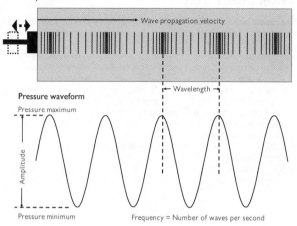

Fig. 1.1 Features of a wave.

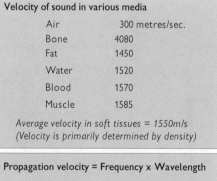

Velocity of sound in various media	
Air	300 metres/sec.
Bone	4080
Fat	1450
Water	1520
Blood	1570
Muscle	1585

*Average velocity in soft tissues = 1550m/s
(Velocity is primarily determined by density)*

Propagation velocity = Frequency x Wavelength

1550 metres/sec. = 1000Hz × 155cm

= 2.5MHz × 0.62mm

= 3.5MHz × 0.44mm

= 5.0MHz × 0.31mm

= 7.0MHz × 0.22mm

Fig. 1.2 Waves and velocity.

Transducer

The transducer (or 'probe') held on the patient's chest transmits ultrasound waves into the thorax and detects echoes returning from the heart and great vessels.

- It contains a bank of very thin slices of a ceramic material that exhibits strong *piezoelectric* properties. This means that it changes its shape when an electric potential is applied and, conversely, generates electricity when mechanically deformed. There are typically 128 slices with total area $2 \times 1cm^2$, each connected by a wire to the machine.
- The frequency that is generated as the crystals vibrate is determined by their mechanical dimensions, in the same way that a bell vibrates when struck by a hammer.
- Transducers for echocardiography typically generate frequencies in the range 1.5–7MHz.
- Since the *piezoelectric effect* is reversible, the same crystal can be used to detect returning echoes from ultrasonic waves it has generated.

Piezoelectricity

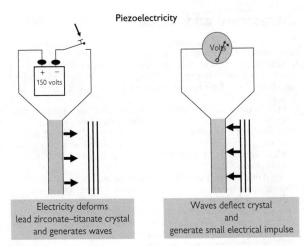

Electricity deforms
lead zirconate–titanate crystal
and generates waves

Waves deflect crystal
and
generate small electrical impulse

Fig. 1.3 Piezoelectric effect.

Ultrasound and tissue

To form an image of the heart, a stream of very brief 'pulses' of ultra-sonic waves, each comprising just a few waves and lasting 1–2μsec (microseconds), is transmitted into the thorax. As each pulse traverses the chest wall and enters the pericardium and the heart, it encounters a succession of interfaces between different types of tissue: blood, muscle, fat, etc.

- A proportion of the incident energy is reflected at each interface, the remainder being transmitted into deeper tissue layers.
- Provided that the interfaces are extensive compared to the ultrasound wavelength, the reflections are *specular* (mirror-like) with the angle of reflection equal to the angle of incidence with respect to a normal to the interface.
- Only if the incident angle is 90° will the reflected waves re-trace the incident path and return to the transducer as an echo. This is not always easy to achieve in practice and limits the quality of signals from many cardiac structures, though the fact that body tissue interfaces are not totally smooth allows return of some echoes even if the interface is not perpendicular to the ultrasound beam.
- The transmitted portion of the ultrasound pulse may then encounter additional interfaces and further echoes return to the transducer.
- The time delay between transmission of an ultrasound pulse and arrival of an echo back at the transducer (round-trip-time) is given by:

    time delay = 2 × interface distance/propagation velocity

- Thus, if the propagation velocity is known and the time delay can be measured, the distance of each echo-generating interface from the transducer can be determined.
- It is important to note that the machine actually measures *time delay* and derives the *distance* from an assumed value for the propagation velocity in soft tissues. It follows that, if the ultrasound passes through an object having different transmission characteristics from soft tissue, e.g. a silicone ball valve prosthesis, the time delay of returning echoes will change and the derived distance measurements will be false.
- The total time for all echoes to return depends on the distance of the furthest structure of interest. If this is 20cm, the round trip time is approximately 260μsec. Only then can a second ultrasound pulse be transmitted, but even so it is possible to send about 3750 pulses each second. This stream of brief pulses is referred to as an *ultrasound beam*.

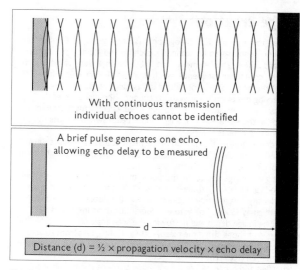

Fig. 1.4 Continuous wave and pulsed wave.

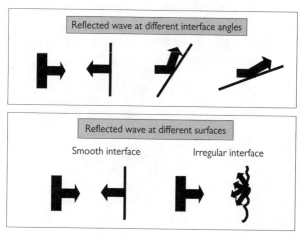

Fig. 1.5 Waves and interfaces.

Image creation

In order to generate 2D tomographic (slice) images of the heart, the ultrasound beam has to be scanned rapidly to and fro across a section of the heart. The crystal elements are activated in a very rapid and very precisely controlled sequence, such that small 'wavelets' from each element merge to form a compound ultrasound wave.

- By varying the electrical activation sequence, the direction of the compound wave can be changed and a sequence forms the sector of an arc, in the same way that a lighthouse beam sweeps across the sea, illuminating objects in its path.
- In order to 'freeze' the motion of the heart at least 25 images per second are required. For a working depth of 20cm, each image comprises about 150 individual scan lines.
- For a given image depth, the maximum number of pulses per second is fixed, and there is a trade-off between the sector angle and image line density. Image frame rate is shown on the display screen and may be as high as $150sec^{-1}$ or as low as $6sec^{-1}$. It can be improved by reducing image depth and narrowing the scan angle.
- Returning echoes strike the piezoelectric crystals, first from structures closest to the transducer, followed in succession by those from more distant interfaces. The minute electrical signals thus generated are amplified and processed to form a visual display showing the relative distances of reflecting structures from the transducer, with the signal intensities providing some information about the nature of the interfaces.

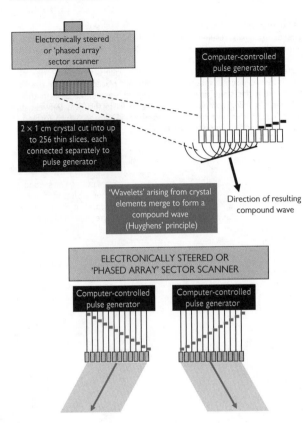

Fig. 1.6 Phased array probes.

2D images

The echo signals resulting from a single ultrasound pulse comprise a sequence of electronic 'blips' representing the intensities of the echo reflections. To facilitate further processing these are digitized, or converted into a series of numbers, whose values represent the echo amplitudes at discrete intervals and which are placed in a digital memory store. From this stage onward, the image is represented by a matrix of numbers, enabling computer processing to fill in the gaps between the original scan lines and create a 'smoothed' 2D image, which forms the visual display on the monitor screen.

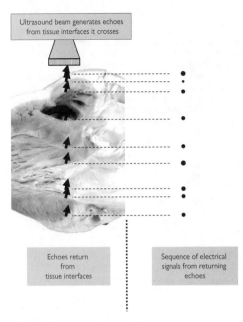

Ultrasound beam generates echoes from tissue interfaces it crosses

Echoes return from tissue interfaces

Sequence of electrical signals from returning echoes

Fig. 1.7 Ultrasound and tissue interfaces.

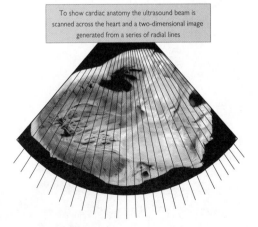

To show cardiac anatomy the ultrasound beam is scanned across the heart and a two-dimensional image generated from a series of radial lines

Fig. 1.8 2D image generation.

M-mode

If the direction of the ultrasound beam is fixed, it interrogates structures along a single axis, a so-called 'ice-pick' or 'needle biopsy' view with tissue interfaces represented as dots on the display screen.

• In order to show motion patterns, a linear sweep is added resulting in a graphic display. This type of display (called M-mode because it demonstrates motion) still offers important benefits.

• It shows data from several cardiac cycles on a single image; it provides temporal continuity making it easier, for example, to identify a structure such as the endocardium from background clutter; and it has far greater temporal resolution (1000 lines/sec compared to 25 lines/sec for a 2D image) making it superior for accurate timing and resolution of rapid movements.

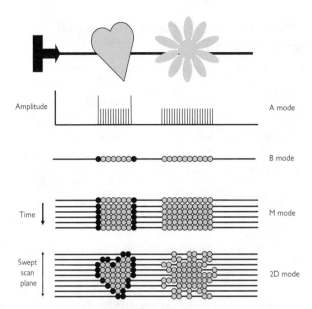

Fig. 1.9 Types of image. A (amplitude) mode traces amplitude of a reflection against distance from probe (of historical interest as one of the first types of ultrasound image). B (brightness) mode represents amplitude as intensity or brightness of a dot. M (motion) mode traces change in brightness over time. 2D images are generated from sweeping across the field of interest.

M-mode images show structures intersected by a stationary ultrasound beam

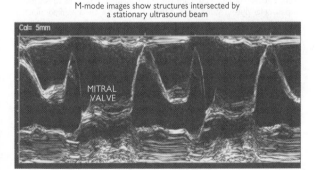

Fig. 1.10 Example of M-mode.

Attenuation, reflection, and depth compensation

Ultrasound waves are quite severely attenuated as they pass through 'spongy' tissues such as fat and muscle. The degree of attenuation depends greatly on the ultrasound frequency.

- At 2.5MHz, approximately half of the amplitude is lost for every 4cm of path length, rising to half per 2cm at 5MHz and half in only 1cm at 7.5MHz. This is a cumulative effect so at 5MHz the wave amplitude reaching a structure 16cm distant is only 1/256, i.e. $(1/2)^8$ of that transmitted.
- The proportion reflected at a tissue interface depends mainly on the difference in density of the tissues. Where there is a large difference, such as an interface with air or bone, most of the incident wave is reflected, creating an intense echo but leaving little to penetrate further to deeper structures. It is for this reason that the operator has to manipulate the transducer to avoid ribs and lungs and that a contact gel is used to eliminate any air between the transducer and the chest wall.
- In contrast, there is relatively little difference in the densities of blood, muscle, and fat, so echoes from interfaces between them are very small—about 0.1% of the incident amplitude.
- The echoes are then further attenuated on the return path to the transducer, with the result that the detected signal is very small indeed. In the case illustrated above, approximately $(1/256) \times (1/1000) \times (1/256)$ or just 1/65,000,000 of the transmitted amplitude!
- Not only is this a very small signal to detect, but the amplification level required would be vastly greater than that needed for the same interface closer to the transducer. To overcome this problem, the machine provides *depth compensation* or *time-gain compensation* (TGC). This automatically increases the amplification during the time echoes from a particular pulse return, so that the last to arrive are amplified much more than the first.
- Most of this compensation is built into the machine, but the user can fine-tune it by means of a bank of slider controls that adjust the amplification at selected depths.
- The reflection and attenuation characteristics of various media can be used to help in their identification. In particular, an interface with air generates a very strong reflection at the proximal boundary, beyond which the air strongly attenuates the beam casting a dark shadow.

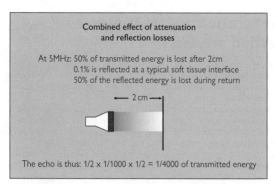

**Combined effect of attenuation
and reflection losses**

At 5MHz: 50% of transmitted energy is lost after 2cm
0.1% is reflected at a typical soft tissue interface
50% of the reflected energy is lost during return

←— 2 cm —→

The echo is thus: 1/2 × 1/1000 × 1/2 = 1/4000 of transmitted energy

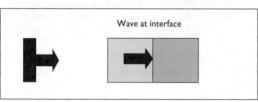

Wave at interface

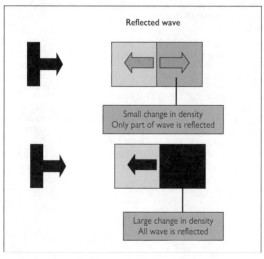

Reflected wave

Small change in density
Only part of wave is reflected

Large change in density
All wave is reflected

Fig. 1.11 Attenuation.

Reverberation and multiple reflection artefacts

The presence of structures with transmission and attenuation characteristics greatly different from those of soft tissue is the cause of reverberation and multiple reflection artefacts, one of the most common sources of misinterpretation of images.

- An ultrasound beam encountering a structure normally generates two echoes—one from each interface. However, the echo returning from the distal interface has to cross the proximal interface, so part of it is again reflected. This process repeats, resulting in multiple images.
- Under normal circumstances this effect is not seen because soft-tissue reflections are so weak. Thus, if the original echo is 0.1% of the incident wave, the secondary echo has undergone two further reflections and is only (0.1% × 0.1% × 0.1%) and too small to register. If, however, the object is a very strong reflector such as a calcified or prosthetic valve with each reflection, say, 10% of the incident wave, then the secondary or higher-order reverberation echoes are strong enough to be detected.
- Another consequence of a high-intensity echo is that it can bounce off the transducer face and back again to the object, creating secondary 'ghost' images.
- The clue to their recognition is that they are always exactly twice as far away from the transducer as a high-intensity echo and, if the primary structure moves a certain distance, the multiple reflection echo moves twice as far.

Clues to avoid and recognize reverberation artefacts

- Always use minimum power consistent with obtaining an image.
- Beware of 'objects' that: (1) are only seen in one imaging plane; (2) do not respect anatomical boundaries, e.g. a valve lying over a chamber wall or a line lying outside the heart; (3) are twice as far from the transducer as intense reflectors; (4) lie on an arc centred at the transducer and include an intense reflection.

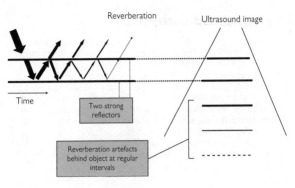

Fig. 1.12 Reverberation artefacts.

Grey scale and compress

- The intensity of an echo depends on the nature of the tissue interface. There is a wide range of echo intensities, with a calcified structure generating an echo many thousands of times more intense than a boundary between, say, blood and newly formed thrombus.
- The limited dynamic range of the display system can only represent a fraction of this range (the difference in light intensity between 'black' ink printed on 'white' paper is only a factor of 30 or so). As a consequence ultrasound images show all intense echoes as 'white', all weak echoes as 'black', and almost no grey tones.
- This can partly be overcome by *compressing* the intensity scale to create a softer image, but at the expense of boundary definition.

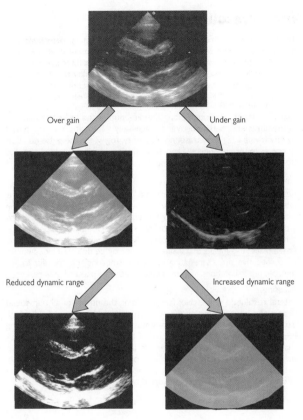

Fig. 1.13 Effects of changes in gain and dynamic range (grey scale) on image.

Image resolution

The quality of all images is affected by processing imperfections and random 'noise'. This is quantified by measuring the *resolution*—how close together two objects can be without their images blurring into one. Resolution in an ultrasound image is limited by inability to generate infinitely brief pulses and spreading of the beam by diffraction.

Axial resolution

'Axial' or 'range' resolution along the direction of the beam is a function of the ultrasound pulse length and is generally <1mm. It can be optimized by employing a higher ultrasound frequency, for which the pulse duration is correspondingly shorter, and by reducing 'ringing' by lowering the transmitted power (*mechanical index*).

Lateral resolution

Resolution at right-angles to the beam direction ('lateral' resolution) is primarily determined by the ultrasound beam width. If two objects are the same distance from the transducer but sufficiently close together that both are illuminated by the beam (or its side-lobes), their echoes return simultaneously and cannot be resolved. As the beam is scanned across the image plane, this means that a single object may be detected by a number of consecutive pulses, resulting in lateral 'smearing' on the display, or multiple representations of a small object such as a pacemaker wire.

Focusing

Lateral resolution is the chief factor limiting the quality of all ultrasound images and is worse than axial resolution by something like a factor of 10. To improve it, the ultrasound beam must be made narrower by focusing it. A plastic lens is fitted on the face of the transducer, in the same way that a glass lens focuses light, though less effectively. Transducers can be constructed with short-, medium-, or long-focus lenses. In addition, the pulsing sequence that steers the beam can be modified to provide additional focusing that can be adjusted by the operator.

Transducer frequency and resolution

Echocardiography transducers tend to range from 2 to 10MHz. Trans-thoracic probes are typically 2–5MHz and transoesophageal probes between 5 and 7MHz. Vascular probes used for peripheral blood vessels are around 10MHz and intravascular probes, which allow imaging in coronary arteries over very small distances, are usually 30–40MHz.

Choice of transducer frequency is determined by the depth of imaging and the resolution required. Low frequency transducers have good penetration but, because of the longer wavelength, poorer resolution. High frequency transducers have good resolution but poor penetration. Therefore, higher frequency transducers with better resolution can be used where less depth is required, e.g. children or transoesophageal echocardiography. Intravascular ultrasound requires very little penetration but very high resolution and therefore uses very high frequencies.

Parallel processing

Although the transducer contains a number of crystal elements to steer
the beam, they act in unison and lateral resolution is constrained by the
scan line density and the beam width. This is not, however, the way in
which the human eye forms an image. Instead of scanning across the field
of view, the scene is flooded with light and image data from it focused on
to the millions of individual receptors that comprise the retina. Impulses
from these are fed simultaneously to the brain, which processes them
simultaneously to form an image of the complete scene. Why cannot an
ultrasound system function similarly? In theory it can, but there are some
major practical limitations. The first is that, because of the difference in
wavelength, to be as effective as an optical lens an ultrasound lens would
have to be several metres in diameter! Secondly, we cannot make transducers with a large number of separate detectors. Thirdly, simultaneous
processing of image data from many detectors ('parallel processing')
requires more computing power.

- Increased computing power already allows imaging systems to have
  two parallel processing paths, and this will undoubtedly increase to
  four or more in time. Even to have two channels provides an
  enormous benefit because, as with two ears, it provides a directional
  capability equivalent to that of a 'stereo' music system.
- In practice the small crystal elements in the transducer are divided into
  two groups. Echoes from objects on the central axis of the beam axis
  arrive simultaneously at the two detector channels, but those from
  off-axis objects reach one detector channel before the other. The
  resulting phase delay allows the computer to assign them to
  corresponding off-axis memory cells. The beam direction is then
  changed. Although objects previously on the beam axis are still
  detected, their echoes are now out of phase, and can be assigned
  to the correct memory location, where they add to those from the
  previous pulse. Several major advantages follow.
  - It is no longer necessary to have a very narrow transmitted beam,
    and to have as many transmitted pulses (scan lines) per image, so
    the frame rate can be increased.
  - By detecting both amplitude and phase data, the total amount of
    information is doubled.
  - The image data in each memory cell are built up over several
    pulses, thus improving sensitivity and reducing noise and allowing
    higher imaging frequencies to be used with consequent improve-
    ment in resolution.

Second harmonic imaging

As ultrasound waves pass deeper into the body, their waveform becomes distorted. This is because soft body tissues are compressed as the positive pressure region of the wave passes through them, causing it to travel faster and, conversely, the negative pressure region of the wave travels more slowly. This change in wave shape can be shown mathematically to be due to the addition of a frequency twice that of the original transmitted frequency (called its *second harmonic*).

- When an ultrasound pulse of, say, 2MHz is transmitted into the body, the echoes that return include both 2MHz and some of its second harmonic frequency (4MHz). By selectively filtering out the original 2MHz frequency, it is possible to form the image exclusively from the 4MHz second harmonic component. Since this arises mainly from the most intense central part of the beam where pressure fluctuations are greatest, and also increases as the waves travel deeper into the body it provides the following important benefits.
  - Harmonic imaging combines the penetration power of a transmitted low fundamental frequency with the improved image resolution of the harmonic and twice the frequency.
  - The harmonic image is preferentially derived from deeper structures, and reduces artefacts from proximal objects such as ribs.
  - The harmonic image away from the central beam axis is relatively weak and thus not so susceptible to off-axis artefacts.
- There is just one problem associated with harmonic imaging. Because the image is now formed from echoes of a single frequency, some 'texture' is lost and it is possible that structures such as valve leaflets may appear artificially thick. Thus, if the quality of the fundamental frequency image is very good, such that second harmonic mode offers little benefit, then it may be better not to use it, but in most patients the improvement in image quality greatly outweighs this minor disadvantage.

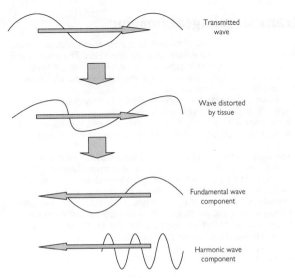

Transmitted
wave

Wave distorted
by tissue

Fundamental wave
component

Harmonic wave
component

Fig. 1.14 Harmonic imaging relies on analysing the harmonics of reflected waves to generate an image.

Transoesophageal imaging

2D imaging from a phased array transducer positioned in the oesophagus has been commercially available since the late 1980s. The transducer is similar in construction to a gastroscope but, in place of the fibre-optic bundle used for light imaging, a miniature ultrasound transducer is mounted at its tip.

- The transoesophageal transducer currently has 64 elements, compared with 128 or 256 for transthoracic transducers.
- Because there is no attenuation from the chest wall, it operates at higher frequencies (up to 7.5MHz) and produces excellent image quality.
- The complete transducer array can be rotated by a small electric motor controlled by the operator to provide image planes that correspond to the orthogonal axes of the heart despite the fact that these are not naturally aligned with the axis of the oesophagus.
- Precautions have to be taken to prevent accidental harm to the patient through heating and the potential for it to apply 150 volt electrical impulses to the back of the heart requires it to be checked regularly to ensure integrity of the electrical insulation.

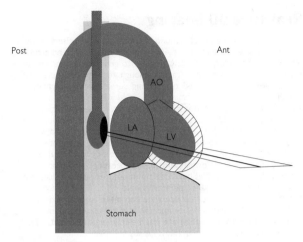

Fig. 1.15 Transoesophageal imaging generates detailed images because the probe lies next to the left atrium inside the oesophagus.

Real-time 3D imaging

If, as well as scanning the ultrasound beam across a linear section of the heart, the entire image plane is scanned up and down, with the echo data fed into a 3D memory array, it is possible to generate a complete 'data-set' of the heart's structures rapidly enough to form real-time images. To achieve this has required overcoming some daunting technological challenges.

- The first is the construction of the transducer. Instead of cutting a crystal into, say, 128 slices, it has to be sliced into some 3000 minute squares, each only 2–3 times the width of a human hair, and a wire attached to each. Even when this is done, the total number of wires is such as to make the connecting cable too unwieldy for clinical use, so the 'front-end' beam forming and image processing have to be controlled by electronics built into the transducer, without making it too large or heavy for the operator to hold.
- The second problem is to process the enormous amount of data in real time. This has involved compromises of frame rate and image depth, with image smoothing and interbeam interpolation but, with increasing computer power, this is rapidly improving.

Displaying the data on 2D video screens is achieved by computer-generated texturing and shadowing to emphasize closer structures and create the impression of a 3D solid, which can be rotated and tilted by a trackball and from which individual 2D sections can be extracted. The clinical possibilities for real-time 3D imaging are enormous, particularly in congenital heart disease, and are only just beginning to be explored.

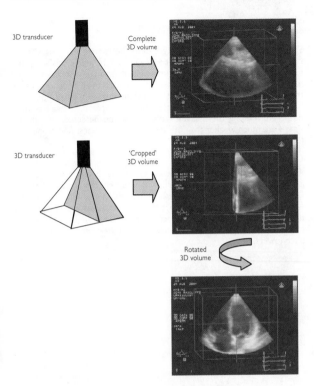

Fig. 1.16 3D transducer allows collection of a 3D dataset that is updated in real time. By cropping the image any image plane can be selected for viewing. In the example above an apical 4-chamber view is produced.

Doppler principles

Specular echoes used to form images of the heart arise from tissue interfaces but, when the ultrasound beam encounters much smaller structures, it interacts with them completely differently: instead of being *reflected* along a defined path, it is *scattered* equally in all directions just as the circular ripples formed when a small stone is thrown into a pond.

Although most of the incident energy is dissipated, a small amount does return along the incident path and can be detected, though the signals are much weaker than the specular image echoes. Red blood cells form ideal scatterers.

Doppler effect

If the blood is moving, the frequency of the backscattered echoes is modified by the Doppler effect. This was first described in 1843 by Christian Doppler, an Austrian mathematician, in relation to light. If a wave source moves towards the observer, the waves are compressed, decreasing the wavelength and increasing the pitch, and, as the source moves away from the observer, the apparent wavelength increases and pitch lowers.

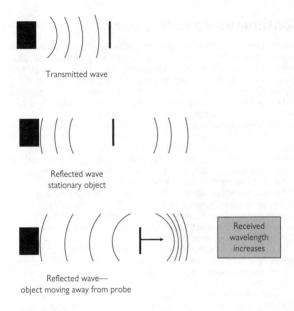

Transmitted wave

Reflected wave
stationary object

Received
wavelength
increases

Reflected wave—
object moving away from probe

Received
wavelength
decreases

Reflected wave—
object moving towards probe

Fig. 1.17 Doppler effect.

Continuous wave Doppler

Instead of the intermittent brief pulses used for imaging, continuous wave Doppler requires transmission of a continuous train of sinusoidal ultrasound waves, with simultaneous reception of the returning backscattered echoes. This is achieved either by using a special, dedicated transducer (commonly referred to as a *pencil probe*) containing two separate crystals, or by assigning the crystal elements in the transducer into two groups, one for transmitting, the other for receiving.

- Backscattered echoes from moving blood, have a slightly different frequency from that transmitted, known as the Doppler shift or Doppler frequency. For a blood velocity of 1m/sec and ultrasound frequency 2.5MHz the Doppler shift is about 3.3kHz, only 0.1%, but readily detected and directly proportional to the blood velocity.

- Blood in an artery does not all flow at the same velocity, due to friction at the walls. Furthermore, with pulsatile flow the velocity is constantly changing resulting in complex flow patterns. The interrogating ultrasound beam does not therefore return just one Doppler shift, but a spectrum of frequencies, like the orchestra tuning up before a performance.

- The machine analyses the complex mix of Doppler shifts and the resulting velocity data are used to generate a spectral Doppler display. The display shows the range of velocities detected at each point in the cardiac cycle, with flow towards the transducer shown above the baseline and flow away from the transducer below it.

- The density of the image shows the amplitude of the signal at each Doppler shift, determined by the number of scatterers and thus the proportion of blood flow at that velocity.

- A line tracing the outer edge of the spectrum shows the peak velocity and a line through the centre of the band approximates to the mean velocity.

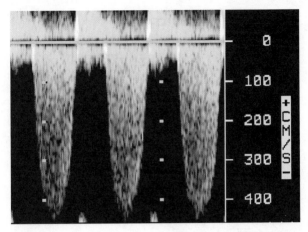

Fig. 1.18 Example of continuous wave Doppler.

Basic fluid dynamics

Volumetric flow

- For steady-state flow (i.e. when velocity is constant) the volume of liquid flowing through a pipe for a given time period (T) is the product of the cross-sectional area of the pipe (A) and the mean velocity (V):

    volume = $A \times V \times T$

- If flow is pulsatile (e.g. blood flow in the circulation) then velocity increases and decreases over time. The product of velocity and time is replaced by use of the *velocity time integral*, ($\int V \cdot dT$).
- This has the dimension of distance (velocity × time = distance). It is called the *stroke distance* and in physiological terms it is the measure of the distance along the artery that an element of the fluid travels during one pumping cycle.

Continuity equation

- If a fluid that is not compressible flows along a rigid-walled pipe, the amount entering one end of the pipe must be the same as that leaving the other end.
- If the diameter of the pipe changes, this still holds true, so a reduction in cross-sectional area is compensated for by an increase in mean velocity. This principle is known as the *continuity equation*.
- The continuity equation is written as: the cross-sectional area of the pipe at position 1 (A_1) multiplied by the velocity at position 1 (V_1) equals the cross-sectional area of the pipe at position 2 (A_2) multiplied by the velocity at position 2 (V_2):

    $A_1 \times V_1 = A_2 \times V_2$

- Provided three of the terms in the equation are known, the fourth can be derived.
- The equation is used, for example, to determine the valve area in aortic stenosis. The orifice is too small and irregular to be measured directly but, if the area of the outflow tract before the valve is measured, together with the velocities across the valve, then the valve area can be calculated.

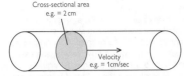

Cross-sectional area
e.g. = 2 cm

Velocity
e.g. = 1cm/sec

Volume = cross-sectional area × velocity × time

e.g. 2 × 1 × 1 = 2cm³

$2 \times 1 \times 2 = 4\text{cm}^3$

After 1 second

After 2 seconds

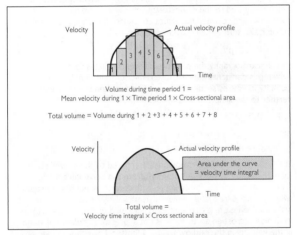

Velocity

Actual velocity profile

Time

Volume during time period 1 =
Mean velocity during 1 × Time period 1 × Cross-sectional area

Total volume = Volume during 1 + 2 + 3 + 4 + 5 + 6 + 7 + 8

Velocity

Actual velocity profile

Area under the curve
= velocity time integral

Time

Total volume =
Velocity time integral × Cross sectional area

Fig. 1.19 Volumetric flow.

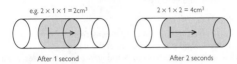

Volume of blood that passes through pipe 1 in fixed time period
must equal volume that passes through pipe 2 in same time period
Area 1 × Velocity 1 = Area 2 × Velocity 2

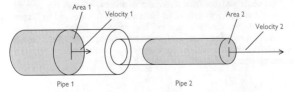

Area 1

Velocity 1

Area 2

Velocity 2

Pipe 1

Pipe 2

Fig. 1.20 Continuity equation.

Bernoulli equation

- Liquid only flows along a pipe if there is a pressure difference between
  its ends. For a fixed pipe diameter, and steady-state flow, only a small
  pressure difference is required to overcome frictional losses but,
  when the pipe becomes narrower, flow velocity increases and the
  additional kinetic (motion) energy it acquires requires a higher
  pressure difference. Neglecting the frictional losses, the relationship
  between pressure and velocity is:

$$P_1 - P_2 = \tfrac{1}{2}\rho(V_2^2 - V_1^2)$$

  V_1, P_1 and V_2, P_2 are the upstream and downstream velocities and pressures, respectively, and ρ is the density of the liquid.
- In most clinical cases of obstructed blood flow (valve stenoses, aortic
  coarctation, restrictive septal defect, etc.) the upstream velocity is
  small compared to the downstream velocity and the difference is
  further magnified when the values are squared, making it admissible
  to omit this term. The equation simplifies to:

$$P_1 - P_2 = \tfrac{1}{2}\rho V_2^2$$

- In echocardiography the pressure difference relates to blood (for
  which ρ is constant), the pressure is measured in mmHg, and
  velocity in metres/second. The equation can then be simplified
  further to the simple and easily memorized:

$$P_1 - P_2 = 4V_2^2$$

  or

  Pressure difference = $4V^2$

- If the upstream velocity is not small compared to the downstream one, then it is not possible to omit it from the Bernoulli equation.
  This situation occurs, for example, with congenital pulmonary stenosis
  where there is frequently a muscular, subvalvular restriction combined
  with a valve lesion. It also applies to very mild obstruction: a velocity
  of 2m/sec across an aortic valve is not a 'pressure gradient' of 16mmHg
  if the velocity in the outflow tract is 1.5m/sec. For echocardiography
  the full equation is:

$$P_1 - P_2 = 4(V_2^2 - V_1^2)$$

Bernoulli and clinical cardiology

The Bernoulli equation is a statement of the Newtonian principle of
conservation of energy applied to fluids and was first derived by Daniel
Bernoulli in the mid-18th century. The simplified Bernoulli equation
was first introduced into clinical cardiology in 1978. As a result
Doppler-derived data almost completely superseded invasive pressure
measurements for evaluation of cardiac lesions.

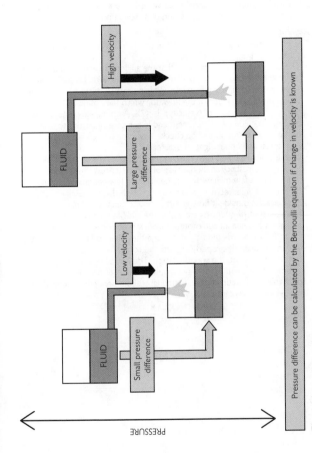

Fig. 1.21 Bernoulli equation.

Limitations of continuous wave Doppler for measuring pressure gradients

Successful application of continuous wave Doppler to measure pressure gradients requires some appreciation of its limitations.

Alignment

The greatest of these limitations is the need to align the ultrasound beam with the direction of blood flow.

- The Doppler equation requires that the angle between the ultrasound beam and the blood flow be known, or that the angle be sufficiently small that its cosine is effectively unity. In practice this means aligning the beam to within 15° of the flow, for which the cosine is 0.97 and the error in the value of (velocity)^2 is <7%. A colour-flow image can be used to guide beam alignment and in the case of aortic stenosis the measurements should be checked by using two conjugate axes (e.g. apical and upper right parasternal).
- It is also necessary to align the beam with the centre of the jet passing through the restriction. In the case of aortic stenosis this is quite small—just a few millimetres diameter and a few centimetres long. Only in this 'inlet jet' is flow laminar, to which the Bernoulli equation is applicable; outside it flow is turbulent and cannot be analysed. The Doppler shift frequencies are within the audible range and the machines provide an audio output from stereo speakers, one responding to flow towards the transducer and the other to flow away from it. When the beam is properly aligned, the sound has a 'hissing' quality but, when it is not, the sound is harsh. The 'pencil probe', which is optimized for continuous wave Doppler and does not provide a potentially distracting image, is strongly recommended for recording high velocity valve jets.

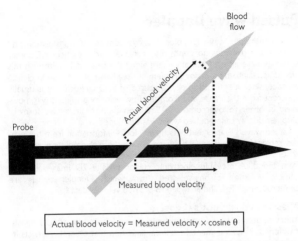

Actual blood velocity = Measured velocity × cosine θ

Fig. 1.22 Relation between angle of ultrasound beam and direction of blood flow.

Pulsed wave Doppler

Since continuous wave Doppler employs continuous transmission and reception, it provides no depth discrimination and a particular Doppler shift may have arisen from anywhere along the beam axis. Although this would appear to be a major problem, it usually is not the case in clinical practice, since identification of the source of a high velocity jet is usually apparent from the image and from the flow velocity profile. It was, however, in order to overcome this limitation that an alternative form of Doppler display called pulsed wave was developed.

Pulsed wave Doppler extracts flow velocity information from the echoes generated during imaging. Mixed in with the high-amplitude, specular echoes arising from tissue interfaces, there are backscattered echoes from blood. A movable electronic cursor on the 2D image allows a 'sample volume' to be selected, from which Doppler signals are extracted, amplified, and analysed to provide velocity data.

Aliasing and Nyquist's theorem

Although pulsed wave Doppler allows spatial localization of flow signals, it suffers from a fundamental technical limitation that severely restricts its clinical use. This is called 'aliasing' and it arises from the fact that there are significant time intervals between the ultrasound pulses. This is an example of *Nyquist's theorem*, which states that, for a wave to be reproduced accurately, it has to be sampled at least twice per cycle. Applied to pulsed wave Doppler, this means that the highest blood velocity that can be detected without ambiguity is that whose Doppler shift is equal to half the pulse repetition frequency (PRF) of the imaging system, which itself is determined by the imaging depth. This is called the *Nyquist limit*.

- The practical effect of aliasing is that the tops of the positive velocities that exceed the Nyquist limit are cut off and displayed as negative velocities, analogous to the stagecoach wheel turning in reverse.
- A simple calculation shows that aliasing occurs at quite modest blood velocities. For a working depth of 15cm, the round-trip time is approximately 200µs and the maximum pulse repetition frequency 5000/sec. The Nyquist limit is thus 2500Hz and, for an ultrasound frequency of 2.5MHz, aliasing begins at only 0.75m/sec.
- Provided that the flow is predominantly towards or away from the transducer, and not bi-directional, the zero velocity baseline can be shifted to favour one direction at the expense of the other, and it is thus possible to increase the aliasing velocity by a factor of up to two, but beyond this nothing can be done.
- When velocities greater than 2 × Nyquist limit are encountered, the display overlaps and it is not possible to tell whether the flow is towards or away from the transducer, let alone measure the velocity. Pulsed wave Doppler does have some limited clinical applications in cases where flow velocity is low, or spatial localization is more important than the peak velocity, but it is generally of no value for quantifying obstructive lesions.

High pulse repetition frequency pulsed wave Doppler

The primary factor determining the aliasing velocity is the pulse repetition frequency, limited by working depth. If the pulse repetition frequency is doubled, instead of Doppler shift data returning only from a single pulse at a specific depth, it will arrive simultaneously from more than one pulse, leading to ambiguity. However, since the pulse repetition frequency has been doubled, so has the aliasing velocity. Although this technique, called 'high pulse repetition frequency' or 'extended range' Doppler, can lead to confusion as to the origin of Doppler signals, by judicious placement of the beam so that the additional sample volumes are not in high-velocity areas, this usually can be avoided.

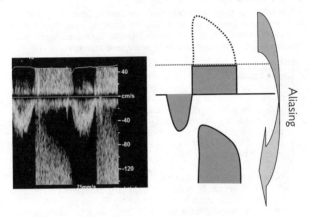

Fig. 1.23 Example of pulsed wave Doppler with aliasing.

Colour flow mapping

The pulsed wave Doppler principle can be extended to detect backscattered echoes, not just from a single 'sample volume' but from a matrix of small 'pixels' on the 2D image or 3D 'voxels' on a real-time 3D image. To analyse the Doppler data in real time imposes burdens on the processing system, and it is not possible to display the full spectral data for numerous sample points simultaneously, but basic velocity information can be provided in the form of a display in which the colour of each pixel indicates the local flow direction and the approximate velocity. The colour flow data are superimposed on the 2D or M-mode image, the standard convention being for flow towards the transducer to be shown as red and flow away from the transducer in blue.

Limitations of colour flow mapping

While colour Doppler has undoubtedly enriched understanding of blood flow within the heart, and is invaluable for detecting valve regurgitation and shunt lesions, it does have severe technical limitations, which must be understood if the images are to be interpreted correctly.

Aliasing

- Colour Doppler is derived from pulsed wave Doppler and suffers from aliasing to an even greater degree, since simultaneous imaging and Doppler lower the effective pulse repetition frequency and aliasing in a colour flow image typically occurs at velocities above 0.5m/sec.
- Aliasing manifests on a colour display as colour inversion: red turning to blue, and vice versa. Thus, for steady flow towards the transducer, a velocity of 0.4m/sec is represented by pale red but, as it increases to 0.6m/sec, it becomes pale blue. At 1.0m/sec (twice the aliasing velocity) the colour display again shows black, and with further increase in velocity red, then blue, and so on. The burden on the system computing power can be reduced by restricting the size of the colour image but, even so, frame rates are significantly reduced.
- Since the Doppler shift is the product of blood velocity and the cosine of the angle between the flow axis and the ultrasound beam, the apparent velocity on a colour display is determined both by the true blood velocity and by the angle at which the flow vector is intersected by the scanning beam. Not only does this mean that constant flow velocity is represented by a range of colours, but it can additionally introduce aliasing at higher velocities.

Turbulent flow (variance mapping)

When flow is turbulent, there is a wide spectrum of local velocities: high and low; forward and reverse. This is indicated on a continuous wave display as broadening of the spectral band, but cannot be indicated by colour Doppler, since it can only display flow velocity at one point and at one time by a single colour. A solution is provided by analysing the time-variance of local velocity so that, when the same pixel detects greatly different velocities in successive images, the display is modified, for example, by showing those pixels in green. This is called variance mapping, but it places further strain on frame rates and aliasing velocity.

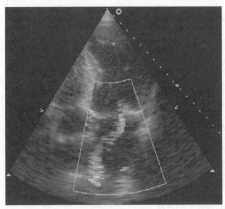

Apical four chamber

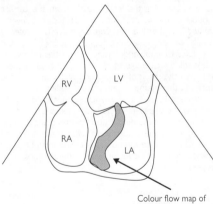

Colour flow map of
mitral regurgitation

Fig. 1.24 Example of colour flow mapping.

Tissue Doppler imaging

All moving objects intersected by the ultrasound beam generate Doppler shifts. For study of blood flow, Doppler signals from moving heart structures such as valve leaflets are removed by selective filtering, since they would generate unwanted artefacts. The filtering is possible because the characteristics of Doppler signals from blood and tissue are markedly different: blood generally has high velocities and relatively low signal amplitude since the red cell scatterers are relatively sparse. Conversely, muscle and valve tissue have much lower velocities, but higher signal amplitudes as the cells are packed together.

• If, instead of removing low velocities, the high velocity signals from blood are filtered out and the velocity and amplification scales suitably adjusted, Doppler signals from tissue motions can be recorded, either as pulsed wave spectral displays or in colour (2D or M-mode).

Strain rate imaging

The disadvantage of all Doppler is that it only detects motion relative to the transducer. Thus, when viewing the left ventricle from the cardiac apex, longitudinal motion of the myocardium is detected, but inward motion of the septum and lateral wall is not. One approach is to select a 'centre of mass', usually on the long axis approximately 1/3 of the distance from mitral annulus to apex, and compute velocities relative to this point. However, it is still the case that motion of a particular element of the myocardium is in part the result of its own contractile function and in part the consequence of other elements pushing and pulling it.

The complex arrangement of layers of myocytes means that each element of viable muscle wall changes its shape in all 3 axes: longitudinal; radial; and circumferential. Strain is the deformation per unit length and is dimensionless; the rate at which the deformation takes place is termed *strain rate*, and longitudinal strain rate can now be derived from Doppler signals in some machines. Since it shows only local deformation, it is independent of extraneous forces.

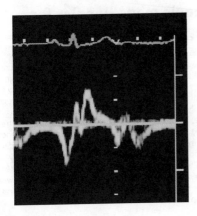

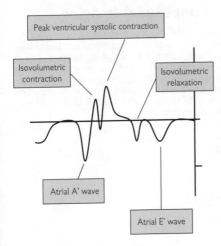

Fig. 1.25 Example of tissue Doppler imaging.

Second harmonic mode Doppler for contrast imaging

Second harmonic imaging was originally developed in order to enhance signals from encapsulated contrast media. These are proprietary products and comprise very small (1–3µm) microspheres of gas contained within a hard outer shell. At very low ultrasound power levels, the microspheres act as conventional scatterers, but with slightly greater power (though still lower than normally used for imaging) the pressure waves distort them and they vibrate, emitting energy at the second harmonic frequency. A display derived from the second harmonic Doppler frequency thus selectively comes from the microspheres and not from surrounding tissue or blood. The addition of contrast greatly enhances the quality of both images of blood-filled cavities and of Doppler signals, giving a clear velocity profile for even very small jets. At higher ultrasound power levels, the microspheres shatter, releasing the contained gas and generating a brief, but very intense, echo.

Power mode (amplitude) imaging

As stated previously, the Doppler shift is determined by velocity, but the intensity of the Doppler signal relates to the number of scatterers within the ultrasound beam. Thus, if there are a lot of scatterers moving in random directions, the net velocity will be zero, but the amplitude of the Doppler signal quite high. Thus, a display showing the amplitude or power of the Doppler signal shows the density of scatterers, regardless of the velocities. This type of display is used, often in conjunction with harmonic mode, in contrast studies.

Is ultrasound safe?

Over half a century of use, involving millions of scans in a wide variety of clinical settings, no case of harm to a patient from diagnostic ultrasound has ever been documented. By any standards the risk:benefit ratio of echocardiography is negligibly low, but there is no such thing as zero-risk and to minimize it the user should always employ the 'ALARA' principle (As Low As Reasonably Achievable) for machine power levels and patient exposure times. Ultrasound at high power levels can be used to coagulate tissues, heat deep muscles, or clean dirty surgical instruments. Potential harmful effects are related to the beam intensity and ultrasound frequency.

Thermal index

- The energy lost through attenuation as the beam passes through tissues is largely converted to heat. The peak intensity as the ultrasound pulse passes may be quite high, but there are large gaps between pulses (pulse duration 2μsec, interval between pulses 200μsec) so the average heating is quite low.
- The term used to express this is the *thermal index*, which is the ratio of the actual beam power to that required to raise the temperature of a specific tissue by 1°C.

Temperature and transoeosophageal echocardiography

A particular issue arises with transoesophageal scanning, where the transducer face is in contact with the oesophagus and local heating could, in the event of a fault within the transducer, cause tissue necrosis. For this reason, the probe tip temperature is monitored and there is an automatic thermal cut-out if it becomes too high.

Mechanical index

Increasing transmitted power causes higher pressure fluctuations as the ultrasound waves travel through tissues. The potential for harm is quantified by the *mechanical index* (MI), a parameter derived by dividing the peak negative wave pressure by the square root of the ultrasound frequency. Most commercial cardiac scanners limit the maximum power to MI = 1.1.

Transthoracic: examination

Patient information

- Transthoracic echocardiography is a simple, non-invasive investigation. The patient can be given simple information on what is intended and how the pictures are created with sound waves.
- They should be aware that they will need to undress to the waist and lie on a bed on their side for around half an hour. If there is a sex discrepancy between echocardiographer and patient there should be the option of a chaperone.
- The operator should be alert to the fact that the patient may find lying in a fixed position on one side for a period of time uncomfortable (e.g. hip or knee problems) and give opportunities for the patient to move or consider alternative imaging positions. Furthermore, the patient may find having the probe pressed against the chest uncomfortable.
- The operator should be aware of any complicating medical problems, such as increased body mass index, chest deformities, lung disease, breast disease, or heart failure, that may make imaging difficult.

Patient preparation

- Ask the patient to undress to the waist and explain that this is 'so you can image the whole of the heart'. A woman may appreciate a pillow case, sheet, or gown to cover her while preparations are in progress.
- Ask the patient to sit on the couch. The ideal position is with them sitting up at 45° supported by the raised head of the couch but rolled over on to their left side. Patients can find the concept of lying on their left side while sitting up confusing. They tend to slide down the bed on rolling over and end up lying down. Demonstrate the position if necessary and explain that they need to lie on their left side to 'bring the heart close to the chest wall'. If the patient is more comfortable lying flat this is an acceptable alternative position.
- Ask them to raise their left arm and place their hand behind their head (some couches have a handle to hold on to). Explain that this is to 'make it easier to get to the heart'.
- Make sure the patient is comfortable as they will need to stay in position for some time.
- Attach ECG electrodes between patient and ultrasound machine and check there is a clear trace on the screen both to time images and trigger loop capture. Aim to have a large QRS complex without artefact. Usually the red electrode is placed by the right shoulder, yellow by left shoulder, and green on the lower chest (usually away from the apex to avoid the imaging window). Alternative positions are with the yellow electrode on the back and/or red in the centre of the chest. Consider more careful skin preparation or changing electrode stickers if the trace is not clear. Some machines allow you to rotate through lead combinations (e.g. I, II, III) to find the best trace. ECG gain can be changed to increase the size of the QRS complexes.
- Enter patient demographic details (and, ideally, details of body size) on to the machine.

Preparing machine and probe

- Set up an ergonomic orientation of machine, patient, and operator. This will depend on your preferred operator position. A standard way is to have the operator sitting behind the patient on the edge of the couch with their right arm holding the probe and wrapped over the patient. The machine is then operated with the left hand. Another standard method is to sit facing the patient holding the probe against the chest wall with the left hand (arm rested on the couch) and with machine operated by the right hand.
- Check transthoracic image settings on machine, with harmonic imaging (if available) and your preferred image post-processing options selected. Set overall gain, compress, and transverse or lateral gain controls to standard positions.
- Make sure there is an ECG tracing on the echo machine and patient details are entered.
- Make sure image storage is possible (to magneto-optical disc, download to image server or videotape).
- Take the appropriate transthoracic probe, apply gel to transducer, and start imaging.

Probe handling and image quality

- The probe should be held in one hand and pressed firmly against the chest wall. Varying the pressure will alter image quality. Ensure sufficient pressure to optimize the image but not too much to make it uncomfortable for the patient. The usual problem while learning is not applying enough pressure to get good image quality.
- A layer of gel ensures good contact between probe and chest wall. It excludes any air (that would degrade image quality). However, too much gel makes it difficult to keep a stable position so, once a layer is established, try not to apply more gel as image quality will not improve.
- The probe has a dot on one side to orientate the probe in your hand with the image on the screen.
- The probe can be moved in multiple directions but the four key movements are: (1) rotation around a point; (2) rocking back and forwards; (3) rocking side to side; and (4) sliding across the chest. Movements needed to improve image quality are usually quite small and, with experience, hand movements are almost subconscious.
- Remember that image quality may be improved by different patient or heart positions. These can be altered by physically rolling the patient a little, one way or the other, readjusting the patient to ensure they are sitting up, or asking the patient to breathe in or out to move the diaphragm (and heart) up or down.
- Imaging well is hard work and requires concentration. If it is proving difficult to find, keep, or return to an image during a study remember a short break can help. Remove the probe from the chest, re-apply gel and start again.

Image optimization

There are four things that can be altered to improve image quality. Check each when you change a view to ensure you have the optimal image. In certain situations a completely different approach is needed, e.g. contrast imaging.

- Contact between probe and chest—this minimizes acoustic loss between probe and heart. Ensure there is a sufficient layer of gel and that you are applying enough pressure on the probe (more pressure might be needed if there is significant fat or tissue under probe).
- Patient position—this can move the heart closer to the probe. Ensure the patient has not slipped out of position. See if rolling the patient slightly, one way or the other, improves the image.
- Cardiac and lung position—these two factors are altered by asking the patient to breath in or out. The heart moves up and down with the diaphragm and any lung tissue between the probe and heart (which contains air and therefore degrades the image) may also move out of the way. Ask the patient to breath in and out slowly. Watch the image. The best image may be at end inspiration or end expiration, or somewhere in between! Ask the patient to hold their breath when the image is at its best.
- Machine settings.
  - Machines usually have *tissue harmonic imaging*, which should routinely be selected.
  - Overall, as well as transverse and lateral, *gains* should be adjusted along with contrast controls (e.g. *compress*) to optimize contrast between blood and myocardium. Newer machines perform all these image optimization procedures automatically just by pressing an *optimization button*.
  - Maximize the frame rate (which determines resolution) while filling the screen with all required information. This can be done by adjusting *depth* to just behind the heart (or area of interest) and reducing *sector width* to the area being studied (particularly important for colour flow mapping and tissue Doppler, which reduce frame rate when switched on but, perversely, require relatively high frame rates to be useful.)

Image acquisition

Standard acquisition

Images are acquired in a standard way—with a set sequence of views (see opposite and pp 86–101). The standard views should always be collected to ensure comprehensive data collection, with additional views when necessary. Even when there is a specific question a full dataset should be acquired to ensure nothing is missed.

Windows

There are three key areas or 'windows' on the chest and abdomen to collect standard images (with additional windows available if needed) (Fig. 2.1). It is normal to image through each window in turn starting with parasternal windows. However, it may be necessary to go back to windows as pathology is found that needs more detailed study.

1. Parasternal window

This window is usually just to the left of the sternum around the 3rd or 4th intercostal space. However, the best position for parasternal views varies with each patient. To find the best window move the probe up or down an intercostal space, and away from or towards the sternum.

2. Apical window

As the name suggests this is at the cardiac apex so normally will be at the bottom left, lateral point of the chest. The apex beat may be felt under the probe. The window should, ideally, be from the true apex to avoid foreshortening. To optimize, ensure probe is lateral enough and move up or down an intercostal space.

3. Subcostal window

This lies below the xiphisternum in the epigastrium. Lie the patient on their back with stomach relaxed (may be easier if the patient bends their legs). Place probe on the abdomen, press it in, and point it back up into the chest so that the image plane tucks under the ribs.

Additional windows

Suprasternal window

This is the suprasternal notch. Lie the patient on their back and raise the chin. Rest the probe in the notch and point it down into the chest.

Right parasternal window

This is often used to look at flow in the ascending aorta. A normal or a stand alone probe can be used. The patient should roll all the way over to lie on their right side. The window is on the right of the sternum usually slightly higher than the equivalent left parasternal window.

Supraclavicular window

This is rarely needed but can be used to look at vascular structures and the aorta. It lies above the clavicles.

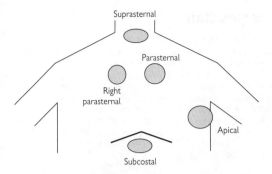

Fig. 2.1 Standard windows for transthoracic echocardiography.

Standard sequence of views

- Parasternal windows
  - Parasternal long axis view
  - (Optional—parasternal right ventricular inflow)
  - (Optional—parasternal right ventricular outflow)
  - Parasternal short axis view (apex)
  - Parasternal short axis view (papillary level)
  - Parasternal short axis view (aortic level)
  - (Optional—right parasternal window)
- Apical window
  - Apical 4-chamber
  - Apical 5-chamber
  - Apical 2-chamber
  - Apical 3-chamber
- Subcostal window
  - Subcostal long and short axis
  - Inferior vena cava
  - (Optional—aorta view)
- Suprasternal window
  - (Optional—aorta view)

Data acquisition

Techniques for each view

In each view, start the study with 2D imaging and then consider whether further echocardiography techniques are required to document the findings. Although a standard minimal dataset acquisition (pp. 86–101) is vital, it is equally important that you analyse and interpret the images as you do the study. It is easy to save a standard set of images for later analysis, but if you only notice pathology after the study you will not have acquired the right images. The preliminary analysis needed to search and identify pathology should be done during the study with detailed confirmation during later reporting. Consider the following in each view:

- colour flow mapping;
- M-mode;
- continuous wave Doppler;
- pulsed wave Doppler;
- tissue Doppler imaging;
- 3D imaging;
- contrast imaging.

In all views 2D and colour flow mapping are used. Most views also use continuous and pulsed wave Doppler as well as occasional M-mode. In some views 3D, contrast, and tissue Doppler imaging may be needed.

Image storage

All images and data must be stored for future reference. With the current ease of storage it is no longer acceptable to perform an echo-cardiogram and only keep handwritten notes, even in emergencies.

Until recently, images were acquired to videotape but now they are usually stored digitally to magneto-optical disc or directly to a main server. Digital storage is usually based on storing a single cardiac cycle loop, triggered off the ECG trace. If the patient has an arrhythmia with variable cardiac cycle length then it may be better to store 3 to 5 beats. It is desirable to have a digital laboratory to store all acquired views. Storage on digital media enables better post-processing and follow-up comparisons.

Parasternal long axis view

The first view. Gives an immediate overall impression of the major valves, left and right ventricles, aorta, and pericardium.

Finding the view

- In the parasternal window hold the probe with the dot pointing to the right shoulder. Adjust probe with slight rotation and rocking.
- The optimal image cuts through the middle of mitral and aortic valves to display left ventricular inflow and outflow. Left ventricular walls lie parallel and straight across screen (anterior border of septum should be same distance from transducer as anterior wall of ascending aorta). Ascending aorta should be a tube with parallel walls.
- Sometimes not all structures can be aligned in a single view; in this situation record several views focused on each detail.

What to record?

- 2D images.
- Colour flow: aortic valve, left ventricular outflow tract, mitral valve.
- M-mode: aortic valve/left atrium, mitral valve, left ventricle.

What do you see?

- *Left ventricle.* Septum (anteroseptal portion), inferolateral (also sometimes called posterior) wall, and cavity are seen. Use 2D (and M-mode) to assess left ventricular size, function, and hypertrophy. Also excellent for left ventricular outflow tract size measurements and evidence of flow acceleration on colour flow. Septal defects may be seen with colour flow.
- *Aortic valve.* Right coronary cusp is at top and non-coronary cusp at bottom. 2D and M-mode can assess movement. Colour flow demonstrates regurgitation.
- *Aortic root.* Entire aortic root, including sinuses, sinotubular junction, and ascending aorta, should be visible for measurement with 2D or M-mode.
- *Ascending aorta.* Slight adjustment by rocking the probe to one side can bring the proximal portion of the ascending aorta into view.
- *Descending aorta.* Seen in cross-section as a circle behind mitral valve. Use as landmark for studying pericardial and pleural fluid.
- *Mitral valve.* A2 and P2 segments usually seen. 2D will pick up movement (prolapse, stenosis, etc.) and tip movement can be documented with M-mode. Use colour flow to identify regurgitation. Vena contracta or flow convergence may be evident.
- *Left atrium.* Left atrial size can be judged and measured with M-mode.
- *Right ventricle.* The right ventricle lies near the probe and can be measured.
- *Pericardium.* Seen anteriorly in front of right heart and posteriorly behind heart. Good view to identify an effusion and measure size.

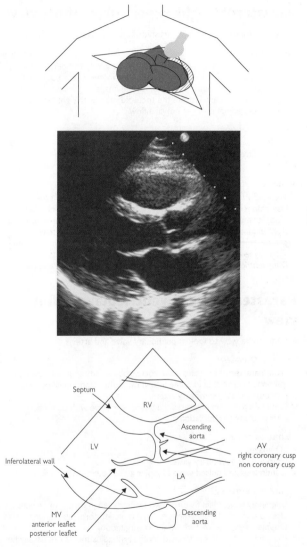

Fig. 2.2 Parasternal long axis view.

Parasternal right ventricular inflow view

A useful extra view to look at tricuspid valve and right ventricular inflow.

Finding the view
• From parasternal long axis view, rock probe slowly to point downwards. The tricuspid valve should come into view. There usually needs to be some slight rotation to optimize the image.
• Optimal images demonstrate the tricuspid valve with right atrium behind and sometimes vena caval inflow.

What to record?
• 2D image.
• Colour flow across the tricuspid valve.
• Continuous and pulsed wave Doppler across the tricuspid valve.

What do you see?
• *Tricuspid valve*. Main feature. Two leaflets seen in centre of screen. Use colour flow to document regurgitation. Jet may be aligned for Doppler measures of inflow and right ventricular systolic pressure.
• *Right atrium*. Lies behind tricuspid valve and slight rotation may demonstrate right atrial appendage, Eustachian valve, and inflow from vena cavae.
• *Right ventricle*. Portion of right ventricle close to tricuspid valve seen.

Parasternal right ventricular outflow view

A useful extra view to look at pulmonary valve and artery.

Finding the view
• From parasternal long axis view, rock probe slowly to point upwards. Pulmonary valve should come into view. Slight rotation will optimize image to include pulmonary artery.
• Optimal image demonstrates the pulmonary valve with pulmonary arterial trunk to bifurcation.

What to record?
• 2D image.
• Colour flow pulmonary valve.
• Continuous and pulsed wave Doppler across pulmonary valve.

What do you see?
• *Pulmonary valve*. Main feature. Two leaflets seen in centre of screen. Use colour flow to document regurgitation. Jet normally aligned for Doppler measures of outflow and regurgitation.
• *Pulmonary artery*. In the far field. With slight adjustments can usually be followed to bifurcation. Can measure size and look for abnormal jets (patent ductus) or thrombus (pulmonary embolus).

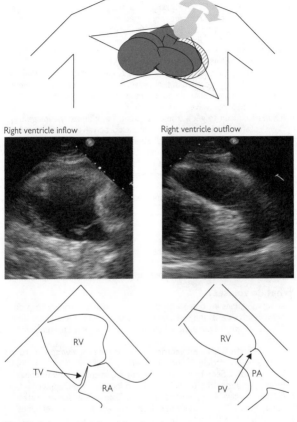

Right ventricle inflow

Right ventricle outflow

Fig. 2.3 Right ventricle inflow and outflow views.

Parasternal short axis (aortic) view

A series of parasternal short axis views are gathered in order to scan through the heart in cross-section. Together they give an impression of left ventricular function, aortic and mitral structure, and the right heart.

Finding the view

- From the parasternal long axis view, rotate the probe around 90° so that the dot points to the left shoulder. Try and rotate from a long axis view with the aortic valve in the centre. Focus on keeping the valve in the centre and you should end up with the classic cross-section through the aortic valve.
- It can be difficult to get a true on-axis cut. To optimize the image try slight rotation around the point until the aortic valve appears circular with the right ventricle wrapped around the valve. Then rock the probe backwards and forwards until the cut is straight.
- Optimal image should have a round aortic valve with 3 cusps evident. The tricuspid valve should be visible on the left and pulmonary valve on the right.
- If all structures are not seen remember to record several views focused on each detail.

What to record?

- 2D images.
- Colour flow: aortic, tricuspid, and pulmonary valve (also sometimes atrial septum).
- Doppler: pulmonary and tricuspid valve.

What do you see?

- *Aortic valve.* Lies in centre with classic Y-shape: left coronary cusp on right, right towards the top, and non-coronary on the left. Use colour flow to identify regurgitation. Left main stem sometimes seen by left cusp.
- *Right ventricle.* Basal right ventricle lies near the probe wrapped around aortic valve. Ventricle can be measured.
- *Tricuspid valve.* Seen to left of aortic valve. Use colour flow to check for regurgitation. May be aligned for continuous wave Doppler.
- *Pulmonary valve.* To right of aortic valve. Colour flow demonstrates regurgitation. Continuous and pulsed wave will document velocities.
- *Left atrium.* Lies behind aortic valve.
- *Interatrial septum.* Septum lies at 7 o'clock and view may be useful to identify septal defects with colour flow.
- *Pericardium.* Seen anteriorly, in front of right heart.

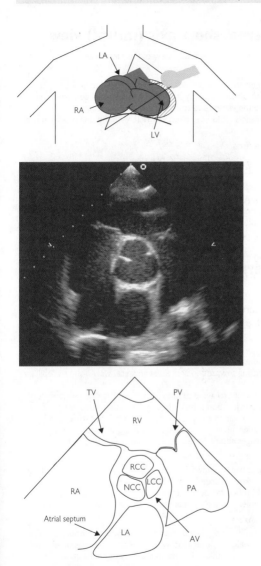

Fig. 2.4 Parasternal short axis (aortic) view.

Parasternal short axis (mitral) view

The classic *en face* or 'fish-mouth' view of the mitral valve.

Finding the view
- From the parasternal short axis aortic view, rock the probe slightly towards the cardiac apex. By starting the parasternal cuts from the aortic valve the views tend to stay 'on-axis'.
- Optimal image should have a left ventricle with the 'fish mouth' mitral valve clearly seen.

What to record?
- 2D images. Consider 2D planimetry if stenosis.
- Consider colour flow across mitral valve, if regurgitation.

What do you see?
- *Mitral valve.* A classic *en face* view of the mitral valve to look at valve morphology (including the separate scallops) and movement. Consider colour flow or 3D imaging if abnormalities. Can also be used to measure valve opening with planimetry.

Parasternal short axis (ventricular) views

The classic short axis views of the left ventricle.

Finding the view
- From the parasternal short axis mitral view, rock probe slightly more towards apex until left ventricle is in cross-section. The papillary level has the bodies of both papillary muscles evident.
- Further rocking towards apex creates an apical view distal to papillary muscles.
- Usually important to avoid off-axis images so that true assessment of left ventricular function is possible. Slight rotation helps bring out the circular ventricular shape. If it is proving very difficult to get a clear image consider moving the probe position slightly within the window.
- Optimal images should have a cross-section of the left ventricle.

What to record?
- 2D images at papillary level for measures: left ventricular size and mass. Consider a view recorded at apical level.
- Consider M-mode measures: left ventricle.
- Tissue Doppler imaging sometimes used in short axis.

What do you see?
- *Left ventricle.* The short axis demonstrates septum, anterior, lateral, and inferior walls (in order clockwise). Use for measures of left ventricular size and thickness and to assess regional function of mid-segments of walls.
- *Right ventricle.* Right ventricle is seen as a crescent around the left ventricle. Use to judge right ventricular size, function, and haemodynamics.

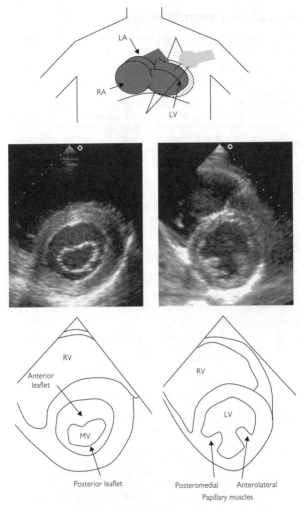

Fig. 2.5 Parasternal short axis (mitral and ventricular) views.

Apical four chamber view

The first, and the main, apical view. Allows assessment of overall left and right ventricular function as well as right and left ventricular inflow.

Finding the view

- In the apical window, hold the probe with the dot pointing towards the couch.
- Probe needs to be as close to the left ventricular apex as possible so alter the image, focusing on obtaining the optimal left ventricle size and shape. The identifying characteristics of the apex are that it moves less than the other walls and is thinner. In a true apical view the left ventricle will be at its longest. Once you have identified the apex optimize the view with rotation and rocking to bring in the right ventricle, left and right atrium, as well as the mitral and tricuspid valve. Exclude the left ventricle outflow and aortic valve by tilting the probe.
- Optimal image should be at apex with both ventricles, both atria, and both mitral and tricuspid valves visible. Septa should be straight down the centre of the image.

What to record?

- 2D images.
- Colour flow mapping: mitral and tricuspid valves.
- Continuous and pulsed wave Doppler: mitral and tricuspid valves.
- Consider Doppler of right upper pulmonary vein.
- Consider tissue Doppler imaging of right and left ventricle as well as 3D datasets. When appropriate use contrast.

What do you see?

- *Mitral valve.* A2 and P2 segments of mitral valve are seen. 2D for movement. Colour flow mapping will show regurgitation (vena contracta, flow convergence, etc.) Doppler well aligned for stenosis and valve inflow. Tissue Doppler of lateral and septal sides of mitral ring may be possible.
- *Tricuspid valve.* Lateral and septal leaflets displayed. As for mitral valve, colour flow, Doppler, and tissue Doppler are possible.
- *Left and right atrium.* Both atria and the interatrial septum can be seen. Pulmonary veins as well as vena cavae may be seen in far field. Use to measure atrial volumes.
- *Left ventricle.* Key view to study global and regional left ventricular function. Septum, apex, and lateral wall are displayed. Good for 2D volume measures if endocardial border is clear. If assessing left ventricular function consider contrast and/or 3D to improve left ventricle data collection. Tissue Doppler of different wall segments is also possible.
- *Right ventricle.* A key view to look at right ventricular size and function. Usually compared relative to left but also tissue Doppler or M-mode of tricuspid free wall annulus can be considered.
- *Pericardium.* Important view to see size and location of pericardial fluid. May also be used for ultrasound-guided pericardiocentesis.

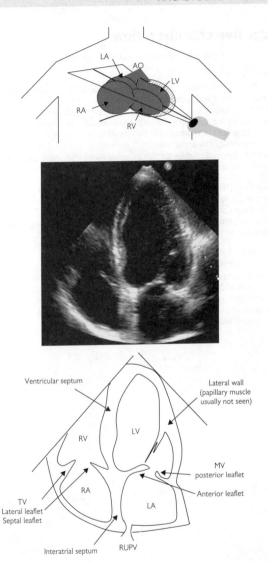

Fig. 2.6 Apical 4-chamber view.

Apical five chamber view

Used to look at left ventricular outflow and aortic valve.

Finding the view

- From the apical 4-chamber view tilt the probe to bring the aortic valve and outflow tract into view.
- Sometimes a better alignment through aortic valve and ascending aorta is obtained by moving probe laterally on chest wall (more into axilla). This foreshortens left ventricle and alters alignment for other valves so use only to study the aortic valve.
- Optimal image looks similar to that of apical 4-chamber view but with the aortic valve evident and ascending aorta in far field.

What to record?

- 2D images.
- Colour flow mapping: aortic valve.
- Continuous and pulsed wave Doppler: aortic valve and left ventricular outflow tract.

What do you see?

- *Aortic valve.* Right and non-coronary cusps (although may not be easy to see). Colour flow demonstrates regurgitation. Continuous wave for stenosis and regurgitation.
- *Left ventricular outflow tract.* Use colour flow mapping for aortic regurgitation or flow turbulence due to obstruction. Best view to place pulsed wave Doppler to assess outflow and obstruction.

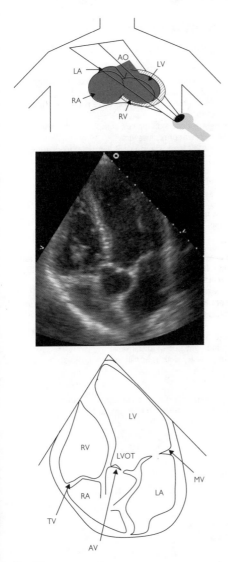

Fig. 2.7 Apical 5-chamber view.

Apical two chamber view

An important view for global and regional left ventricular assessment.

Finding the view

- From the apical 4-chamber view, rotate the probe around 90° anti-clockwise. Watch the picture and try and keep the mitral valve in place. If the apex of the ventricle changes you were probably not at the apex and are foreshortening.
- Keep rotating until right ventricle disappears completely but before left ventricular outflow tract comes into view.
- Optimal image contains left ventricle (no right ventricle) from apex, centred in the image. Mitral valve is cut through the commissure. Left atrium is in far field and left atrial appendage may be visible.

What to record?

- 2D images.
- Consider colour flow and Doppler measures across mitral valve.
- Consider tissue Doppler imaging of ventricle.

What do you see?

- *Left ventricle.* Inferior wall on left, and anterior wall on right. Good for regional assessment. Use plane for ventricular volume measures and tissue Doppler of wall segments.
- *Mitral valve.* Ideal image is of a commissural view with P3, A2, and P1 segments visible from left to right. Colour flow and Doppler measures are possible as well as assessment of the long axis of the mitral valve ring.
- *Left atrial appendage.* Sometimes visible as a curved finger pointing towards probe around right side of mitral valve.
- *Coronary sinus.* The coronary sinus is usually seen in cross-section on the left of the mitral valve.

Adaptation of view

- *Right ventricle.* Slight tilting of probe to point forwards can scan into a two chamber view of right ventricle (not a standard view).

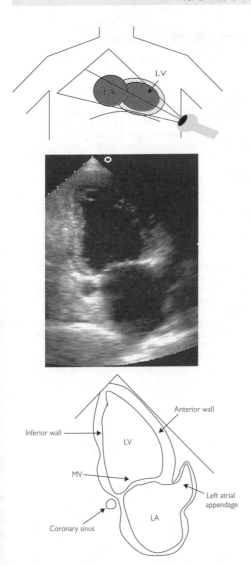

Fig. 2.8 Apical 2-chamber view.

Apical three chamber view

Similar to the parasternal long axis view but includes left ventricular apex.

Finding the view

- From the apical 2-chamber view continue rotating the probe anti-clockwise to around 135° from the 4-chamber view.
- Watch the picture and keep the mitral valve in place, rotating until the left ventricular outflow tract and aortic valve come into view.
- Optimal image contains left ventricle from apex straight down the screen with mitral valve, left atrium, left ventricular outflow tract, and aortic valve in far field.

What to record?

- 2D images.
- Consider tissue Doppler imaging of ventricle.
- Consider colour flow and Doppler measurements across aortic valve as may be well aligned.
- Consider colour flow and Doppler measures across mitral valve.

What do you see?

- *Left ventricle.* Good view to assess septum on right of image and apex and inferolateral (posterior) wall on left of image.
- *Aortic valve.* Right coronary cusp is on right and non-coronary cusp on left. Colour flow will demonstrate regurgitation and valve is usually aligned for Doppler measurements.
- *Mitral valve.* A2 and P2 segments of valve seen and can consider colour flow and other Doppler measures if not enough detail from other views.
- *Left atrium.* Atrium lies behind mitral valve.

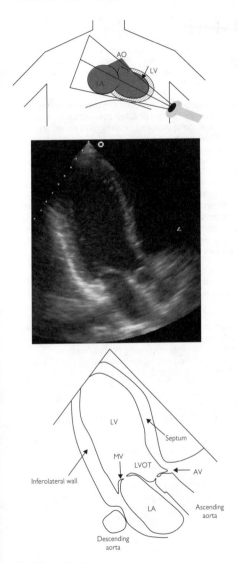

Fig. 2.9 Apical 3-chamber view.

Subcostal views

Very useful views to study pericardial effusions, assess right ventricular inflow, and screen for septal defects. Also, alternative window for equivalent of parasternal views if parasternal window not possible.

Finding the view

- In the subcostal window have the probe flat and pressed into the stomach so that the imaging plane is directed upwards under the ribs.
- With slight rotation and tilting back and forward you will find the heart. You will need to increase the depth. If it is difficult to get an image, ask the patient to take a breath in. This drops the diaphragm and often brings the heart into view. Once you have found the heart, optimize the image with gentle movements of the probe.
- Optimal image will look like a 4-chamber view but from the side. Both ventricles and both atria should be seen with the atrial and ventricular septa aligned horizontally across the screen. Both mitral and aortic valves should be evident.
- The probe can also be rotated 90° in this view to create a short axis subcostal view. By tilting back and forward this can be used to look at left and right ventricles and the pulmonary valve.

What to record?

- 2D images.
- Colour flow mapping: tricuspid valve and septa (atrial and ventricular).

What do you see?

- *Right ventricle.* Close to probe and both free wall and septum are seen. Wall thickness can be measured. The septum is flat across the screen so good alignment for colour flow mapping of septal defects.
- *Right atrium.* Good view to look at right ventricular inflow as close to probe. May see Eustachian valve and entry of inferior vena cava. Because of horizontal alignment of interatrial septum an ideal view for colour flow mapping of atrial septal defects and Doppler alignment to quantify flow across defects.
- *Tricuspid valve.* Close to probe and can be used for colour flow mapping of regurgitation.
- *Pericardium.* Excellent view to assess size and depth of effusion when planning pericardiocentesis as probe in position of a subxiphisternum approach.
- *Left ventricle.* In far field. Septum and lateral wall are seen.
- *Mitral valve.* In far field and little extra information provided.
- *Left atrium.* Little extra information provided about left atrium.

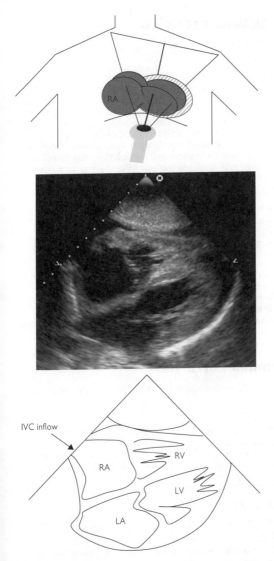

Fig. 2.10 Subcostal view.

Inferior vena cava view

Essential to assess right atrial pressure.

Finding the view
- From the subcostal view rotate the probe anticlockwise.
- Keep the right atrium in the centre of the image and focus on the atrium as you rotate the probe. The opening of the inferior vena cava should become more obvious. As you rotate the probe the inferior vena cava should open out into a long tubular structure horizontally across the screen. If you are worried it may be the aorta, not the inferior vena cava, use pulsed wave Doppler to demonstrate continuous, low velocity venous flow rather than pulsatile, high velocity aortic flow.
- Optimal image is of the inferior vena cava like a railway track across the screen perhaps seen opening into right atrium. Hepatic veins emptying into inferior vena cava may also be seen.

What to record?
- 2D images with inspiration and expiration (a 5 beat loop may be required).
- M-mode measures with respiration.
- Consider pulsed wave Doppler in aligned hepatic veins.

What do you see?
- *Inferior vena cava.* Use to measure diameter and whether it reduces in size with inspiration (normally should do).
- *Liver and hepatic veins.* These can be seen draining into the inferior vena cava and may be aligned for Doppler measures. If right atrial pressures are high they may be dilated.

Abdominal aorta view

Not an essential view but interesting! A simple screening test for aortic aneurysm.

Finding the view
- From the subcostal inferior vena cava view tilt the probe out of the plane of the inferior vena cava. The aorta should come into view and look very similar to the inferior vena cava. It usually lies to the left of the inferior vena cava and slightly deeper. Confirm it is aorta with pulsed wave Doppler to demonstrate arterial flow.
- Optimal image is of the aorta like a 'railway track' across the screen.

What to record?
- 2D images.

What do you see?
- *Aorta.* May see wall thickening, aneurysm, or even gross mobile thrombus and plaque.

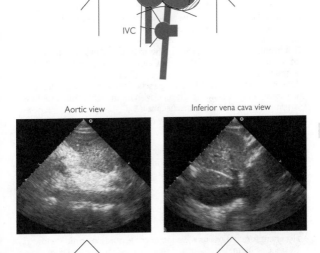

Aortic view

Inferior vena cava view

Fig. 2.11 Subcostal abdominal aorta view (left) and inferior vena cava view (right).

Suprasternal view

A view to look at size of aorta and aortic flow for coarctation or aortic regurgitation.

Finding the view

- In the suprasternal window have the probe pointing, slightly rotated, into the chest behind the sternum. The dot on the probe should be towards the left shoulder. Use light pressure (with extra gel to maintain contact between probe and skin if necessary) as it can be uncomfortable.
- Tilt probe back and forward until the arch comes into view then rotate to maximize the curve of the arch. Colour flow may help identify flow in the aorta.
- Optimal image has distal ascending aorta, arch, and proximal descending aorta with origin of the left subclavian on the right, and potentially origin of left carotid and brachiocephalic.

What to record?

- 2D images.
- Doppler of flow in ascending and descending aorta.
- Consider colour flow mapping around arch and subclavian artery (looking for jets associated with patent ductus arteriosus, coarctation, or obstruction).

What do you see?

- *Aortic arch.* Curves through picture and can be measured.
- *Ascending aorta.* Can be difficult to see clearly but can provide alignment for continuous wave Doppler measures in aortic stenosis.
- *Descending aorta.* Usually better seen than ascending aorta. Size can be measured and is aligned for Doppler studies of aortic flow to grade aortic regurgitation or coarctations.
- *Left subclavian artery.* Easiest branch to see and important landmark for isthmus (common site of dissection and coarctation).

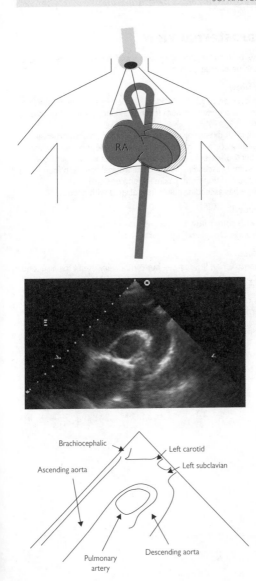

Fig. 2.12 Suprasternal view.

Right parasternal view

An extra view to look at ascending aorta and judge severity of aortic stenosis but can be difficult to find.

Finding the view

• Roll patient over on to right side. Place probe on right side of sternum pointing down and under sternum (both stand alone and 2D probes can be used).
• Adjust probe in all directions looking for Doppler across aortic valve and up ascending aorta. If using stand alone Doppler probe look for the aortic spectral pattern and if using a 2D probe use colour flow mapping to identify ascending aorta. Once a signal has been found keep adjusting probe position until maximal Doppler signal.
• Optimal image has ascending aortic flow aligned with probe.

What to record?

• 2D images with colour flow to demonstrate aorta.
• Continuous wave Doppler of flow through aortic valve.

What do you see?

• *Ascending aorta.* Often little to see but can be very useful for a second measure of an aortic gradient if there is concern that it is being under-estimated. The alignment of flow through the aortic valve for Doppler measures is often better in the right parasternal view than in the apical or suprasternal views.

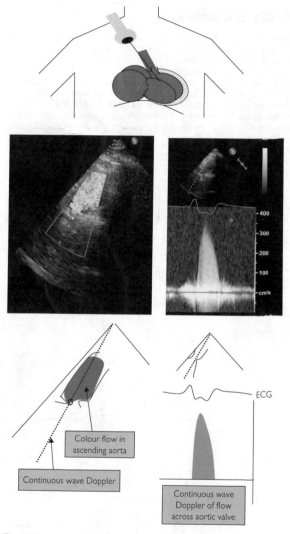

Fig. 2.13 Right parasternal view. Used to measure flow across aortic valve and in ascending aorta.

Standard examination

The minimal sequence of views and measurements needed to perform a study can be standardized to ensure collection of a *minimal dataset*. Minimal datasets are published by bodies of experts as a guide to what information should be collected.

On the following pages is a graphic description of a standard examination in the order of data collection, accompanied by tables for each view summarizing a minimal dataset (in bold). The tables are adapted from those published by the British Society of Echocardiography Education Committee. Information in italics in the tables is additional data that is collected when appropriate to describe pathology.

Abbreviations are on pp. xi–xiii.

Quality of echocardiographic recordings

The quality of echocardiographic recordings is based on the following criteria.
- Is the dataset complete, i.e. a full standard examination and minimal dataset?
- Are all the recordings obtained from the appropriate imaging points, i.e. correct apical position, etc.?
- Is image quality good, i.e. are the views appropriately recorded, correct gain and depth, etc.?

Image quality

2D/3D imaging is best judged on endocardial border definition. Look at the proportion of the border that is clearly seen in the three apicall views. Judge image quality as:
- good if >80% of the border is seen in the three apical views;
- poor if the endocardium is not visible.

Image quality is moderate if endocardial border is visible but less than 80%. For stress echocardiography good image quality is required and there should be a maximum of two segments not seen in any view.

Spectral Doppler should be judged as:
- good if the cursor position is displayed, there is good alignment (with the angle between flow and beam <30°), and the spectrum has a clear envelope;
- poor if the angle between flow and beam is >30° or the spectrum is incomplete.

Only good spectral Doppler tracing should be used for quantitative analysis.

Colour flow mapping should be judged as:
- good if the flow of interest is aligned with the probe and gain settings are correct (just below the level that produces background noise). If for flow convergence, the baseline has been shifted;
- poor if the flow is not aligned or gain settings are incorrect.

For assessment of regurgitation colour flow mapping must be good. When used to align spectral Doppler then suboptimal settings may be sufficient.

Parasternal long axis view

2D IMAGE
Can be used for measurements
Acquire right ventricle
inflow and outflow views if required

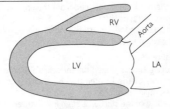

COLOUR FLOW
1. Aortic valve
2. Mitral valve

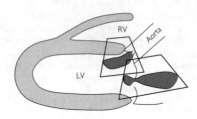

M-MODE (see tracings opposite)
1. Aortic root and left atrium
2. Mitral valve movement (trace not shown)
3. Left ventricle size
Measurements are edge to edge

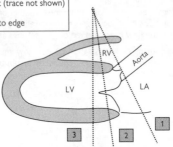

Dataset—parasternal long axis views

Modality	Structures	Measure	Calculate
2D	LV cavity, size, function	LVDd/s, IVSd/s, LVPWd/s	FS
	RV cavity, size, function		
	LA size	LAs	
	Aortic root, AV appearance, function	*Annulus; root, ascending*	
	MV appearance, function	*MV annulus*	
M-mode	LV cavity size, wall thickness	LVDd/s, IVSd/s, LVPWd/s	FS
	RV cavity size	RVd	
	MV	*± es separation*	
	AV/aortic root/LA size	LAs, root	*LA : Ao cusp separation*
CFM	MV inflow/MR		
	LVOT/AR (VSD)	AR width	*AR : LVOT*

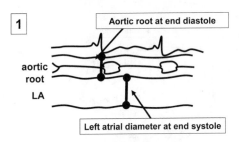

1

Aortic root at end diastole

aortic root

LA

Left atrial diameter at end systole

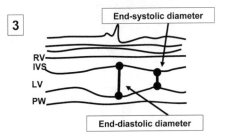

3

End-systolic diameter

RV
IVS
LV
PW

End-diastolic diameter

Parasternal short axis view—ventricle and mitral

2D IMAGE
Assess LV function and regional abnormalities
Assess RV
Can be used for M-mode or 2D measures of LV size and function

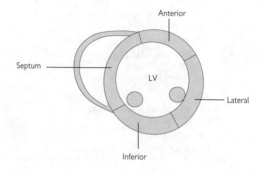

2D IMAGE
Assess mitral valve morphology
Consider colour flow across mitral valve and planimetry

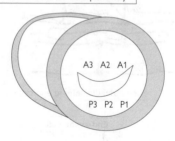

Dataset—parasternal short axis views, Part 1

Modality	Structures	Measure	Calculate
Mitral valve			
2D	**MV appearance, function**	*MVA planimetry*	
	LV size, wall thickness, function		
	RV cavity size, function		
CFM	*MV inflow, MR (VSD)*		
Papillary muscles			
2D	**LV size, wall thickness, function**		*FS*
	RV size, wall thickness, function		
CFM	*(VSD)*		
Apical			
2D	**LV size, wall thickness, function**		
CFM	*(VSD)*		

Parasternal short axis view—aortic valve level

2D IMAGE
Assess tricuspid, aortic, and pulmonary valve morphology
Can measure right ventricle size

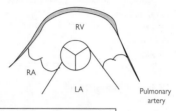

COLOUR FLOW
Assess tricuspid, aortic, and pulmonary valve
Can assess atrial septum

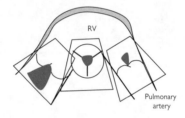

DOPPLER
Use continuous wave to assess pulmonary regurgitation and stenosis
Pulsed wave Doppler can measure right ventricle outflow
Continuous wave can be used at tricuspid valve to assess regurgitation

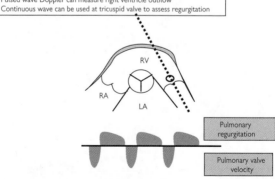

Dataset—parasternal short axis view, Part 2

Modality	Structures	Measure	Calculate
Aortic valve			
2D	LA, atrial septum		
	RA		
	TV appearance, function		
	RV cavity size, function		
	PV, PA	PV annulus	
	AV appearance, function		
CFM	SVC, RUPV, atrial septum		
	TV inflow, TR		
	RVOT, PS, PR, PA (PDA)		
PW	RVOT	Vmax, vti, Vmean	
CW	TR	Vmax	PAs pressure
	PS	Vmax, Vmean	Pmax, Pmean
	PR	Vmax, PRed	PAd pressure

Apical views—four chamber

2D IMAGE
Assess LV size, thickness, function, and regional wall motion
Assess RV size and function
Look at mitral and tricuspid morphology

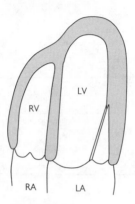

COLOUR FLOW
Assess mitral and tricuspid valves

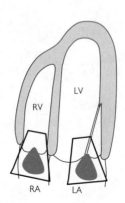

Dataset—apical 4-chamber, Part 1

Modality	Structures	Measure	Calculate
2D	LV cavity size, wall thickness, function		
	RV cavity size, function		
	LA size	Area/vol	LA vol index
	RA size	Area/vol	RA vol index
	MV appearance, function		
	TV appearance, function		
CFM	TV inflow/TR		
	MV inflow/MR		

Apical views—four chamber, Doppler

DOPPLER–MITRAL VALVE
Use PW at mitral valve tips to assess left ventricle inflow
Use CW across valve to assess mitral regurgitation

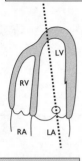

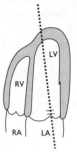

E and A waves of inflow

Mitral regurgitation

DOPPLER–TRICUSPID VALVE
Assess tricuspid regurgitation with CW across valve to estimate right ventricle pressure

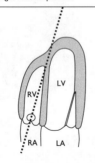

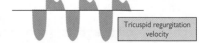

Tricuspid regurgitation velocity

Dataset—apical 4-chamber, Part 2

Modality	Structures	Measure	Calculate
PW	LV inflow (MV tips)	E, A, *DET, IVRT*	E:A ratio
CW	MS	*Vmax, Vmean, P1/2*	*Pmax, Pmean, MVA*
	MR		
	TS	*Vmax, Vmean*	*Pmax, Pmean*
	TR	**Vmax**	**PAs pressure**

Apical views—five chamber

2D IMAGE
Identify left ventricle outflow

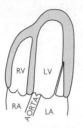

COLOUR FLOW
Assess aortic regurgitation

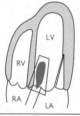

DOPPLER—AORTIC VALVE
Use PW to measure LVOT velocity
Use CW to measure velocity across valve and assess regurgitation

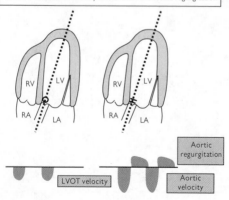

Dataset—apical 5-chamber

Modality	Structures	Measure	Calculate
2D	LV cavity size, wall thickness, function		
	LVOT; AV appearance, function		
CFM	LVOT, AV		
PW	LVOT	vti, Vmax, Vmean	Pmax, Pmean
CW	LVOT, AS	Vmax, Vmean	Pmax, Pmean
	AR	DET	

Apical views—two and three chamber

2D IMAGE
Assess LV function and regional abnormalities
Assess mitral valve morphology

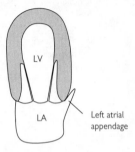

LV

LA

Left atrial
appendage

2D IMAGE
Assess LV function and regional abnormalities
Assess mitral and aortic valve morphology
Can use Doppler at aortic and mitral valves

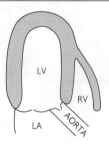

LV

RV

LA

AORTA

Dataset—apical 2-chamber

Modality	Structures	Measure	Calculate
2D	LV cavity size, wall thickness, function		
	MV appearance, function		
CFM	LV inflow, MR		
PW	LV inflow (MV tips)	E, DET, A (IVRT)	E:A ratio
CW	MS	Vmax, Vmean	Pmax, Pmean
	MR		

Dataset—apical 3-chamber

Modality	Structures	Measure	Calculate
2D	LV cavity size, wall thickness, function; LVOT; AV appearance, function		
CFM	LV inflow, MR, LVOT, AV		
PW	LV inflow (MV tips)	E, DET, A (IVRT)	E:A ratio
	LVOT	vti, Vmax, Vmean	SV, CO, Pmax, Pmean
CW	MS	Vmax, Vmean	Pmax, Pmean
	MR		
	LVOT, AS	Vmax, Vmean	Pmax, Pmean
	AR	DET	

Subcostal and suprasternal views

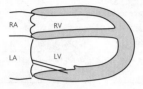

2D IMAGE
Assess right heart and look for pericardial effusion

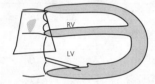

COLOUR FLOW
Assess atrial and ventricular septum

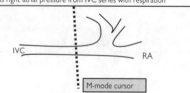

2D and M-MODE –INFERIOR VENA CAVA
Assess right atrial pressure from IVC series with respiration

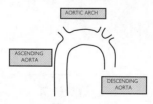

2D IMAGE and DOPPLER-AORTA
Use Doppler in descending aorta to assess aortic regurgitation

Datasets—subcostal views

Modality	Structures	Measure	Calculate
Subcostal 4-chamber			
2D	**4-chamber structures**		
CFM	**Atrial septum, 4-chamber structures**		
Subcostal short axis			
2D	**IVC, Hep. V (modified view)**, *atrial septum, SAX structures, desc. aorta (modified view)*		
M-mode	**IVC respiratory variation**		
CFM	*SAX structures, atrial septum, IVC, Hep. V*		
PW	*Hep. V, desc. aorta*		

Dataset—suprasternal views

Modality	Structures	Measure	Calculate
2D	*Arch*		
CFM	*Arch, coarctation, PDA*		
PW	*Desc. aorta*	*Flow reversal*	
CW	*Asc. aorta (AS)*	*Vmax, Vmean*	*Pmax, Pmean*
	Desc. aorta (coarct.)	*Vmax, Vmean*	*Pmax, Pmean*

Transthoracic: anatomy and pathology

Mitral valve

Normal anatomy

The mitral valve has two leaflets (anterior and posterior). The posterior is long and thin and forms a crescent around the wider anterior leaflet. The surface area of both leaflets is approximately equal but the distance between mitral ring and coaption line is shorter on the posterior leaflet. Each leaflet has 3 scallops, which meet each other along the coaption line. They are named: A1, A2, A3 (anterior) and P1, P2, P3 (posterior). P1 and A1 are adjacent to the anterolateral commissure and A3 and P3 nearest the right heart. Below the valve are two papillary muscles: a larger anterolateral (usually a single trunk) and a smaller posteromedial (often 2–3 distinct trunks). These support chordae tendinae: 1st order attached to leaflet tips; 2nd order to undersurface of leaflets; and 3rd order run directly from ventricular wall to leaflet undersurface. Chordae from both papillary muscles attach to both leaflets. The valve leaflets are supported by the mitral valve annulus, which divides the left atrium and ventricle, and is a fibrous elliptical structure.

Normal findings

Views

- The mitral valve can be seen in most views. Parasternal long axis and parasternal short axis (mitral valve level) views are particularly useful to look at valve motion and structure.
- The three apical views offer the ability to scan through the mitral valve in multiple planes and do Doppler measurements.

Findings

- Parasternal long axis. Segments of the anterior leaflet (A2—nearest the left ventricular outflow tract) and posterior leaflet (P2) are seen as thin structures uniform in echogenicity. The posteromedial papillary muscle may be seen attached to the posterior wall.
- Parasternal short axis. At the mitral valve level, all three segments of each leaflet are seen and the 2 commissures. This creates the classic 'fish mouth' appearance. At the midlevel of the left ventricle the bodies of the two papillary muscles can be seen.
- Apical 4-chamber view. The A2 and A1 segments of the anterior leaflet are shown on the left and the P1 segment of the posterior leaflet on the right. The mitral valve annulus is usually slightly out of line with the tricuspid valve annulus (the tricuspid annulus is normally up to 1cm closer to the right ventricular apex).
- Apical 2-chamber view. The P1 and P3 segments are seen either side of the A2 segment of the anterior mitral valve leaflet.
- Apical 3-chamber view. The A2 and P2 segments are visualized similarly to the parasternal long axis view.

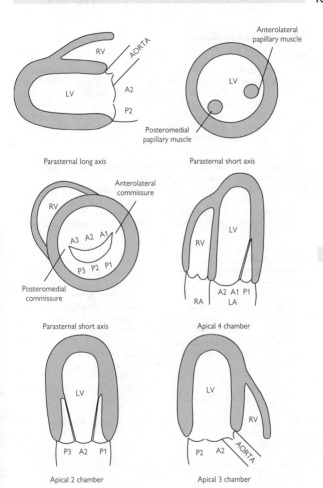

Fig. 3.1 Standard echocardiography views of mitral valve.

Mitral stenosis

General

The commonest cause of mitral stenosis is still rheumatic disease. Systemic lupus erythematosus is a rare cause and congenital mitral stenosis is very rare. Clinically, atrial myxoma and cor triatriatum may mimic mitral stenosis. Mitral annular calcification is common in the elderly and can involve the entire posterior part of the annulus. Occasionally, annular calcification can extend to the base of the leaflets leading to stenosis but more commonly leads to regurgitation.

Assessment

- Echocardiography should be used to diagnose stenosis and describe probable aetiology based on appearance.
- Severity should be graded according to: valve area; pressure gradient across the valve; changes to left atrium, left ventricle, and right heart.
- The examination should also be used to look for associated valvular lesions (in particular rheumatic aortic disease) and complications such as endocarditis.

Appearance

Comment on the valve.

- Mobility of base of leaflet compared to tips. In rheumatic disease the tips tend to be restricted so the valve appears to '*dome*'. This may also be referred to as a '*hockey stick*' or '*elbowing*' appearance.
- Thickening or calcification of leaflets, annulus, and subvalvular apparatus.
- Evidence of fusion of the commissures. Use a short axis view.
- Chordae—thickening, shortening, calcification.

Comment on associated features.

- Associated valvular lesions (aortic rheumatic disease).
- Left atrium.
  - Usually grossly enlarged. Give measurement.
  - Spontaneous left atrial contrast (associated with significant stenosis and suggests very slow atrial blood flow or stasis).
- Right heart
  - Tricuspid regurgitation and right ventricular pressure.
  - Right ventricle and atrial size.
- Left ventricular function.

Differentiation of rheumatic mitral stenosis from calcification

In rheumatic disease (in contrast to degenerative mitral valve disease):

- thickening comes first with calcification later;
- leaflet thickening affects the commissures and leaflet edges, whereas mitral annular calcification tends to spare the leaflet tips;
- there is subvalvular involvement with shortening of chordae;
- combination of loss of leaflet mobility due to commissural fusion and chordal shortening and tethering leads to 'doming' or 'hockey-stick' appearance of, in particular, the anterior leaflet.

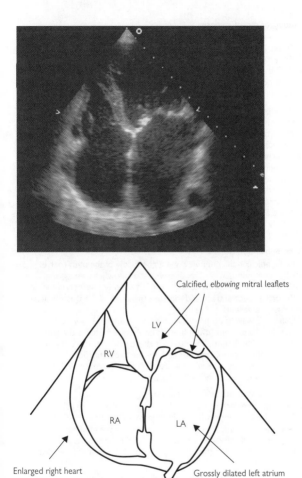

Calcified, *elbowing* mitral leaflets

LV

RV

RA

LA

Enlarged right heart

Grossly dilated left atrium

Fig. 3.2 Apical 4-chamber view demonstrating rheumatic mitral stenosis with doming, calcified valve. The left atrium is grossly dilated.

Grading of mitral stenosis
- Grade stenosis as mild, moderate, or severe based on *valve area* (Table 3.1). Use *planimetered* measurements and *pressure half-time* (P1/2 time) across the valve. Also, report the actual measures.
- Back this up with assessment of *pressure gradient* across the valve.
- Comment on associated changes that support your assessment. Include changes to the *left atrium* and *right-sided pressures*.

Planimetry
- In parasternal short axis view, angle the probe to the mitral valve level.
- Move the probe back and forth until you are sure you at the level of the *leaflet tips*. If the plane is too basal, MS will be underestimated.
- 3D echocardiography (if available) at the parasternal short axis level is very effective at demonstrating the 'mouth' of mitral stenosis to ensure planimetry is at the leaflet tips.
- Record a loop and scroll through to find the maximum opening in diastole (Fig. 3.3).
- Trace along the *inner edge* of the leaflets. This may be difficult in heavily calcified valves so comment if there is a lot of calcification.
- Report the surface area of the orifice.

Pressure half-time
- In the apical 4-chamber view get a good view of the mitral valve.
- Align continuous wave Doppler with the inflow jet through the stenosis. Try and minimize any angle between the beam and the jet.
- Record a spectral trace and measure the slope of the diastolic flow across the valve (Fig. 3.4).
- Use the E-wave if both E-wave (diastolic filling) and A-wave (atrial systole) are present (often there is no A-wave because the patient is in atrial fibrillation). If the trace is slightly curved with a steep start (a '*ski-slope*'), ignore the start and use the flatter portion.
- The machine automatically reports P1/2 time and mitral valve area where MV area (in cm^2) = 220/P1/2 time (in msec)

Mean transmitral valve diastolic pressure gradient
- Use the same technique/recording as used for pressure half-time.
- Trace the Doppler profile of the transmitral diastolic flow. The machine automatically reports the mean pressure gradient.
- Pressure gradient varies significantly with the filling time. If the patient is in atrial fibrillation this will vary so report the mean of 2–3 beats.

Problems with P1/2 time and pressure gradient

- Quantification based on P1/2 time assumes normal LV patho-physiology. Significant changes in LV compliance (e.g. LV hypertrophy) or pathology that increases LV pressure during diastole (e.g. AR) shorten the P1/2 time. MV area is underestimated.
- Normal atrial pathophysiology is also assumed. An atrial septal defect with left to right shunt shortens the P1/2 time (as blood also leaves from left to right atrium) and MV area is overestimated. Conversely, a right to left shunt will lengthen the P1/2 time.

Table 3.1 Parameters to determine severity of mitral stenosis

	MILD	MODERATE	SEVERE
MV area (cm²)	2.2–1.5	1.5–1.0	<1.0
MV P1/2 time (msec)	100–150	150–220	>220
Mean pressure gradient (mmHg)	<5	Variable	>10
TR velocity (m/sec)	<2.7	Variable	>3
PA pressure (mmHg)	<30	Variable	>50

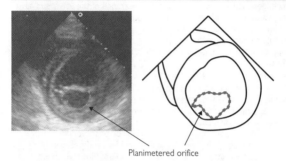

Planimetered orifice

Fig. 3.3 Planimetered mitral valve orifice in parasternal short axis.

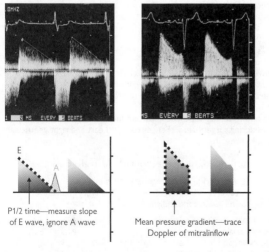

P1/2 time—measure slope of E wave, ignore A wave

Mean pressure gradient—trace Doppler of mitralinflow

Fig. 3.4 Pressure half-time and mean pressure gradient.

Mitral regurgitation

Mitral regurgitation is common. A trace of 'physiological' mitral regurgitation is seen in up to 50% of people with normal cardiac anatomy. Pathological mitral regurgitation can be caused by changes in the leaflets (e.g. endocarditis, myxomatous change), subvalvular apparatus (e.g. papillary muscle rupture), or mitral annulus (e.g. left ventricular dilatation).

Assessment

- Mitral regurgitation is easily identified with colour flow placed over the mitral valve and left atrium in parasternal long axis and apical views.
- Once identified a wider study of the appearance of the valve, subvalvular apparatus, and left ventricle should be used to determine aetiology and impact on cardiac function.
- Severity should be judged by combining measurements from all main Doppler modalities (colour flow, continuous and pulsed wave) and 2D echocardiography.

Appearance

- Map the *regurgitant jet* with colour flow in parasternal and apical views. Establish the shape and pattern. Comment on the following.
  - Where the regurgitation passes through the valve, e.g. central, by a commissure or through a perforation.
  - The direction of eccentric jets (anterior or posterior). Anteriorly directed suggests a posterior leaflet problem and posteriorly directed suggests an anterior leaflet problem. Note which left atrial wall the jet entrains against and how far back it goes.
  - If there are several jets, comment on each one.
  - Spectral Doppler and colour M-mode can define the timing of regurgitation, e.g. confined to a short period after valve closure (closing volume) or to late systole (often found in mitral valve prolapse).
- In parasternal and apical views use M-mode and 2D to look at both *valve leaflets*. Comment on:
  - movement, evidence of prolapse, calcification, masses, vegetations.
- Look at *subvalvular apparatus*. Comment on:
  - papillary muscle and chordae with reference to shortening, rupture.
- Report *associated features*:
  - left atrial size, left ventricular size and function (important when considering surgery), any changes to right heart and right ventricular systolic pressure.

Physiological, mild, or trace (trivial) regurgitation

It is reasonable to decide mitral regurgitation is *mild* or *trivial* if:
- jet is small (jet area <4 cm^2 or <20% left atrial area) and central;
- no flow convergence zone is displayed.

To call mitral regurgitation *physiological* make sure:
- valve morphology is normal;
- the regurgitation has a short duration (typically post valve closure);
- it is mild or trivial (as above).

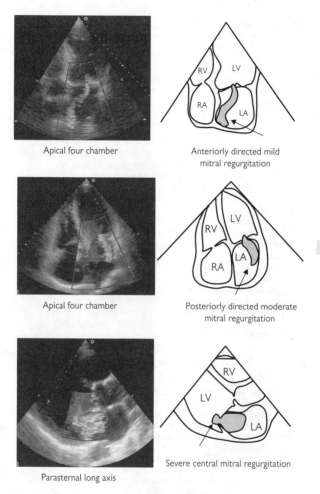

Apical four chamber

Anteriorly directed mild
mitral regurgitation

Apical four chamber

Posteriorly directed moderate
mitral regurgitation

Parasternal long axis

Severe central mitral regurgitation

Fig. 3.5 Colour flow mapping of mitral regurgitation with eccentric and central jets.

Grading severity
- Gauge severity as mild, moderate, or severe based on the combination of *jet area*, *vena contracta*, *flow convergence (PISA)* and changes in *systolic pulmonary vein flow* (if technically possible) (Table 3.2).
- Gross pathology, e.g. a flail leaflet, points to severe regurgitation.
- Once you have an impression of severity use *continuous wave Doppler waveform density*, changes in left ventricular *mitral inflow*, and left ventricular function to support your assessment.
- You can provide further quantification of regurgitation with measurement of *effective regurgitant orifice* area (EROA), *regurgitant volume*, and *regurgitant fraction*.

Colour Doppler jet area
- Establish an apical image that includes the whole left atrium.
- Using colour flow mapping, optimize the image to include the whole regurgitant jet. Set Nyquist limit at 50–60cm/sec.
- Record a loop and scroll through to reach the frame with the maximum jet size.
- Trace the regurgitant jet. Trace the border of the left atrium. If there are multiple jets add the separate jet areas together.
- Report the absolute size of the jet and the size relative to the size of the left atrium (percentage).
- Grade the severity but bear in mind the following.
  - If the jet area relative to left atrium suggests the regurgitation is mild or moderate but the left atrium is very large (>70mm^2) then grade it as moderate or severe, respectively.
  - If the jet area suggests the regurgitation is moderate or severe but the regurgitation is not pansystolic then class it as mild or moderate, respectively.

Problems with jet area to gauge severity

Correlation between jet area and severity of mitral regurgitation is poor and the measurement should be used only in combination with the other methods. This is because of the following.
- The regurgitant jet area includes turbulent (aliased) flow signals as well as laminar velocities in the same direction as the mitral regurgitation jet. Movement of blood already in the left atrium that moves with the regurgitant jet (entrainment) is therefore included.
- Jet area can be artificially changed. Reducing the scale increases the area because the lower filter setting means lower velocities are displayed. Try and use average scale settings (50–60cm/sec) and ensure the same setting on follow-up scans.
- Eccentric jets are underestimated as they flatten out against walls and go out of plane.

Table 3.2 Assessment of severity of mitral regurgitation

	SPECIFIC SIGNS OF SEVERITY	
	MILD	SEVERE
Jet (Nyquist, 50–60cm/sec)	<4cm² or <20% LA; small & central	>40% LA; large & central or wall impinging & swirling
Vena contracta	<0.3cm	>0.7cm
PISA r (Nyquist, 40cm/sec)	None/minimal (<0.4cm)	Large (>1cm)
Pulmonary vein flow	—	Systolic reversal
Valve structure	—	Flail or rupture
	SUPPORTIVE SIGNS OF SEVERITY	
	MILD	SEVERE
Pulmonary vein flow	Systolic dominant	
Mitral inflow	A-wave dominant	E-wave dominant (>1.2m/sec)
CW trace	Soft & parabolic	Dense & triangular
LV & LA	Normal size LV if chronic MR	Enlarged LV & LA if no other cause

Report as MODERATE if signs of regurgitation are greater than MILD but there are no signs of SEVERE regurgitation.

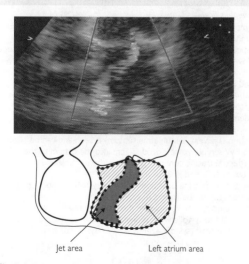

Jet area   Left atrium area

Fig. 3.6 Colour jet area and area of left atrium as marker of severity.

Vena contracta
- Obtain a clear view of the colour flow through the mitral valve in parasternal long axis or apical 4-chamber views.
- If necessary, scan along the commissural line to ensure you have the point of regurgitation through the valve.
- Zoom in on the colour flow through the mitral valve.
- Record a loop and scroll through to identify the image with maximal flow through the valve.
- The vena contracta is the narrowest region of the regurgitant jet (usually just below the valve in the left atrium).
- Report the diameter. >0.7cm suggests severe regurgitation.
- A parasternal short axis view just below the mitral valve level can be used and cross-sectional area of the regurgitant jet recorded. The cross-sectional area is one way of measuring the effective regurgitant orifice area (EROA).

Problems with vena contracta as marker of severity

This method is simple and thought to be independent of haemodynamics, driving pressure, and flow rate. However, low colour gain, poor acoustic windows, or failure to assess multiple jets can underestimate the vena contracta. A high colour gain, irregular shape of jet, or atrial fibrillation can lead to overestimation.

Flow convergence (PISA, proximal isovelocity surface area) See p. 118.

Pulmonary venous flow
Normally blood flows from the pulmonary veins throughout the cardiac cycle. As mitral regurgitation becomes more severe, left atrial pressure increases more rapidly during systole and reduces the amount of blood that can flow from the pulmonary vein (blunted systolic pulmonary vein flow). With severe regurgitation atrial pressures are high and blood starts to be forced back into the veins (reversed systolic pulmonary flow).
- Obtain an apical 4-chamber view with enough depth to see the back of the left atrium.
- Try to identify the pulmonary vein orifices on the back of the left atrium. With transthoracic echocardiography, often only the right upper pulmonary vein (by the atrial septum) is seen and can be aligned.
- Place the PW sample volume around 1cm into the ostium of the vein.
- A good spectral tracing confirms you are in the right place.
- Look at the systolic and diastolic components.
  - If they are in opposite directions with the systolic component going away from the probe report *reversed systolic flow*.
  - If in the same direction, measure the height of the two waves and comment if the systolic wave is *blunted* relative to diastolic or the relation is normal (systolic slightly larger—*systolic dominant*).

Problems with pulmonary venous flow

Any pathology that increases left atrial pressure can blunt pulmonary vein flow. If systolic flow reversal is present then this is very specific but not very sensitive for severe regurgitation.

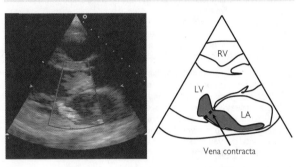

Fig. 3.7 Vena contracta: narrowest part of jet as passes through valve.

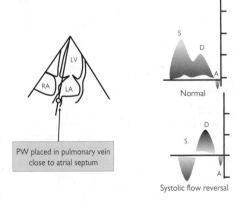

Fig. 3.8 Measuring pulmonary vein flow.

Mitral inflow

As regurgitation becomes more severe the amount of blood forced into the left atrium during systole increases. This increased volume of blood increases left atrial pressure. Therefore, blood leaves the atrium more quickly at the start of diastole, i.e. peak early diastolic velocity increases.

- In an apical 4-chamber view place the pulsed wave Doppler cursor at the mitral valve tips.
- E wave >1.2m/sec is indicative of severe mitral regurgitation.
- However, a hyperdynamic circulation or even minor degrees of mitral stenosis can also increase E-wave amplitude. If the A-wave is dominant, severe mitral regurgitation is virtually ruled out.

Continuous wave Doppler intensity/shape

- In an apical 4-chamber view place the continuous wave Doppler through the mitral valve orifice and record a spectral trace.
- Make a qualitative judgement about the density of the systolic regurgitant waveform relative to the mitral inflow density. If they are the same this suggests there is as much blood flow into the atrium during systole as back into the ventricle during diastole and regurgitation is severe. (Peak velocity allows calculation of *regurgitant orifice area* (p. 118)).

Regurgitant volume/regurgitant fraction

The principle behind the *regurgitant volume* is that the amount of blood that flows through the mitral valve into the left ventricle during diastole (assuming there is no aortic regurgitation to fill the left ventricle as well) should equal the amount of blood that leaves the left ventricle during systole. The amount of blood leaving through the aortic valve in systole can be calculated and subtracted from the amount flowing across the mitral valve in diastole. The difference is the volume flowing back through the incompetent mitral valve. *Regurgitant volume* is not usually calculated as accuracy depends on accurate measures of the outflow tract and mitral valve area. The mitral ring is difficult to assess because it is not circular and changes throughout the cardiac cycle. To measure do the following.

- In apical 4-chamber view record pulsed wave at the mitral valve (it is controversial whether the sample volume should be at annulus or valve tip level). Trace the vti. Estimate mitral valve cross-sectional area (CSA). Use annulus width and assume a circular orifice (alternatively measure the annulus in two perpendicular planes and calculate area as an oval).

  Mitral inflow volume = vti × CSA mitral valve

- In apical 5-chamber view record pulsed wave in left ventricular outflow and measure vti. Measure outflow tract diameter in parasternal long axis and estimate cross-sectional area (assuming it is circular).

  LV outflow volume = vti × CSA left ventricular outflow.

- Mitral regurgitant volume is: MV inflow volume − LV outflow volume.
- Regurgitant fraction (<20% mild; >50% severe regurgitation) is:

  Mitral regurgitant volume/mitral inflow volume

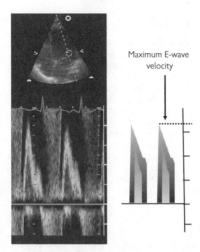

Fig. 3.9 Maximum E-wave velocity >1.2m/sec—severe regurgitation.

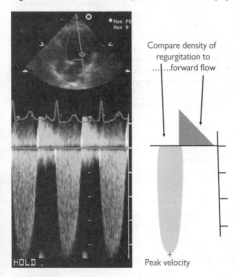

Fig. 3.10 Severe regurgitation is suggested if density of regurgitation is similar to forward flow. Peak velocity can be used with PISA to calculate effective regurgitant orifice area (p. 118).

PISA (proximal isovelocity surface area)

PISA or *flow convergence zone* is a measurement of how much blood travels through a valve. It has been applied in several situations (e.g. aortic regurgitation, mitral stenosis) but is validated for assessment of mitral regurgitation. If regurgitation is mild, only blood near the valve moves towards the atrium. With severe regurgitation blood further away in the ventricle moves backwards. An impression of how far this *flow convergence zone* extends into the ventricle is obtained by looking at the velocity of blood flow in the ventricle with colour flow mapping. To quantify the distance you use the principle that at a certain velocity the colour flow will alias (change colour). The further away this change in colour, the more blood is being funneled back through the mitral valve, and the more severe the regurgitation. In 3D the aliasing layer is a coloured hemisphere sitting on the mitral valve. The *PISA* refers to the surface area of the hemisphere (Fig. 3.11) and correlates to the *regurgitant flow*.

Assessment

- Get a good image of the mitral valve (usually the apical 4-chamber view is best) and ensure you are in the plane of the regurgitant jet.
- Check what the colour scale is set to, i.e. aliasing velocity, $v_{aliasing}$. You can use this velocity if the flow convergence is obvious but to optimize the colour contrast at the boundary layer it is normal to shift the zero of the baseline so that the aliasing velocity is 40cm/sec.
- Acquire a loop of the cardiac cycle and scroll through to identify the mid-systolic hemisphere shell. (Fig. 3.11).
- Measure the radius (r) from valve orifice to point of colour change. If the colour flow is obscuring the valve orifice on your loop, place a caliper at the aliasing zone; then suppress the colour flow and position the second cursor on the valve.
- Report severity based on the parameters below.

Grading severity

- *Radius* (r). A simple approach is just to record r with the aliasing velocity set at 40cm/sec. Severe mitral regurgitation is present if r >1cm and mild if <0.4cm.
- *Regurgitant flow*. Regurgitant flow is calculated as $2\Pi r^2 \times v_{aliasing}$ and has been validated against angiographic grades of regurgitation. Clinically it is normally used with the continuous wave Doppler velocity to measure orifice area.
- *Effective regurgitant orifice area (EROA)*. Regurgitant flow can be combined with the peak CW velocity (p. 116) to calculate EROA.

   EROA = regurgitant flow/peak velocity on CW

   EROA: 0–20mm^2, mild; 20–40mm^2, moderate; >40mm^2, severe.

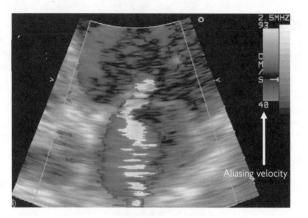

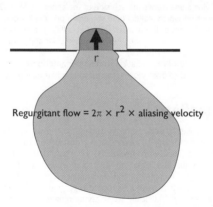

Regurgitant flow = $2\pi \times r^2 \times$ aliasing velocity

Fig. 3.11 Calculation of regurgitant flow in mitral regurgitation using the principle of proximal isovelocity surface area. Note the zero baseline shift to get an aliasing velocity of 40cm/sec and measurement of radius from valve orifice to edge of aliasing boundary.

Mitral valve prolapse

Early studies suggested a high prevalence of up to 20% for mitral valve prolapse but revised criteria for diagnosis have lead to more conservative estimates of around 2%. The key to the change is the differentiation of an anatomically normal valve that bows more than normal from a thickened valve, classically with myxomatous degeneration, that truly prolapses. This is important because it is only the latter patients who have clinical complications. Prolapse can be seen with M-mode but 2D is usually preferred to identify the condition.

- Study the valve in the parasternal long axis view.
- Comment on leaflet thickening or abnormal appearance.
- Report mitral valve *prolapse* if one or both leaflets entirely crosses the plane of the mitral valve annulus back into the left atrium during systole and the tip is >2mm into the left atrium. If the tip is within the plane of the annulus and there is no more than trivial regurgitation then this can be reported as *bowing*, without prolapse (Fig. 3.12).
- The leaflet position relative to the valve plane is determined precisely by drawing a line between each side of the annulus (Fig. 3.13).
- Comment on which leaflets (and scallops if possible) prolapse and check if any part of the prolapsing leaflet is flail (see below).
- Report any associated changes in the subvalvular apparatus (papillary muscle or chordae rupture).
- Report degree of regurgitation (remember anterior leaflet prolapse will be related to posteriorly-directed regurgitation and vice versa).

Flail leaflets

Flail leaflets usually occur due to damage to the subvalvular apparatus. This can be secondary to degeneration, destruction by endocarditis, or ischaemia associated with myocardial infarction. The extent of the flail can vary from just the leaflet tip (due to chordae failure) through to the whole valve (usually papillary muscle rupture). The degree of flail associates with the severity of the associated regurgitation. This can vary from mild to severe and clinically from asymptomatic to haemodynamically unstable.

- Report a flail leaflet/leaflet scallop/leaflet tip if part of the leaflet points back into the left atrium in systole rather than towards the ventricle.
- Comment on which leaflet is affected. If you can see, mention how extensive and which scallop.
- There will be regurgitation so report severity.
- Assess both papillary muscles and the chordae to look for ruptures. To look at the subvalvular apparatus use a combination of views— parasternal long and short axis, all the apical views (2-chamber view can be good to see both papillary muscles), and subcostal views.
- Report related findings according to suspected clinical aetiology. e.g. regional wall motion abnormalities and left ventricle function in myocardial infarction, vegetations in endocarditis.

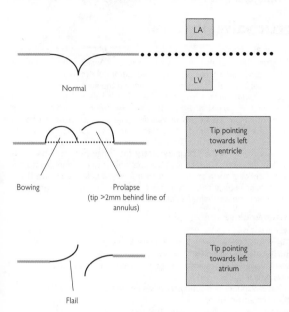

Fig. 3.12 Definitions of normal, prolapsing, and flail.

Posterior leaflet prolapse behind line of annulus

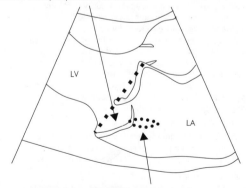

Flail leaflet would point back into atrium

Fig. 3.13 Example of a prolapsing posterior mitral leaflet seen in a parasternal long axis view with superimposed figure of a flail element.

Aortic valve

Normal anatomy

The aortic valve has three cusps of similar size, which close to form a Y shape. Each cusp tip has a small thickened nodule (*nodule of Arantius*). The cusp edges usually overlap by 2–3mm and the lines where they meet are called *commissures*. Closure of the cusps is referred to as *coaption* and opening as *excursion*. Around each cusp are outpouchings of the aortic root called the *sinuses of Valsalva*. The sinuses create a pool of blood above the valve in diastole that improves blood flow down the coronaries and ensures a tight seal. Cusps and associated sinuses are named according to the coronary artery that originates from the sinus (right, left, and non). Above the valves the bulging sinuses merge into the tubular ascending aorta at the *sinotubular junction*. Below the valve is the *left ventricular outflow tract* made up of the *membranous interventricular septum*, *anterior mitral valve leaflet*, and *anterior left ventricular wall*.

Normal findings

Views

- The minimal views are: parasternal long axis, parasternal short axis (aortic valve level), and apical 5-chamber.
- Aortic valve velocities are also obtained from the *right* parasternal view, which can be used for detailed assessment of aortic stenosis.
- Apical 3-chamber and subcostal views provide alternative windows to study the aortic valve.
- Suprasternal view allows measurement of flow in the aorta for assessment of aortic regurgitation.

Aortic valve

- Parasternal long axis: two cusps are seen (usually right coronary by septum and non-coronary by mitral valve). The leaflets open to lie parallel to the aorta and close to form two curved lines.
- Parasternal short axis (aortic valve level): all three cusps are seen (left cusp on the right, right cusp at the top, and non-coronary cusp on the right). This is the classic Y-shape view. The left main coronary artery may be seen and helps identify the left coronary cusp.
- Apical 5- and 3-chamber: the valve is aligned for Doppler measures and two cusps are seen (usually non-coronary cusp next to atrium and right coronary cusp next to septum).

Sinuses of Valsalva and sinotubular junction

- Parasternal long axis: the sinuses bulge to the right of the valve and the sinotubular junction is the point where the ascending aorta starts.
- Parasternal short axis (aortic valve level): sinuses surround each cusp.

Left ventricular outflow tract

- Best seen and measured in parasternal long axis. It is formed by the septum and anterior mitral valve leaflet. Usually around 2cm wide and roughly circular.

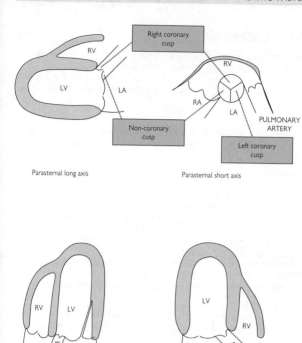

Parasternal long axis

Parasternal short axis

Apical 5 chamber

Apical 3 chamber

Fig. 3.14 Key views to study the aortic valve.

Aortic stenosis

Aortic stenosis is common. Aortic valve thickening occurs in 25% of people aged over 65 and severe stenosis occurs in 3% aged over 75. In the West, the predominant cause is calcific degenerative disease. A bicuspid valve occurs in 2% of the population. Rheumatic disease is now uncommon.

Assessment

The echocardiographic study is aimed at determining the appearance of the valve, the grade of stenosis, the effect on the left ventricle, and the presence of associated disease.

Appearance

Comment on the following.

- Degree and distribution of thickening. The term *aortic sclerosis* describes valve leaflet thickening (>2mm) without significant stenosis.
- How many functional cusps (two in a bicuspid valve, three in rheumatic or calcific degenerative disease; Fig. 3.15).
- Is the closure line central (calcific degenerative or rheumatic disease) or eccentric (bicuspid valve).
- Motion: normal or reduced? Systolic bowing (bicuspid or rheumatic)?
- Commissural fusion (rheumatic disease).
- Associated rheumatic mitral stenosis suggests a rheumatic aetiology.

Grading severity

Grade aortic stenosis from *velocity* across the valve, *pressure gradient*, and *effective orifice area* (calculated from *continuity equation*) (Table 3.3).

Table 3.3 Parameters to assess severity of aortic stenosis

	MILD	MODERATE	SEVERE
Peak velocity (m/sec)	2.0–3.0	3.0–4.0	>4.0
Peak gradient (mmHg)	<35	35–65	>65
Mean gradient (mmHg)	<20	20–40	>40
Valve area (cm^2)	2.0–1.5	1.0–1.5	<1.0

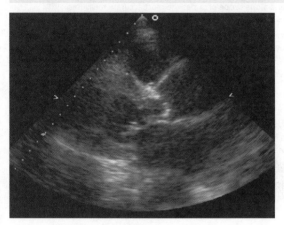

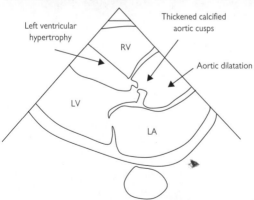

Fig. 3.15 Parasternal long axis demonstrating calcified aortic valve.

Aortic peak velocity
- In apical 5-chamber view (or 3-chamber) align the continuous wave Doppler, from the apex, through the aortic valve, into the aorta. Spend some time looking for the maximum velocity.
- Record several beats and measure the peak velocity on the spectral trace with the greatest velocity. This can be affected by the filling time so ignore ectopic or post-ectopic beats and in atrial fibrillation average two or three beats (Fig. 3.16).
- Repeat the measurement in at least one other approach (e.g. supra-sternal or right parasternal). Report maximum velocity found. The stand alone probe provides the most accurate measures.

Peak pressure gradient
The peak gradient is usually automatically calculated by the machine from the *peak velocity*. The relation between the two is very simple (the simplified Bernoulli equation):

peak gradient = $4 \times$ peak velocity^2

The equation is less accurate if the peak velocity is <3.0m/sec and the long form of the Bernoulli equation can be used:

peak gradient = $4 \times (v_2^2 - v_1^2)$

where v_2 = peak aortic velocity and v_1 = peak left ventricular outflow tract velocity.

Mean pressure gradient
To obtain the mean pressure gradient trace the continuous wave spectral trace of flow through the aortic valve (Fig. 3.16) and the machine will automatically calculate the *vti* (velocity time integral) and *mean pressure gradient* (mean pressure across the valve during systole).

Effect of other diseases on diagnosing and grading stenosis

- Moderate or severe aortic regurgitation will increase transaortic flow and may lead to overestimation of the grade of stenosis if using peak gradient. The continuity equation remains valid and should be used.
- Left ventricular dysfunction can be associated with lower transaortic and left ventricular outflow tract velocities and therefore underestimation of peak gradient. The continuity equation remains valid and should be used.
- A subaortic membrane or septal hypertrophy may occasionally be mistaken for valvular stenosis. Use pulsed wave Doppler in different positions in the left ventricular outflow tract to identify whether the blood starts to accelerate below or at the level of the valve.
- Examine the aorta for dilatation of the ascending aorta (commonly associated with bicuspid aortic valve, but also with calcific degenerative disease). If a bicuspid valve is suspected, use the suprasternal window to look for associated aortic coarctation.
- Pulmonary hypertension is common in severe aortic stenosis and is associated with a high operative risk. Estimate pulmonary artery pressure and assess the right ventricle.

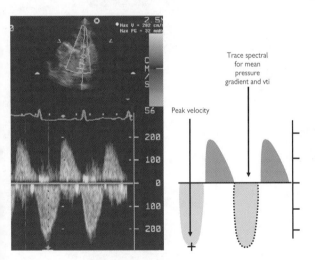

Fig. 3.16 Continuous wave in an apical view to measure velocities.

Effective orifice area/valve area

The continuity equation is based on the principle that the volume of blood that flows through the left ventricle outflow tract during 1sec must equal the blood through the aortic valve during 1sec.

- Obtain the continuous wave Doppler trace through the aortic valve (Fig. 3.16) and record the *peak velocity* and vti$_{(VALVE)}$.
- In an apical view, record pulsed wave Doppler in the left ventricle outflow tract. Trace the waveform and record peak velocity and vti$_{(LVOT)}$ (Fig. 3.17).
- In the parasternal long axis view zoom in on the left ventricle outflow tract and measure the diameter. Record the maximum edge-to-edge diameter just below the insertion of the aortic valve leaflets.
- Calculate the cross-sectional area of the left ventricle outflow tract:

    Area LVOT $= \pi \times$ (LVOT diameter/2)^2

- Put the figures into the rearranged continuity equation:

    Valve area $=$ (Area LVOT $\times$ vti$_{(LVOT)}$)/vti$_{(VALVE)}$

Although the equation can be calculated with peak velocity, vti should be used.

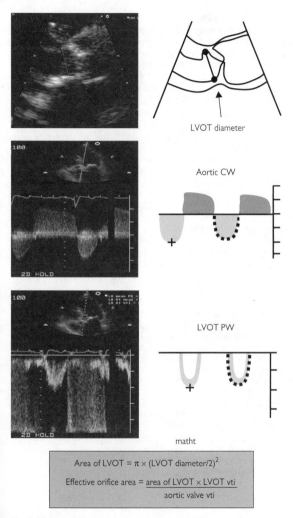

LVOT diameter

Aortic CW

LVOT PW

matht

$$\text{Area of LVOT} = \pi \times (\text{LVOT diameter}/2)^2$$

$$\text{Effective orifice area} = \frac{\text{area of LVOT} \times \text{LVOT vti}}{\text{aortic valve vti}}$$

Fig. 3.17 Two views and three measures are needed for continuity equation. Use a parasternal long axis view to measure LVOT diameter (top). In an apical 5-chamber view measure CW Doppler across the aortic valve (middle) and PW Doppler in the LVOT (bottom).

Effect on the left ventricle

Left ventricular hypertrophy or concentric remodelling (relative wall thickness >0.45 without hypertrophy (see p. 180)) are usual in compensated severe aortic stenosis. The left ventricle can also dilate if there is high wall stress as a result of severe pressure load, excessive fibrosis, or another cause of left ventricle dysfunction (e.g. myocardial infarction).

• During assessment of aortic stenosis also report a full evaluation of the left ventricle (function (p. 164) and hypertrophy (p. 180)).

A common dilemma in the relation between the left ventricle and aortic stenosis is whether any left ventricular dysfunction is secondary to the stenosis or another pathology (e.g. ischaemia). Also, an apparently small gradient or a decline in gradient may be secondary to impaired left ventricle function. The continuity equation remains accurate and should be used to assess valve area.

• If the mean gradient is <30mmHg (suggesting mild to moderate stenosis) but the valve area calculated by the continuity equation is <1.0cm^2 (suggesting severe stenosis) then a dobutamine stress echocardiogram can be considered to differentiate:
  • end-stage severe aortic stenosis;
  • moderate aortic stenosis associated with left ventricle dysfunction from another cause (e.g. myocardial infarction or myocarditis).

Dobutamine stress echocardiography

Give low-dose dobutamine intravenously (5 then 10, if necessary 20mcg/kg/min in 5min stages). Aim for a 10% increase in heart rate or 20% increase in left ventricle outflow tract or aortic valve vti. If the patient also has coronary artery disease, ischaemia may occur at very low levels of stress in the presence of aortic stenosis. Therefore carefully monitor wall motion and left ventricle size to look for evidence of ischaemia during the study (see Chapter 6, 'Stress echocardiography').

There are two things to look for during the study. The first is to determine whether severe aortic stenosis is present or not. The second is to determine whether the impaired left ventricle is able to increase output (*ventricular reserve* is present). This is important because the risk of mortality following aortic valve replacement for severe aortic stenosis is approximately 5% if contractile reserve is present and 35% if absent.

• Severe aortic stenosis is defined by:
  • mean gradient >30mmHg at any time during dobutamine stress;
  • valve area <1.2cm^2 throughout the infusion.
• Ventricular reserve is present if there is:
  • a rise in vti by >20% during the study.

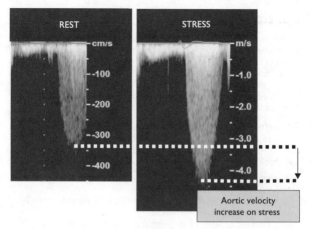

Fig. 3.18 Stress echocardiography in a patient with aortic stenosis and impaired left ventricle function. Velocities during stress are consistent with a mean gradient of >30mmHg (severe aortic stenosis) and the increase in vti is >20%, suggesting preserved ventricular contractile reserve.

Aortic regurgitation

Aortic regurgitation is easily seen with colour flow mapping over the aortic valve. The technique has 95% sensitivity and 100% specificity. Small traces of central regurgitation (felt not to be clinically significant) are seen more frequently with increasing age of patient. Below 40 years they are present in <1%, but by 60 years in 10–20%, and over 80 years in most people. Aortic regurgitation can occur due to changes in the aortic root or aortic valve (Table 3.4).

Assessment

Use colour flow mapping to identify and describe any aortic regurgitation. The study should then look for probable aetiology, grade severity, and check for associated problems.

Appearance

- Map the regurgitation with colour flow.
  - Look at the jet in all views and establish the shape and pattern of the regurgitation.
  - Comment on whether the regurgitation is through the valve (*valvular*) or around the side (*paravalvular*).
  - If valvular comment on whether it is central, eccentric along a commissure or even through a perforation (often easiest to see in parasternal short axis).
  - Comment on whether the jet lies in the centre of the left ventricular outflow tract or passes eccentrically down one of the walls. If eccentric comment on which wall it entrains against.
- Use a systematic approach to establish cause based on the clinical situation.
  - Look at the aortic root. In the parasternal long axis, measure aortic root dimension, look for a dissection flap. In parasternal short axis look at the aortic root for evidence of thickening or abscess.
  - Look at the aortic valve. In parasternal long axis look for evidence of abnormal valve motion/prolapse, vegetations, calcification/rheumatic changes. In parasternal short axis look at number of cusps.
  - Look at the rest of heart. Evidence of congenital abnormalities, e.g. ventricular septal defect.

Table 3.4 Causes of aortic regurgitation

Aortic valve
- Degeneration: calcific
- Infectious: endocarditis, post rheumatic fever
- Congenital: bicuspid valve; associated with other congenital abnormalities

Aortic root dilatation
- Hypertension
- Dissection/aneurysm
- Medial necrosis
- Trauma
- Congenital: Marfan's, Ehlers–Danlos, osteogenesis imperfecta
- Inflammatory: rheumatoid arthritis, systemic lupus erythematosus, syphilis, Reiter's syndrome, giant cell arteritis, ankylosing spondylitis

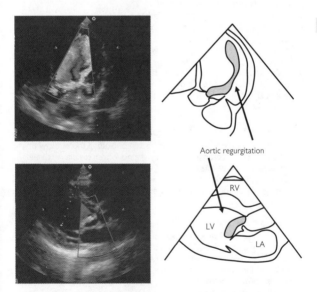

Fig. 3.19 Examples of colour flow mapping of aortic regurgitation. Top figure is a 5-chamber view of severe regurgitation with a long, broad jet. Bottom figure shows mild regurgitation in a parasternal long axis view.

Grading severity

Assess regurgitation as *mild*, *moderate*, or *severe* based on *jet width*, *vena contracta*, and *flow in descending aorta* (Table 3.5). Once you have an impression of the severity use *pressure half-time* and *left ventricular function* to develop your assessment. If you want further clarification there are a range of other measures that have been tried and can help.

Vena contracta

• In parasternal long axis look at the colour jet through the valve.
• The vena contracta is *'the narrowest part of the jet below the flow convergence'region'*, i.e. the narrowest point of the jet as it passes through the valve. This should represent the regurgitant orifice and is relatively accurate even for eccentric jets.
• Measure the jet with calipers and report the absolute measurement. Severe regurgitation is associated with width >0.6cm (Fig. 3.20).
• The same measurement can be done in cross-section in parasternal short axis view, although it is difficult to know if you are at the right level.

Jet width as proportion of outflow tract

• Measure the *vena contracta* (jet width).
• Suppress the colour and measure the width of the left ventricular outflow tract at the same point.
• Report the jet width as a percentage of left ventricular outflow tract. Severe regurgitation is suggested by a jet that is >65% of outflow tract.
• Jet size assessed in parasternal short axis can also be used (although technically more difficult and does not supply more information). Report area relative to left ventricular outflow tract area in the same view.

Problems with jet width to assess aortic regurgitation

• Eccentric jets tend to 'entrain' or 'flatten out' along the outflow tract wall they are directed against. They are no longer circular in three dimensions and will have different widths depending on the view.
• Changes in gain and colour scale will affect jet width so control settings should be kept relatively constant (50–60cm/sec), especially for follow up.

Descending aortic flow

• In the suprasternal view produce an image of the aortic arch and descending aorta. (Fig. 3.21, p. 137).
• Place the pulsed wave Doppler cursor in the centre of the descending aorta and look at the spectral trace.
• Flow is normally below the line for virtually all of systole and diastole, i.e. blood is moving down the aorta.
• Look at flow during diastole. Some flow may be above the line at the start of diastole. However, in severe regurgitation all flow during diastole is back towards the heart as a large volume of blood flows back into the ventricle. If this is seen, report *reversed holodiastolic aortic flow*.

Table 3.5 Parameters to determine severity of aortic regurgitation

	SPECIFIC SIGNS OF SEVERITY	
	MILD	SEVERE
Vena contracta	<0.3cm	>0.6cm
Jet (Nyquist, 50–60cm/sec)	Central, <25% of LVOT	Central, >65% of LVOT
Descending aorta	No or brief early diastolic flow reversal	

	SUPPORTIVE SIGNS OF SEVERITY	
	MILD	SEVERE
Pressure half-time	>500msec	<200msec
Descending aorta	—	Holodiastolic flow reversal
Left ventricle (only for chronic lesions)	Normal LV	Moderate or greater LV enlargement (no other cause)

Report as MODERATE if signs of regurgitation are greater than MILD but there are no features of SEVERE regurgitation.

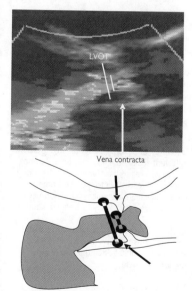

Fig. 3.20 Parasternal long axis with vena contracta and left ventricular outflow tract diameter marked.

Pressure half time (P1/2 time)
- In the apical 5-chamber view, or apical 3-chamber, align the continuous wave Doppler through the aortic regurgitation jet (identified with colour flow mapping). Try and ensure the Doppler passes through the regurgitant orifice of the valve and the length of the jet (for eccentric jets the view may need to be adjusted or be off axis).
- Look at the spectral trace. The regurgitant jet will be seen as a broad trace with a flat, sloped top above the baseline that co-incides with diastole on the ECG.
- Look at the density of the waveform compared to the systolic forward waveform. Similar density suggests severe regurgitation.
- Measure the peak velocity (usually 4–6m/sec).
- Measure the slope of the flat part of the curve. The *deceleration slope* (the slope of the curve) and *pressure half time* (time for pressure to fall across the valve by a half) are usually calculated automatically. The two measures are generally correlated.
- Report the *pressure half time*. <200msec indicates the pressure between the aorta and left ventricle equalizes very quickly in diastole (usually due to a large regurgitant volume) and suggests severe regurgitation. The corresponding value for *deceleration slope* is >400cm/sec^2. For deceleration slope the larger the number the steeper the slope.

Left ventricle
Serial studies of changes in left ventricle size are useful to monitor progression of aortic regurgitation and help decide timing for intervention.
- Assessment can be based on standard measures of left ventricular size (p. 166).
- A left ventricular end-diastolic dimension of >7cm and/or left ventricular end-systolic dimension of >4.5 cm are markers of severe chronic aortic regurgitation.

Acute or chronic regurgitation? P1/2 time and left ventricle

P1/2 time is most useful as a marker of severity in acute regurgitation. With chronic regurgitation, left ventricular function and aortic compliance change to accommodate larger regurgitant volumes. This slows down the equalization in pressure and leads to a longer P1/2 time.

Other things that differentiate acute from chronic regurgitation are:
- cause: dissection and endocarditis are more likely to be associated with acute regurgitation;
- in acute severe regurgitation the left ventricle is usually of normal dimension and thickness, with vigorous function; in chronic severe regurgitation there has been time for dilatation and possibly eccentric hypertrophy of the left ventricle.

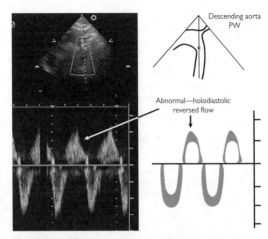

Fig. 3.21 A suprasternal view with pulsed wave Doppler placed in the descending aorta. The spectral trace shows reversed holodiastolic flow.

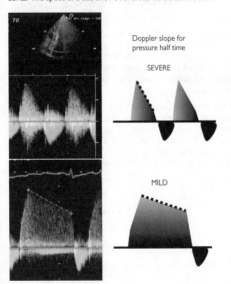

Fig. 3.22 Continuous wave traces from an apical 5-chamber view to measure pressure half time.

Other possible measures

The *length and surface area of the jet* have been used to judge severity. A rough estimation can be made as to whether the jet reaches the end of the anterior mitral valve leaflet (moderate) or extends into the body of the left ventricle (severe). Originally this was done using pulsed wave Doppler to identify the jet. Colour flow jet area is highly dependent on control settings because the boundary layers have low velocity. Also eccentric jets may be long and thin as they track along structures.

Regurgitant volume can be calculated because the blood flow out of the left ventricle across the aortic valve in systole should be the same as the blood flow into the left ventricle during diastole. The diastolic component will be comprised of blood flow across the mitral valve plus any blood that has regurgitated back into the left ventricle across the aortic valve. Both flow across the aortic valve in systole and mitral inflow can be calculated. Aortic regurgitant flow will be the difference between the two. However, the measure is inaccurate if there is any significant mitral regurgitation as this reduces the blood flow through the aortic valve in systole. It is also very dependent on accurate measures of mitral valve area and left ventricular outflow diameter. The principle is the same as that used for determining regurgitant volume in mitral regurgitation and the same measures (mitral valve inflow and left ventricular outflow tract flow) are used. See p. 116 for how to do the measurements.

Regurgitant volume = LVOT flow − mitral valve inflow

Interestingly, the stroke volume should be the same at any valve in the heart if it is competent and there is no shunt so, if measurements are difficult at the mitral valve, the pulmonary or tricuspid could be used.

Theoretically, the *proximal isovelocity surface area (PISA)* methods can be used at any regurgitant valve although they are only usually practical and validated for the mitral valve (p. 118).

Colour M-mode. If the M-mode cursor with colour flow is placed below the valve in a parasternal long axis view then the position of the regurgitation within the outflow tract and timing during diastole (e.g. late diastole due to aortic leaflet prolapse or mild regurgitation in early diastole) can be studied. Measurements of jet width and left ventricular outflow tract can also theoretically be done with the same tracing.

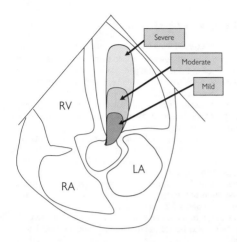

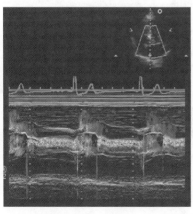

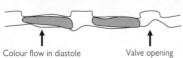

Colour flow in diastole   Valve opening

Fig. 3.23 Additional measures to assess aortic regurgitation: length of jet extending into the ventricle based on an apical 4-chamber view (top figure) and colour M-mode in a parasternal long axis view to demonstrate the regurgitant flow in the outflow tract during diastole (bottom figure).

Other aortic valve disease

Bicuspid and quadricuspid valves

The aortic valve can occur with fewer or more than three cusps. Bicuspid valves are seen in 2% of the population and quadricuspid valves in 0.04% of the population. Five cusps have also been reported, although this may often be secondary to endocarditis. Sometimes valves have three cusps but are functionally bicuspid because of fusion of two cusps along a commissure. Bicuspid valves are often associated with aortic stenosis and multiple cusps with aortic regurgitation.

It is very easy to make a tricuspid valve appear bicuspid in a parasternal short axis view if the plane is slightly off axis. If you suspect a bicuspid valve make sure this is consistent in several views. Clues to a valve being truly bicuspid include the following.

• Leaflets of unequal size. True congenital bicuspid valves occur because of failure of separation of the right and non-coronary cusp or failure of separation of the right and left coronary cusps.
• An atypical orientation of the commissure in the parasternal short axis. This will either lie roughly horizontal (between 10 and 4 o'clock) or roughly vertical.
• Abnormal valve motion (best seen in a parasternal long axis view). The valve typically domes with the valve opening off centre.

When assessing a bicuspid valve report: the suspected cause, e.g. true congenital or due to valve fusion; degree of calcification (they are more prone to degeneration); associated functional problems (regurgitation and stenosis); associated congenital problems (they are linked with coarctation of the aorta); and associated changes to the aorta (e.g. dilatation or dissection).

Lambl's excrescences

These are thin strands attached to the aortic cusps several millimetres long. They are also seen on the mitral valve. They are not clinically significant although their relevance will depend on the clinical situation as it is important not to miss endocarditis vegetations.

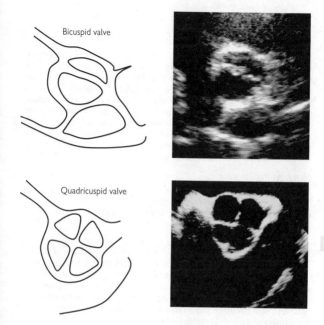

Fig. 3.24 Examples of bicuspid and quadricuspid aortic valves.

Tricuspid valve

Normal anatomy

The tricuspid valve has three cusps of unequal size: anterior (largest); posterior; and septal (smallest). Their anatomy is very variable. The free margins of the cusps are attached to chordae tendinae, which are, in turn, attached in groups to three papillary muscles that project from the septum and right ventricular free wall. Chordae from each papillary muscle attach to all leaflets. The valve has an annulus and valve ring with a normal area of 5–8cm^2. The valve allows free flow of blood from the right atrium during diastole but closes as systole increases the intraventricular pressure. Abnormalities of the tricuspid valve must not be overlooked, especially in mitral valve disease.

Normal findings

Views

The best views are: parasternal short-axis (aortic valve level), right ventricular inflow, apical 4-chamber, and subcostal views.

Findings

- Parasternal short axis (aortic valve level). The tricuspid valve lies to the right of the aorta. The anterior leaflet is seen on the left and septal is closest to the atrial septum. In all views the tricuspid leaflets demonstrate wide diastolic opening and a normal coaptation in systole.
- Right ventricular inflow. This gives a very good view of the posterior (on the left) and anterior (on the right) leaflets as well as the right atrium, right ventricle, and, sometimes, the inferior vena cava, coronary sinus, and Eustachian valve.
- Apical 4-chamber. The anterior and septal leaflets are seen (septal nearest the septum). In this view the tricuspid annulus should lie closer to the apex (up to 1cm) than the mitral annulus. This plane also provides a good view of the right heart.
- Subcostal 4-chamber. This view allows good access to images of the right atrium, atrial septum, and inferior vena cava. The tricuspid valve (anterior and septal leaflets) is usually clearly seen similar to the apical 4-chamber view.

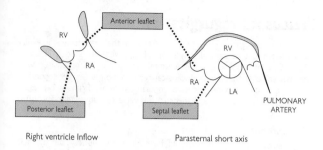

Right ventricle Inflow   Parasternal short axis

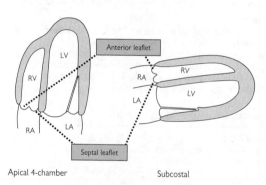

Apical 4-chamber   Subcostal

Fig. 3.25 Key views to study the tricuspid valve.

Tricuspid regurgitation

Tricuspid regurgitation is common. Because the leaflets are irregular a small amount of central, physiological regurgitation is seen in up to 70% of normal individuals. Physiological regurgitation is associated with normal valvular anatomy. Pathological regurgitation is usually secondary to right ventricular and tricuspid annular dilatation. Primary causes of tricuspid regurgitation are changes to the valve or subvalvular apparatus (Table 3.6).

Assessment

'Physiological' regurgitation should be commented upon. Transthoracic echocardiography should aim to establish the aetiology of pathological tricuspid regurgitation and provide a quantitative estimate of severity. The assessment must also include evaluation of the right-sided chambers.

Appearance

- Look at the regurgitant jet with colour flow Doppler in several views and comment on the direction and size of the jet.
- Report abnormal valve appearance (restricted motion and thickening of carcinoid, vegetations of endocarditis or valve rupture)
- Report right heart size and function (p. 210) and assess right ventricular systolic pressure (p. 148).

Table 3.6 Causes of tricuspid regurgitation

Valve and apparatus
- Infection: endocarditis, rheumatic heart disease
- Congenital: Ebstein's anomaly
- Metabolic: carcinoid
- Connective tissue disease
- Subvalvular: chordal rupture, papillary muscle dysfunction

Right heart
- Pulmonary hypertension
- Right heart failure with lung pathology
- Ischaemic heart disease
- Pulmonary valve disease
- Cardiomyopathy
- Volume overload
- Pacing lead

Table 3.7 Parameters to assess severity of tricuspid regurgitation

	MILD	SEVERE
Jet (Nyquist, 50–60cm/sec)	<5cm^2	>10cm^2
Vena contracta	—	>0.7cm
PISA r (Nyquist 40cm/sec)	<0.5cm	>1cm
Hepatic vein flow	Normal	Systolic reversal
Valve structure	Normal	Abnormal
CW trace	Soft & parabolic	Dense & triangular
RV/RA/IVC	Normal size	Usually dilated

Report as MODERATE if signs of regurgitation are greater than MILD but there are no features of SEVERE regurgitation.

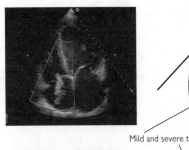
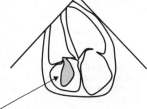

Mild and severe tricuspid regurgitation

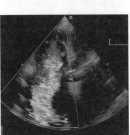
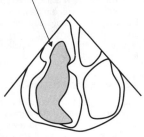

Fig. 3.26 Colour flow mapping of tricuspid regurgitation in apical 4-chamber views with examples of mild (top) and severe (bottom) regurgitation.

Grading severity

The methods to grade severity are borrowed directly from those used for mitral regurgitation. Assessment of tricuspid regurgitation tends to be more subjective with less clinical need for accuracy. Judge severity on *jet area*. Support your impression with *vena contracta*, *flow convergence* (PISA), *continuous wave density*, and *contour*. There are also changes in *hepatic vein flow*, which are equivalent to changes in pulmonary vein flow seen in mitral regurgitation (Table 3.7, p. 145).

Jet area
- In the apical 4-chamber view obtain an image that includes the entire right atrium and the main plane of the regurgitant jet.
- Record a loop and scroll through to a frame with the largest jet. Trace around the jet and report the area. Greater than $10cm^2$ suggests severe regurgitation.

Vena contracta
- In the apical 4-chamber view place colour flow over the tricuspid valve and obtain a plane that demonstrates the regurgitant orifice.
- Zoom in on the valve and measure the vena contracta (narrowest diameter of the colour flow jet as it passes through the valve). Greater than 7mm suggests severe regurgitation (Fig. 3.28).

Continuous wave Doppler waveform
- In the apical 4-chamber, parasternal short axis, or right ventricular inflow views drop the continuous wave through the tricuspid valve aligned with the regurgitant jet.
- Report the signal intensity relative to the antegrade flow and comment on the waveform (parabolic or triangular). Triangular and dense suggests severe regurgitation.

Hepatic vein flow
- In a subcostal view place the pulsed wave Doppler cursor in a hepatic vein that aligns with the probe and record a spectral tracing of flow. Normally flow through both systole and diastole is towards the right atrium. In severe tricuspid regurgitation the rise in right atrial pressure leads to flow away from the right heart during systole. Report systolic flow reversal if seen.

Pacemakers and tricuspid regurgitation

Tricuspid regurgitation is more common with a pacemaker lead (both temporary and permanent) because it disrupts leaflet coaption. Tricuspid regurgitation velocity, however, will not be affected as this is determined by right ventricular systolic pressure.

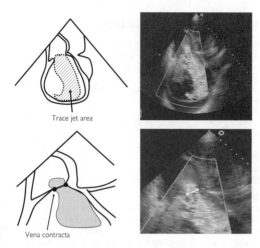

Fig. 3.27 Measure jet area (top) and support your assessment with a vena contracta (bottom) or PISA measurement.

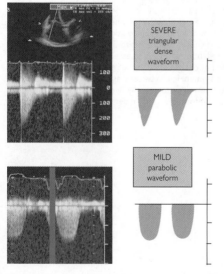

SEVERE
triangular
dense
waveform

MILD
parabolic
waveform

Fig. 3.28 Density and shape of Doppler can give clue to severity.

Right heart haemodynamics

The most widely reported haemodynamic measure in echocardiography is *right ventricular systolic pressure*. This is partly because it has a broad clinical relevance and partly because it is easy to measure as it uses tricuspid regurgitation—found in 70% of individuals.

The measurement is based on the velocity of regurgitant blood at the tricuspid valve. This can be used to calculate the pressure gradient across the valve—the higher the pressure in the right ventricle relative to the right atrium, the higher the velocity of regurgitant blood. To calculate right ventricular systolic pressure *right atrial pressure* must be added to the pressure gradient. Fortunately, there are both clinical (jugular venous pressure, JVP) and echocardiographic methods (inferior vena cava and right atrial size) to estimate right atrial pressure. Using all these measures echocardiography can also report *pulmonary artery systolic pressure*.

Right atrial pressure

- JVP can be used but requires accurate clinical assessment with the patient lying at 45°. The measure lacks accuracy if very low or very high and is directly affected by moderate to severe TR.
- A floating constant of 5, 10, or 15mmHg provides most accuracy over a range of pathologies. The constant is chosen based on the pattern of changes in *right atrial size*, *IVC*, and *TR severity* (Table 3.8).
  - Assess right atrial size from an apical 4-chamber view (p. 228). Report as normal, dilated, or very dilated.
  - Assess the IVC from a subcostal view. Measure the diameter (<1.7cm is normal, except in athletes when diameter can be 2–3cm) and check for respiratory variation by asking the patient to sniff. Inferior vena cava should reduce in size by around 50%.
  - Tricuspid regurgitation severity is assessed routinely (p. 146).
- If accurate assessment of right atrial pressure is not possible then a constant of 10 (or 14) mmHg can be used as an estimate of right atrial pressure. This method will systematically overestimate right systolic ventricular pressure at low levels and underestimate it at high levels.

Table 3.8 Parameters to assess right atrial pressure

	Right atrial pressure (mmHg)		
	5	**10**	**15**
Right atrium	Normal	Dilated	Very dilated
TR	Mild	Moderate	Severe
TR velocity (m/sec)	<2.5	2.5–4	>4
IVC	Normal, <1.7cm	Dilated	Dilated; no respiratory variation

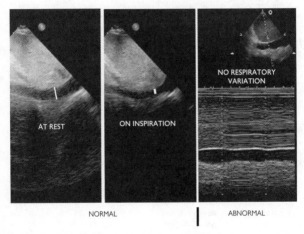

NORMAL | ABNORMAL

Fig. 3.29 The 2D images demonstrate normal respiratory variation of the inferior vena cava and the M-mode trace demonstrates lack of variation.

Tricuspid velocity and right ventricular systolic pressure
- In apical 4-chamber, parasternal short axis, or right ventricular inflow view, align continuous wave through the tricuspid valve regurgitation.
- Record a spectral trace and measure the peak velocity (Fig. 3.29). Based on the simplified Bernoulli equation (p. 38):

$$\text{pressure gradient} = 4 \times \text{peak velocity}^2$$

$$\text{Right ventricular systolic pressure} = \text{tricuspid pressure gradient} + \text{right atrial pressure}$$

Pulmonary artery systolic pressure
- By subtracting the pressure gradient across the pulmonary valve (p. 160) from *right ventricular systolic pressure* you can calculate *pulmonary artery systolic pressure*. Because the gradient is usually small and right atrial pressure is estimated, *right ventricular systolic pressure* is often reported as *pulmonary artery systolic pressure*.

Pulmonary artery diastolic pressure
- The velocity of the pulmonary valve regurgitant jet (p. 150) can be used to quantify the pressure gradient (using the Bernoulli equation) between the pulmonary artery and right ventricle during diastole.
- Add right ventricular diastolic pressure (assumed to be *right atrial pressure*, p. 148) to the pulmonary valve pressure gradient to calculate *pulmonary artery diastolic pressure*.

Mean pulmonary artery pressure
- To calculate *mean pulmonary artery pressure* use pulmonary artery systolic and diastolic pressure in the equation:

$$(\text{diastolic pressure} + \text{systolic pressure})/3$$

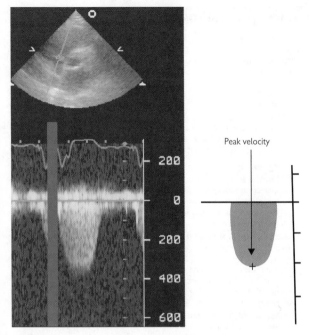

Fig. 3.30 A parasternal short axis view has been used to obtain a continuous wave Doppler trace across the tricuspid valve to measure peak velocity and derive a pressure gradient.

Tricuspid stenosis

Tricuspid stenosis is rare. The commonest cause is rheumatic heart disease with coexistent mitral stenosis. Other causes include: carcinoid syndrome, right atrial tumour, and obstruction of right ventricular inflow tract (large atrial thrombus or large vegetations).

Assessment

Appearance

Comment on:
- leaflet thickening or calcification;
- leaflet motion: classically restricted with doming of one or more leaflets in diastole (especially the anterior leaflet).

Grading severity

- Determine severity on the transvalvular gradient.
  - Use continuous wave Doppler aligned across the tricuspid valve in an apical 4-chamber view.
  - Measure peak velocity and calculate peak gradient using the Bernoulli equation.
- Severe tricuspid stenosis is associated with a valve area of less than 1cm^2 or a mean gradient of >7mmHg.
- Pressure half time cannot be used to measure valve area as the appropriate constant for the tricuspid valve has not been determined.
- Severity can also be assessed from tricuspid valve area. This can be calculated using the continuity equation. A pulsed wave Doppler vti can be taken at the level of the valve annulus and the cross-sectional area of the tricuspid annulus calculated based on the annulus diameter and the assumption that the orifice is circular. These measurements can then be combined with the continuous wave vti across the valve.

TV area = (annulus PW vti × area of annulus)/valve CW vti

Table 3.9 Parameters to assess tricuspid stenosis

	MILD	MODERATE	SEVERE
Mean gradient (mmHg)	<4	4–7	>7
Valve area (cm²)	–	–	<1

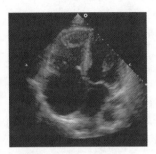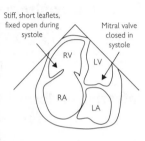

Fig. 3.31 An apical 4-chamber view demonstrating carcinoid heart disease causing tricuspid stenosis.

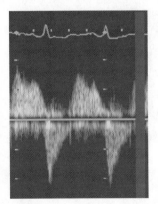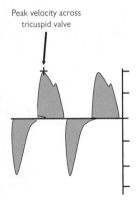

Fig. 3.32 Continuous wave Doppler is used in an apical 4-chamber view to record peak and mean velocity across the tricuspid valve. This can be used to estimate a gradient in tricuspid stenosis.

Tricuspid valve surgery

Tricuspid valve surgery—replacement or annuloplasty—is rarely required because it affords little functional improvement. However, it may be considered in severe tricuspid regurgitation with haemodynamic consequences or when associated with mitral valve disease.

Carcinoid syndrome

Characterized by the release of 5-hydroxytryptamine from a metastasizing tumour resulting in thickened and shortened tricuspid leaflets with severe tricuspid regurgitation. The pulmonary valve may also be involved and the right atrium and right ventricle are frequently dilated.

Infective endocarditis

Right-sided endocarditis is uncommon except in intravenous drug users, patients with indwelling catheters, or those with ventricular septal defects. There may be associated left-sided lesions.

Ebstein anomaly

A congenital anomaly of the tricuspid valve with apical displacement of one or more leaflets. This diagnosis should be considered when the distance between the mitral and tricuspid valve planes is >1cm. There is enlargement of the right atrium and tricuspid regurgitation.

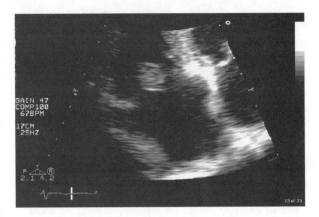

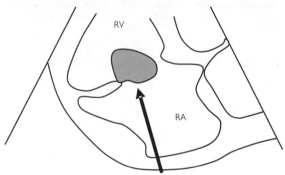

Vegetation on tricuspid valve

Fig. 3.33 A zoomed apical 4-chamber view to highlight a vegetation on the tricuspid valve.

Pulmonary valve

Normal anatomy

The pulmonary valve consists of three leaflets: anterior; left; and right. It develops alongside the aortic valve. The right heart and pulmonary artery then twist around the left heart and aorta. The valve lies at the junction of the right ventricular outflow tract and the pulmonary trunk.

Normal findings

Views

- There are limited views of the pulmonary valve. The best views are the parasternal short axis (aortic valve level) and the right ventricular outflow. Subcostal short axis views (at the aortic valve level) can also be used but are similar to the parasternal short axis view.

Findings

- Parasternal short axis (aortic valve level). This provides a view of the tricuspid valve, right ventricle, and pulmonary valve wrapped around the aortic valve. The pulmonary valve lies on the right and this view can be used to align Doppler through the right ventricular outflow, pulmonary valve, and pulmonary artery.
- Right ventricular outflow. In some people this provides excellent views of the pulmonary valve, pulmonary artery, and bifurcation. This view can also be used for alignment of Doppler.

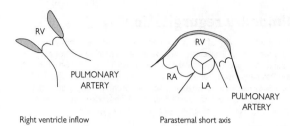

Right ventricle inflow   Parasternal short axis

Fig. 3.34 Key views to assess the pulmonary valve.

Pulmonary regurgitation

Colour flow mapping of the pulmonary valve identifies small regurgitant jets in most people. These can often be quite eccentric. Pathological causes of regurgitation are similar to those for tricuspid regurgitation (Table 3.6, p. 144). Primary valve problems include: rheumatic heart disease, infective endocarditis, carcinoid, iatrogenic (post-valvotomy), congenital (following surgery for tetralogy of Fallot, leaflet absence). Secondary causes are due to dilatation of the pulmonary artery (e.g. pulmonary hypertension, Marfan).

Assessment

Appearance

- Map the regurgitation with colour flow in the parasternal short axis and right ventricular outflow views. Comment on size, site of regurgitation, and direction.
- Pulmonary regurgitation is commonly at one edge of a commissure and can appear to lie next to the aorta. This should not be confused with an aorta–pulmonary communication, which would have flow throughout the cardiac cycle instead of just during diastole.
- Comment on any visible valve pathology (e.g. thickening, vegetation).

Grading severity

- Criteria for assessment are borrowed from aortic regurgitation but assessment is more qualitative.
- Grade severity as *mild*, *moderate*, or *severe* based on the following.
  - Jet length and width relative to outflow tract.
  - Continuous wave regurgitation intensity and shape. Increased slope of the Doppler signal (deceleration time) suggests severe.
  - Abnormal pulmonary artery anatomy suggests more severe regurgitation.
  - Flow across pulmonary valve relative to systemic circulation and evidence of right ventricular dilatation.
  - Holodiastolic flow reversal in the main pulmonary artery (equivalent to aortic flow reversal) suggests severe regurgitation.
- Comment on changes to the right heart—right ventricular dilatation and right ventricular volume overload.

Table 3.10 Parameters to assess pulmonary regurgitation

	MILD	SEVERE
Jet size on CFM	<10mm long	Large with wide origin
CW density & shape	Soft & slow	Dense & steep
Pulmonary valve	Normal	Abnormal
Pulmonary artery flow	Increased	Greatly increased compared to systemic circulation
Right ventricle size	Normal	Dilated

If features suggest more than MILD regurgitation but no features of SEVERE, grade as MODERATE.

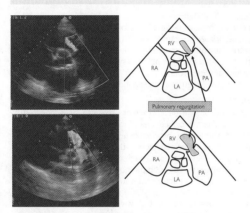

Fig. 3.35 Colour flow mapping of pulmonary regurgitation in parasternal short axis views. Mild (top) and severe (lower) regurgitation.

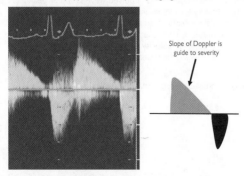

Fig. 3.36 Doppler features to assess pulmonary regurgitation.

Pulmonary stenosis

Pulmonary stenosis is usually valvular and congenital (e.g. related to rubella, Noonan's, or tetralogy of Fallot). The valve usually has fusion of several cusps to form a funnel. Pulmonary stenosis can also occur due to stenosis of the main pulmonary artery (e.g. following rubella, post-surgical banding of the pulmonary artery) or subvalvular problems (e.g. congenital in association with valvular stenosis, tetralogy of Fallot, and transposition of the great arteries).

Assessment

Appearance

- Comment on the valve.
  - Thickened, calcified leaflets.
  - Motion: doming of valve leaflets in systole and restricted motion.
- Comment on associated structures.
  - Right ventricular outflow tract and evidence of narrowing.
  - Post-stenotic dilatation of the pulmonary artery.
  - Right ventricular hypertrophy.
  - Functional tricuspid regurgitation secondary to pressure overload.

Grading severity

Grade severity based on the peak gradient. This can be supported by calculating the valve effective orifice area (Table 3.11).

- In the parasternal short axis (aortic valve level) or right ventricular outflow view measure the velocity across the pulmonary valve with continuous wave Doppler aligned through the right ventricular outflow tract, pulmonary valve, and common pulmonary artery.
- Report velocity and gradient across the valve (calculated with the simplified Bernoulli equation). Mean gradient and pulmonary valve vti can be obtained by tracing the spectral waveform (Fig. 3.37).
- The continuity equation can be used to measure effective orifice area of the pulmonary valve. In the parasternal short axis view record a right ventricular outflow tract (RVOT) pulsed wave Doppler peak velocity or vti (velocity$_{(RVOT)}$). Measure the outflow tract diameter at this point and calculate a cross-sectional area assuming it is circular (cross-sectional area$_{(RVOT)}$). Then use the continuity equation including these measures and the peak velocity or vti from continuous wave across the valve (velocity$_{(PV)}$). Pulmonary valve cross-sectional area equals:

$$[\text{velocity}_{(RVOT)} \times \text{cross-sectional area}_{(RVOT)}]/\text{velocity}_{(PV)}$$

Table 3.11 Parameters to determine severity of pulmonary stenosis

	MILD	MODERATE	SEVERE
Peak gradient (mmHg)	10–25	25–40	>40
Valve area (cm^2)	>1.0	0.5–1.0	<0.5

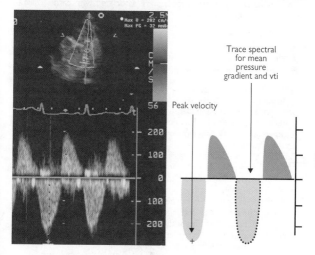

Fig. 3.37 Severity of pulmonary stenosis can be assessed in a similar way to assessment of aortic stenosis. In this example a continuous wave Doppler trace has been obtained from a parasternal short axis view. The peak velocity can be used to calculate a gradient or be used in the continuity equation.

Left ventricle

Normal anatomy

The left ventricle is a cavity with muscular walls that contains the papillary muscles and their chordal attachments. The anatomical characteristics of the chamber size and thickness can vary significantly with pathology, and many cardiac and systemic processes are associated with cardiac dilatation or hypertrophy.

Normal findings

Views

The left ventricle is seen in virtually all windows. The minimal views are parasternal long and short axis and the apical 4-, 2-, and 3-chamber views.

Findings

- Parasternal long axis. The basal and mid-segments of the septum and posterior wall (in some publications it is also referred to as the inferolateral wall) are visible. This view is used for linear measures of wall thickness and cavity dimensions. The left ventricular outflow tract can also be assessed.
- Parasternal short axis. By angling the probe back and forth, the whole of the left ventricle can be scanned in cross-section. The key ventricle views are mid-ventricle (mid-papillary) and apical. The mid-ventricle level is used for linear and area measures of walls and cavity. Regional wall motion abnormalities can also be assessed in (in clockwise order) septum, anterior, lateral, and inferior walls.
- Apical 4-chamber. Provides best views of apex, septum (on left), and lateral (on right) walls for regional assessment. Suitable for tracing ventricular area and left ventricular length.
- Apical 2-chamber. Focuses on inferior (on left) and anterior walls (on right).
- Apical 3-chamber. The parasternal long axis view but from the apex. Looks at posterior (inferolateral) wall and septum.
- Subcostal provides an alternative view of the left ventricle but is not essential.

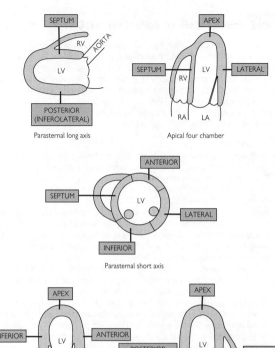

Fig. 3.38 Key views to assess the left ventricle with walls marked.

Left ventricular assessment

Accurate left ventricular assessment (diameters, volumes, wall thickness, mass, and function) is critical in clinical practice. Measurements can be altered by virtually all cardiovascular pathologies. The most common indication for echocardiography is evaluation of left ventricular function, with ejection fraction being the most sought parameter. Assessments are frequently visually estimated but there is significant interobserver variability and dependence on interpreter skill. Quantitative measures are recommended to ensure diagnostic accuracy.

Assessment

- Start with an overview of the ventricle in all views (parasternal and apical) and gather an impression of appearance, size, and function.
- Comment on obvious structural changes:
  - ventricular shape, aneurysms, wall thinning, wall hypertrophy, wall character ('speckling', etc.).
- Report quantitative measures of size (p. 166) and a general summary: *normal, mild, moderate,* or *severe* dilatation; *normal, mild, moderate,* or *severe* hypertrophy. If hypertrophy, give an idea of the pattern based on appearance and *relative wall thickness*, i.e. *eccentric, concentric, asymmetric (septal, apical)* (p. 180).
  - 2D and M-mode quantification of left ventricular size and mass have been well validated but both have advantages and disadvantages.
  - M-mode measures in parasternal views are widely used. They are very dependent on M-mode alignment and take no account of left ventricular shape or regional wall motion abnormalities. The alignment problem is reduced with 2D guided or direct 2D-measures.
  - In general, left ventricular shape changes are best accounted for by using the volumetric *biplane Simpson's* method for volumes and the *truncated ellipsoid* method for left ventricular mass. These methods should therefore be used to provide accurate assessment of left ventricular volume and mass, respectively.
  - Reference ranges are dependent on gender and body habitus. Ideally, height and weight should be recorded and body surface area used to correct left ventricular dimensions.
- Using the measures of left ventricular size, report a quantitative assessment of systolic function (e.g. *ejection fraction*) and summarize as *normal* systolic function or *mild, moderate,* or *severe* systolic dysfunction (p. 188).
- From apical and parasternal views look at changes in regional wall motion (*normal, hypokinesis, akinesis, dyskinesis, aneurysmal*). Report abnormalities (p. 194).
- When relevant, assess and report *left ventricular diastolic function* from changes in mitral valve inflow and tissue Doppler imaging (p. 198).
- Finally, ensure you have reported fully pathologies that might relate to the changes you have identified in the left ventricle (e.g. valve disease).

Left ventricular size

Because it is difficult to quantify a 3D structure using 2D imaging, the techniques that have developed rely on measuring the ventricle in standard places. The measures are then reported directly (*linear methods*) or used in mathematical equations to model an assumed shape for the ventricle (*volumetric measures*). In principle, the more measures of the left ventricle in the more planes the more accurate the assessment. Conversely, the fewer measures the more assumptions have to be made and the more likely it is that regional pathology is overlooked. Sometimes—such as in a normal heart—simple linear measures are adequate. However, if there is pathology accuracy is required.

Linear measures
M-mode
This is based on change in size in a single plane at the mid-ventricle level in a parasternal view (Fig. 3.39). Recent guidelines suggest this should be a parasternal short axis view.
- Optimize a parasternal long axis view with the septum and posterior wall lying parallel (or a parasternal short axis mid-ventricle view).
- Drop the M-mode cursor through opposing walls so that it intersects both at right angles. In the long axis view the cursor should lie at the level of the mitral valve tips (some guidelines suggest chordal level).
- Look at the M-mode trace and identify the two walls. Measure from edge-to-edge where the walls are closest together (peak systole) and furthest apart (end diastole). Report the *left ventricular systolic* and *end-diastolic* diameters.
- The M-mode trace from a parasternal long axis view can also be used to measure septal and posterior wall thickness at end diastole.

2D-imaging
This follows the same principle as M-mode but relies on clear 2D images.
- Record a loop of an optimized parasternal long axis or short axis (mid-ventricle) view. Scroll through to identify the end-diastolic frame (largest ventricle).
- Measure from endocardial border to endocardial border in a line at right angles to each wall (Fig. 3.40). In the long axis view the line should pass through the MV tips. Report the *left ventricular end-diastolic diameter*.
- Scroll through the loop to identify the end-systolic frame (smallest ventricle) and, using the same technique, measure *left ventricular end-systolic diameter*.

Normal ranges depend on technique, sex, and body size

Systematic differences between techniques mean 'normal' ranges vary (Table 3.13). For instance, direct 2D measures tend to produce slightly smaller measures than M-mode. Also, normal ranges depend on the sex and size of the person. Always report the method you used and demographic data.

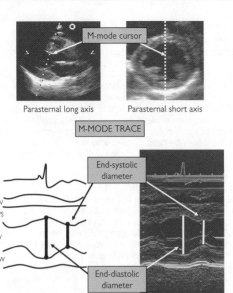

Fig. 3.39 Measurements using M-mode in parasternal views.

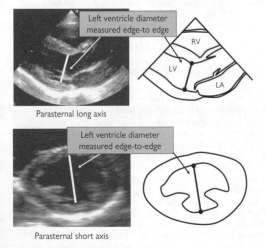

Fig. 3.40 Examples of 2D measures in parasternal views.

Volumetric measures

Simpson's method

Simpson's method is based on the principle of slicing the left ventricle from apex down to mitral valve annulus into a series of discs. The volume of each disc is then calculated (using the diameter and thickness of each slice). All the disc volumes are added together to provide the total left ventricular volume. If done in a single plane (based on apical 4-chamber view) it is assumed the left ventricle is circular at each level. Accuracy is improved by using diameters in two perpendicular planes (biplane—apical 4- and 2-chamber) so that the disc surface area is more precisely defined. Although this can be done 'by hand' by measuring the diameter at multiple levels, in reality, you trace the outline of the ventricle and the machine or off-line software automatically calculates the volume.

- In the apical 4-chamber view obtain a clear image of the left ventricular cavity with a clear endocardial border.
- Record a loop and scroll through to find the end-diastolic image (usually just before the aortic valve opens or on the R-wave of the ECG). This image should have the largest left ventricular volume.
- Trace around the endocardial border going from one side of the mitral valve annulus to the other and joining the two ends with a straight line. Record the *left ventricular end-diastolic volume*.
- Measure the length of the left ventricle from apex to middle of mitral valve. Depending on the machine, identification of the apex may be automatic after tracing the border. Record *left ventricular long axis*.
- Scroll through the loop again and find the smallest left ventricular volume at end-systole (usually just before the mitral valve opens or on the T-wave of the ECG). Trace around the endocardial border, as before, and record *left ventricular end-systolic volume*.
- The method above will provide single plane measures of left ventricular volumes. For biplane measures repeat the process for diastolic and systolic images using an optimized apical 2-chamber view.

Avoid foreshortening. Ensure a clear endocardial border

- Accurate left ventricular volume measurements require an unforeshortened ventricle. Foreshortening leads to underestimation of volume and changes ventricular shape. Foreshortening can usually be avoided by moving more lateral ± one intercostal space further down. 3 pointers to be confident you have identified the true apex:
  - apex is fixed and does not move towards the base in systole;
  - apical myocardium is thinner than the rest of the ventricle;
  - the view is the one with the longest ventricle (if apical view).
- If the endocardial border is not clear, volumes will be overestimated. Clear definition is particularly important to see regional wall motion abnormalities. Endocardial definition can be enhanced by machine controls to improve grey levels (such as harmonic imaging, gain, contrast) or probe position (increased pressure, better contact, slight changes in window). If these factors make no difference, intravascular contrast agents provide excellent border definition.

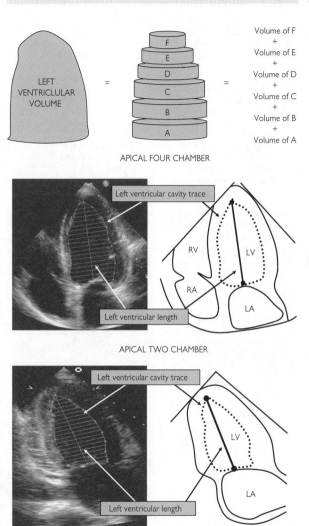

APICAL FOUR CHAMBER

APICAL TWO CHAMBER

Fig. 3.41 Biplane Simpson's method for measurement of left ventricle cavity size.

Area length equation

This method can be used if apical definition is poor and it is difficult to trace the border. It is based on an equation that models a 'bullet-shaped' ventricle (and therefore does not take account of regional abnormalities). For the equation you need the length of the ventricle and the cross-sectional area at the mid-papillary level.

• Obtain a clear parasternal short axis (mid-ventricle level) view with good endocardial border definition and record a loop.
• Trace around the endocardial border in the end-diastolic frame to obtain the *end-diastolic cross-sectional area*.
• In an apical 4-chamber view record the distance from the middle of the mitral valve annulus to the left ventricular apex at end-diastole and record the *end-diastolic left ventricular long axis length*.
• Ventricular volume at *end-diastole* is then:

(5 × cross-sectional area in parasternal SAX × ventricular length)/6

• Ventricular volume at *end-systole* can be measured in exactly the same way but using parasternal and apical images frozen at end-systole.

3D imaging

3D image acquisition has the advantage of taking into account variation in ventricular shape in all directions rather than just the two of biplane measurements. Real-time 3D imaging makes this a clinical possibility. It is dependent on capturing the whole left ventricle within the 3D-probe sector and still requires images to have good endocardial border definition.

• A 3D image set is acquired from the apex. The border can then be traced in two 2D planes. The rest of the border is tracked automatically from the 3D dataset to create a volume rendered outline of left ventricular volume throughout the cardiac cycle.

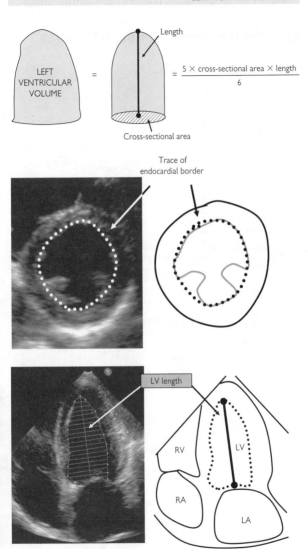

Fig. 3.42 Area length equation based on measurement of cross-sectional area and left ventricle length.

Left ventricular size: normal ranges

Table 3.12 Ranges for measurements of LV size. (Adapted from Recommendations for chamber quantification: a report of the American Society of Echocardiography Guidelines and Standards Committee and the Chamber Quantification Writing Group, developed in conjunction with the European Association of Echocardiography. *J Am Soc Echocardiogr* 2005; **18**: 1440–63.)

Part 1, Values for women

	WOMEN			
	NORMAL	MILD	MODERATE	SEVERE
LV dimension				
LV d diameter, cm	3.9–5.3	5.4–5.7	5.8–6.1	>6.1
LV d diameter/BSA, cm/m^2	2.4–3.2	3.3–3.4	3.5–3.7	>3.7
LV d diam/height, cm/m	2.5–3.2	3.3–3.4	3.5–3.6	>3.7
LV volume				
LV d vol, mL	56–104	105–117	118–130	>130
LV d vol/BSA, mL/m^2	**35–75**	**76–86**	**87–96**	**>96**
LV s vol, mL	19–49	50–59	60–69	>69
LV s vol/BSA, mL/m^2	**12–30**	**31–36**	**37–42**	**>42**
Linear method: fractional shortening				
Endocardial, %	27–45	22–26	17–21	<17
Mid-wall, %	15–23	13–14	11–12	<11
2D method				
Ejection fraction, %	**>54**	**45–54**	**30–44**	**<30**

BSA, Body surface area; d, diastolic; s, systolic.
Bold rows identify best validated measures.

Table 3.12 (cont.)

Part 2, Values for men

	MEN			
	NORMAL	MILD	MODERATE	SEVERE
LV dimension				
LV d diameter, cm	4.2–5.9	6.0–6.3	6.4–6.8	>6.8
LV d diameter/BSA, cm/m²	2.2–3.1	3.2–3.4	3.5–3.6	>3.6
LV d diam/height, cm/m	2.4–3.3	3.4–3.5	3.6–3.7	>3.7
LV volume				
LV d vol, mL	67–155	156–178	179–201	>201
LV d vol/BSA, mL/m²	**35–75**	**76–86**	**87–96**	**>96**
LV s vol, mL	22–58	59–70	71–82	>82
LV s vol/BSA, mL/m²	**12–30**	**31–36**	**37–42**	**>42**
Linear method: fractional shortening				
Endocardial, %	25–43	20–24	15–19	<15
Mid-wall, %	14–22	12–13	10–11	<10
2D method				
Ejection fraction, %	**>54**	**45–54**	**30–44**	**<30**

BSA, Body surface area; d, diastolic; s, systolic.
Bold rows identify best validated measures.

Left ventricular thickness and mass

All measurements of left ventricular mass are based on the principle of estimating the difference between the epicardial and endocardial left ventricular volumes and then calculating the mass of this 'shell' using the known myocardial density (i.e multiplication of the volume by 1.05). The measurement techniques are the same as for quantification of left ventricular size (p. 164). However, they are applied to obtain both a cavity volume and a total volume. Measurements are done at end-diastole.

Linear measures of wall thickness can be reported directly or used to estimate mass based on simple formulae but do not take account of changes in left ventricular geometry. Volume measures are preferred.

Linear measures

Interventricular septum and posterior wall thickness

The simplest and most widely used assessments of left ventricular thickness are *interventricular septum* and *posterior wall thickness* from M-mode or 2D images. They are reported as wall thickness and used with ventricular diameter to estimate *relative wall thickness* (p. 178).

- In a parasternal long axis or parasternal short axis (mid-papillary level) drop an M-mode cursor through the ventricle perpendicular to the walls at the level of the mitral valve leaflet tips.
- Identify the lines that relate to the septum and posterior wall and measure the thinnest part (end-diastole).
- Measurements can also be done directly from parasternal 2D images, frozen in end-diastole. Measure with calipers from edge to edge.

Volume measures from linear measures

Teichholz method or prolate ellipse of revolution

Left ventricular mass can be estimated from linear dimensions (see above) using a 'prolate ellipse of revolution' formula. Traditionally, this was based on M-mode measures. The equation uses cubed measurements so slightly off-axis views or small errors in diameter are amplified into large differences in volume. The method takes no account of abnormal left ventricular morphology and is rarely used now.

- In parasternal long axis or parasternal short axis (mid-papillary level) views obtain measures of *left ventricular end-diastolic diameter* (LVEDD), *interventricular septum thickness* (IVS), and *posterior wall thickness* (PWT).
- In an apical 4-chamber view obtain a measure of *end-diastolic left ventricular length* (from apex to middle of mitral valve annulus).
- LV mass is usually automatically calculated using the formula:

$$[0.8 \times (\textbf{1.05} \times ((\textbf{LVEDD} + \textbf{PWT} + \textbf{IVS})^3 - (\textbf{LVEDD})^3))]+0.6 \text{ g}$$

(the constants (0.8 and 0.6) improve the accuracy of the basic equation (in bold) in studies based on post-mortem hearts).

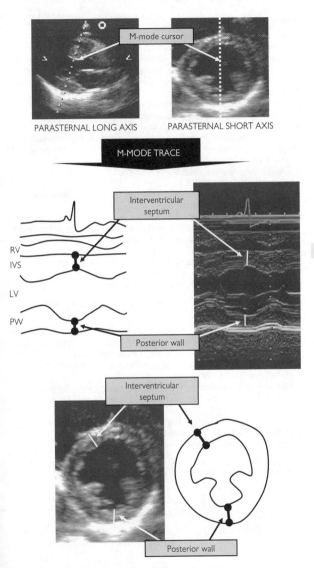

Fig. 3.43 Position for linear measures of left ventricular thickness.

Volume measures

There are two validated methods available for estimating left ventricular mass based on the *area-length* formula and the *truncated ellipsoid model*. Both methods use the same set of measurements in end-diastole—*total ventricular* and *cavity* area (short axis view, mid-papillary level) and *left ventricular length* (apical 2-chamber view)—and only vary in the equation they use to estimate volumes.

- Obtain a clear parasternal short axis view (mid-ventricle level) with good endocardial and epicardial border definition.
- Record a loop and scroll through to the end-diastolic frame.
- Trace around the endocardial border and record the *endocardial* or *left ventricular cavity* cross-sectional area. Do not include the papillary muscles in the tracing.
- Trace around the epicardial border and record the *epicardial* or *total* cross-sectional area.
- Myocardial area is the difference between the *total* cross-sectional area and the *cavity* cross-sectional area.
- In a non-foreshortened apical 2-chamber view record a loop and iden- tify the end-diastolic frame (when the ventricle is largest). Measure the distance from apex to the middle of the mitral valve annulus. Record the *left ventricular length*.
- The machine or off-line software will automatically calculate left ventricular mass from these measurements.
- The truncated ellipsoid equation for a volume is:

$$8 \times (\text{cross-sectional area in parasternal short axis})^2/(3 \times \pi \times \text{LV length})$$

Other volume measures

It is possible to use a biplane Simpson's method (p. 168) to calculate mass. The accuracy of the technique is dependent on obtaining a clear epicardial border in both planes but, unlike other methods, will take account of regional wall motion abnormalities or asymmetric variation in wall thickness.

- Measure total end-diastolic left ventricular volume using Simpson's method by tracing the *epicardial* border in apical 4- and 2-chamber views.
- Subtract *left ventricular end-diastolic volume* assessed with Simpson's method from this total volume. Multiply the difference by 1.05 to obtain a left ventricular mass.

In the same way *3D imaging* can be used to determine mass based on measurement of end-diastolic volume and total volume (p. 170).

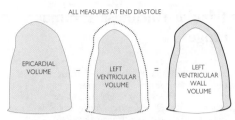

ALL MEASURES AT END DIASTOLE

LEFT VENTRICLE WALL VOLUME × MYOCARDIAL DENSITY (1.05) = LEFT VENTRICLE MASS

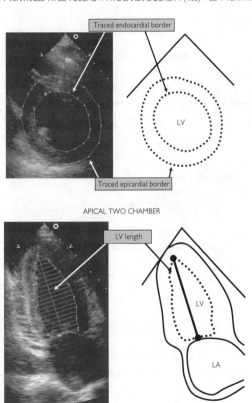

Fig. 3.44 Measures for volume assessment of left ventricular mass.

Left ventricular thickness and mass: normal ranges

Table 3.13 Ranges for measurements of LV mass. (Adapted from Recommendations for chamber quantification: a report of the American Society of Echocardiography Guidelines and Standards Committee and the Chamber Quantification Writing Group, developed in conjunction with the European Association of Echocardiography. J Am Soc Echocardiogr 2005;18:1440–63.)

Part 1, Values for women

	WOMEN			
	NORMAL	MILD	MODERATE	SEVERE
Linear method				
LV mass, g	67–162	163–186	187–210	>210
LV mass/BSA, g/m²	**43–95**	**96–108**	**109–121**	**>121**
LV mass/height, g/m	41–99	100–115	116–128	>128
LV mass/height², g/m²	18–44	45–51	52–58	>58
Relative wall thickness, cm	0.22–0.42	0.43–0.47	0.48–0.52	>0.52
Septal thickness, cm	**0.6–0.9**	**1.0–1.2**	**1.3–1.5**	**>1.5**
Posterior wall thickness, cm	**0.6–0.9**	**1.0–1.2**	**1.3–1.5**	**>1.5**
2D method				
LV mass, g	66–150	151–171	172–182	>182
LV mass/BSA, g/m²	**44–s88**	**89–100**	**101–112**	**>112**

BSA, Body surface area.
Bold rows identify best validated measures.

Table 3.13 (cont.)

Part 2, Values for men

	MEN			
	Normal	Mild	Moderate	Severe
Linear method				
LV mass, g	88–224	225–258	259–292	>292
LV mass/BSA, g/m²	**49–115**	**116–131**	**132–148**	**>148**
LV mass/height, g/m	52–126	127–144	145–162	>163
LV mass/height², g/m²	20–48	49–55	56–63	>63
Relative wall thickness, cm	0.24–0.42	0.43–0.46	0.47–0.51	>0.51
Septal thickness, cm	**0.6–1.0**	**1.1–1.3**	**1.4–1.6**	**>1.6**
Posterior wall thickness, cm	**0.6–1.0**	**1.1–1.3**	**1.4–1.6**	**>1.6**
2D method				
LV mass, g	96–200	201–227	228–254	>254
LV mass/BSA, g/m²	**50–102**	**103–116**	**117–130**	**>130**

BSA, Body surface area.
Bold rows identify best validated measures.

Left ventricular hypertrophy

The clinical importance of left ventricular mass relates to identification of pathological left ventricular hypertrophy. Left ventricular hypertrophy can occur secondary to other pathology (e.g. aortic valve disease or hypertension) or be a primary problem with the myocardium (e.g. hypertrophic cardiomyopathy, infiltrative cardiomyopathy). With hypertrophic cardiomyopathy there may be asymmetric changes with septal or apical changes. Physiological hypertrophy is also found (e.g. athletes or in pregnancy) that is thought to be reversible. In the elderly there is sometimes septal angulation and thickening that creates the impression of septal hypertrophy but left ventricular mass is usually unchanged.

Assessment

If hypertrophy is present base further assessment on: (1) a description of the pattern (global or asymmetric); (2) a description of severity using overall mass and mass relative to ventricular size; (3) characterization of related pathology (e.g. valve disease or outflow tract obstruction) and unusual appearances (e.g. speckling texture of amyloid, localized hypertrophy of tumour).

Appearance

- Using all views make a qualitative judgement of hypertrophy. Parasternal short axis view is good for seeing concentric hypertrophy. Parasternal long axis and apical 5-chamber views pick up septal hypertrophy. Apical and subcostal views can look for apical hypertrophy. Report the pattern and, if asymmetric, wall thickness measures at different points.
- A commonly reported abnormal texture is amyloid 'speckling'. This can be influenced by contrast and gain settings. Localized hypertrophy with abnormal echolucency might suggest malignant infiltration.

Grading severity

Left ventricular mass can be clinically graded into 4 categories: (1) normal; (2) increased relative wall thickness with increased mass (concentric left ventricular hypertrophy); (3) increased mass with normal relative wall thickness (eccentric left ventricular hypertrophy); or (4) normal mass with increased relative wall thickness (concentric remodelling). Concentric changes suggest pressure overload (e.g. due to aortic stenosis or hypertension). Eccentric changes suggest volume overload (e.g. due to aortic regurgitation). Grade severity by reporting overall mass and/or wall thickness, and relative wall thickness.

- Overall severity. Table 3.13 (pp. 178–9) provides a guide to grading hypertrophy based on mass and wall thickness measures.
- Relative wall thickness. Use left ventricular posterior wall thickness (PWT) and left ventricular end-diastolic diameter (LVEDD). Relative wall thickness is calculated as:

$$(2 \times PWT)/LVEDD$$

- If relative wall thickness is >0.42 report concentric hypertrophy.
- If relative wall thickness is <0.42 report eccentric hypertrophy.

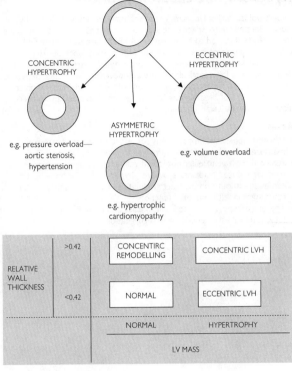

Fig. 3.45 Patterns of hypertrophy.

Hypertrophic cardiomyopathy

Hypertrophic cardiomyopathy describes marked left ventricular hypertrophy secondary to specific genetic abnormalities. There are multiple gene defects that lead to hypertrophy and more are being identified. The responsible genes commonly control muscle fibre function. The hypertrophy can be of many different patterns and towards the end of the disease process left ventricular failure can develop. The classic pattern is of marked septal hypertrophy associated with significant outflow obstruction. Symptoms of breathlessness, however, may also be due to reduced diastolic left ventricular function.

Assessment

- If hypertrophic cardiomyopathy is suspected report the pattern and measures of *wall thickness*, *relative wall thickness*, and *mass*.
- Assess the left ventricular outflow at rest and consider looking for exercise-induced gradients. However, hypertrophic cardiomyopathy can exist without outflow tract gradients and symptoms may be due to changes in left ventricular function.
- Therefore, report left ventricular systolic and diastolic function and look at mitral valve function and regurgitation.

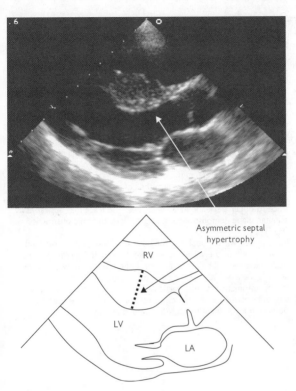

Fig. 3.46 Parasternal long axis view demonstrates septal hypertrophy.

Left ventricular outflow

Historically, *M-mode* has been used to demonstrate outflow obstruction.

- Systolic anterior motion of mitral valve is seen with M-mode placed through the mitral leaflets. It is considered severe (i.e. obstructive) if the leaflet touches the ventricular septum or the outflow tract is narrowed by the anterior mitral valve leaflet for >40% of systole.
- Obstruction tends to be in mid to late systole leading to a drop in flow through the aortic valve towards the end of systole. Therefore, an M-mode trace through the aortic leaflets can demonstrate early closure of the valve and the valve may appear to flutter as flow drops.

Doppler should be used as the main method to quantify obstruction.

- In an apical 5- or 3-chamber view place colour flow mapping over the outflow tract. This may demonstrate turbulent, high velocity, flow (an irregular scattering) in the outflow tract.
- In the apical 5-chamber view align the continuous wave Doppler through the outflow tract, aortic valve, and aorta. Record a spectral trace to obtain peak and mean velocities. The trace may appear as a scimitar shape demonstrating the classic, late, dynamic obstruction (Fig. 3.48).
- Place pulsed wave Doppler at the bottom of the outflow tract and move it towards the valve. If the gradient is due to hypertrophy the peak velocities will be present in the outflow tract below the valve and the trace will start aliasing due to the high velocities.
- In a symptomatic patient—particularly if symptomatic on exercise— without obstruction, an exercise stress protocol can be used and outflow tract gradient measured at peak exercise.

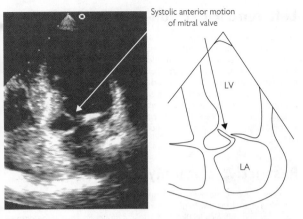

Fig. 3.47 Apical 4-chamber view demonstrates systolic anterior motion of mitral valve.

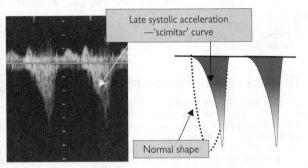

Fig. 3.48 Scimitar-shaped spectral trace characteristic of late systolic acceleration.

Left ventricular non-compaction

Left ventricular non-compaction is an inherited condition characterized by marked trabeculation usually within the left ventricular apex. This leads to impaired ventricular function and can be a substrate for left-sided thrombi and arrhythmias. To identify non-compaction left-sided contrast agents are usually required. In apical views the trabeculation is seen as a partially contrast-filled layer. Report the thickness of the trabeculation relative to the myocardium. A ratio of >2.1 non-compacted (trabeculations) myocardium to compacted (normal) myocardium at end-systole suggests left ventricular non-compaction. Magnetic resonance imaging aids diagnosis.

Restrictive cardiomyopathy

True restrictive cardiomyopathy is rare and tends to occur due to infiltrative disease such as amyloidosis. Symptoms develop due to myocardial thickening and stiffening leading to diastolic dysfunction. Late in the disease systolic dysfunction can develop as contractile function diminishes.
• A full assessment of the left ventricle (size and mass, systolic and diastolic function) is needed for diagnosis. Classic appearance is normal systolic function and cavity dimensions but abnormal diastolic function with varying increases in wall thickness.
• The usual diagnostic conundrum is differentiation from constrictive pericarditis. Techniques such as tissue Doppler imaging and mitral inflow are useful and described in the pericardium section on p. 240.

Dilated cardiomyopathy

Dilated cardiomyopathy describes left ventricular dilatation and impaired function and can be accompanied by right ventricular dilatation. There can be many underlying causes, such as ischaemic heart disease, tachycardia-induced, metabolic conditions (e.g. hyperthyroidism, phaeochromocytomas), post-partum, or post-myocarditis. The term idiopathic dilated cardiomyopathy is used if no underlying cause is identified. Echocardiography should provide information on ventricular size and function and be used for follow up to gauge recovery or deterioration.

Myocarditis

Myocarditis occurs due to a viral infection either acutely or as a post-viral phenomenon. It is characterized by acute onset left ventricular global systolic dysfunction that can range from mild to fatal. Echocardiography should identify normal ventricular dimensions but a global reduction in function. This may evolve into a dilated cardiomyopathy. A pericardial effusion may also develop. Recovery is assessed by repeated echocardiography to determine changes in left ventricular function.

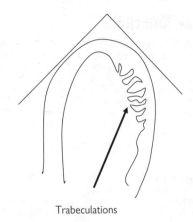

Trabeculations

2D IMAGE

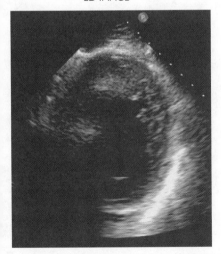

Fig. 3.49 An apical 4-chamber view demonstrating lateral wall trabeculation. The abnormal trabeculations of left ventricular non-compaction can be highlighted with contrast or colour flow mapping.

Left ventricular function

Assessment of left ventricular function is one of the most frequently requested echocardiography studies, with ejection fraction the most sought after parameter. This is driven by several issues. The number of patients presenting with dyspnoea and possible congestive heart failure is increasing, there is clear prognostic significance to the parameter of ejection fraction, and it is used to guide therapy (especially decisions for device therapy in heart failure and surgery for valve disease). Remember that congestive heart failure is a clinical diagnosis and, even before clinical signs are evident, abnormalities of left ventricular function may be apparent. Early detection is critical to prevent progression of heart failure.

Assessment

An assessment of left ventricular function should be comprehensive. Table 3.14 outlines the techniques for a complete examination. Not all will be felt necessary for all patients and selection should be based on the clinical indication for the study. However, the minimal requirements are an assessment of:
- left ventricular size and shape;
- systolic function, including regional differences;
- diastolic function.

Table 3.14 Assessment of left ventricular function

- **Global systolic function.**
  - Subjective evaluation of size, shape, regional and global function.
  - Measurement of left ventricular volumes/dimensions, ejection fraction (Simpson's).
  - Doppler. Volumetric measurements, dP/dt in patients with mitral regurgitation.
  - New techniques for myocardial function (strain, strain rate).
  - Left ventricular response to exercise stress.
- **Left ventricular shape and wall stress.**
- **Regional systolic function.**
  - Subjective evaluation of segmental function, wall motion score.
  - Myocardial contrast enhancement.
- **Diastolic function.**
  - Transmitral flow categorization.
  - Strategies for recognition of pseudonormal filling.
  - Left atrial size (area or volume).
  - Annular tissue Doppler (E/E′).
  - Response to Valsalva manoeuvre.
  - Others (pulmonary vein flow, mitral flow propagation).
- **Synchrony.**
  - M-mode intraventricular delay.
  - Doppler assessment of interventricular delay.
  - Tissue Doppler imaging.

Global systolic function

Left ventricular systolic evaluation is commonly performed by eye. Although the eyeball of an experienced reader is equivalent to the track-ball, the desirability of visual assessment is dependent on the circumstances. Visual assessment alone is appropriate in an emergency but inappropriate in most circumstances when elective decisions are being made. Global systolic function should be quantified. The standard approaches are detailed below and the most accurate (and therefore the preferred methods) are based on volumetric measures (p. 168).

2D measures

Ejection fraction

This represents the fraction of blood within the left ventricle that is ejected in one cardiac cycle. To calculate, use the end-diastolic (LVEDV) and end-systolic (LVESV) volumes (p. 168). The ejection fraction is:

$$\frac{LVEDV - LVESV}{LVEDV} \times 100\%$$

Linear measures (p. 166) of left ventricular size (left ventricular end-diastolic diameter (LVEDD) and left ventricular end-systolic diameter (LVESD)) are notoriously inaccurate but, if the only measures available, ejection fraction is:

$$\frac{LVEDD^3 - LVESD^3}{LVEDD^3} \times 100\%$$

Fractional shortening (fractional area change)

Fractional shortening and fractional area change represent summary measures of changes in left ventricular size in mid-cavity. *Fractional shortening* is based on the standard linear measures (p. 166):

$$\frac{LVEDD - LVESD}{LVEDD} \times 100\%$$

Fractional area change uses end-diastolic (LVEDA) and end-systolic (LVESA) cavity cross-sectional area traced in parasternal short axis (mid-ventricle level) view (to measure area see p. 170):

$$\frac{LVEDA - LVESA}{LVEDA} \times 100\%$$

Stroke volume and cardiac output

The volume of blood that forms the ejection fraction (LVEDV – LVESV) represents the *stroke volume*. Normally this is around 75–100mL.

If the mitral valve is competent then this can be multiplied by heart rate to calculate *cardiac output*. Normally this is around 4–8L/min.

These measures vary with body size and should be divided by body surface area (body surface area = sq root(height(m) × weight(kg)/36)) to give a *stroke volume index* (normally 40–70mL/m^2) and *cardiac index* (normally 2.5–4L/min/m^2), respectively.

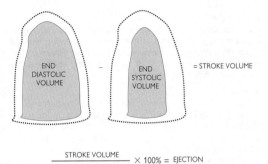

Fig. 3.50 Principle of ejection fraction. This can also be estimated from linear measures.

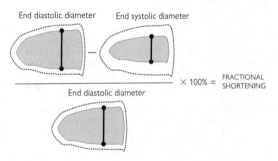

Fig. 3.51 Principle of fractional shortening based on linear measures.

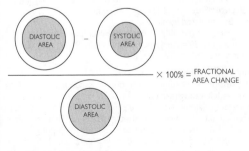

Fig. 3.52 Principle of fractional area change.

Doppler evaluation

Doppler is less useful for systolic function evaluation. Measurements of stroke volume are more commonly written about than performed, and depend on accurate outflow tract measures (errors of which are squared to calculate area). Measurement of dP/dt can be a useful extra measure in patients with severe mitral regurgitation.

Stroke volume

Doppler evaluation of stroke volume is based on the measurement of blood flow through the left ventricular outlet tract during a cardiac cycle.

- In apical 5-chamber view record a pulsed wave Doppler in the outflow tract and trace the shape. Record the velocity time integral (vti).
- In a parasternal long axis view, zoom the left ventricular outflow tract (LVOT) and measure the width (edge to edge, just below aortic valve).
- Stroke volume is the area of the outflow tract ($\pi \times$ (LVOT diameter/2)^2) multiplied by the outflow tract vti.
- Cardiac output is stroke volume multiplied by heart rate.
- Normal cardiac output = 4–8L/min.
- Normal stroke volume = 75–100mL.

dP/dt

dP/dt describes the rise in intraventricular pressure during early systole. The change in pressure is determined by systolic contraction so the faster the rise the better the left ventricular systolic function. Theoretically this should be less dependent than ejection fraction on the loading condition of the heart. It can only be measured if there is significant mitral regurgitation.

- In an apical 4-chamber view align the continuous wave Doppler through the mitral valve and the associated regurgitant jet.
- Record a spectral trace at a sweep speed of 100mm/sec to broaden the tracing. Set the scale to focus on the 0–4m/sec range.
- Measure the time taken for the velocity of the regurgitant jet to rise from 1 to 3m/sec (the measure has been standardized for this pressure rise from 4 to 36mmHg). The machine or software will normally automatically calculate dP/dt if the 1 and 3m/sec points are marked, although it can be calculated by hand.
- dP/dt >1200mmHg/sec (roughly <27msec between points) relates to normal function and <800mmHg/sec (roughly >40msec) is severely depressed function.

Left ventricular outflow vti

To gain an impression of whether cardiac output is *normal*, *low*, or *high* measure vti in the left ventricular outflow tract using pulsed wave Doppler from an apical 5-chamber view. In the general population if the heart rate is between 60 and 100 then normal range is 18–22. This technique can also be applied to assess right ventricular output using pulsed wave Doppler in the right ventricular outflow tract in a parasternal short axis view. Normal value should be 76% (or three-quarters) of left ventricular outflow vti (i.e. 14–17).

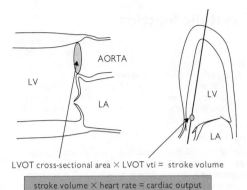

LVOT cross-sectional area × LVOT vti = stroke volume

stroke volume × heart rate = cardiac output

Fig. 3.53 Stroke volume can be used as a Doppler-based assessment of left ventricle function.

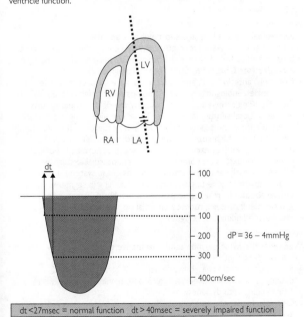

dt <27msec = normal function   dt > 40msec = severely impaired function

Fig. 3.54 dP/dt measures the rise in intraventricular pressure. A mitral regurgitant jet has been assessed with continuous wave Doppler in an apical 4-chamber view.

Regional systolic function

Although regional changes can occur in cardiomyopathies, the most common cause of regional left ventricular dysfunction is coronary artery disease. Regional abnormalities are usually assessed by eye and are dependent on operator experience. Basic assessment is of wall movement in coronary artery territories. This should be refined to gauge movement of wall segments and can then be semi-quantified with wall motion scores. There are fully quantitative methods although not yet in routine clinical practice.

Qualitative assessment

The key to reporting regional dysfunction is to use a standard system to segment the heart. The standard 16-segment model of the American Society of Echocardiography (septal, lateral, anterior, and inferior at the apex, as well as anteroseptal and posterior segments at the base and mid-papillary muscle level) is still widely used, although the American Heart Association has moved to a 17-segment model (which includes a true apical segment) to encourage similar segment models between imaging techniques (p. 197).

Wall motion

- Record parasternal long and short axis and, apical 4-, 3-, and 2-chamber views. Avoid foreshortening and ensure a clear endocardial border (see p. 168). Enhance the border with left-sided contrast agents if needed (see Chapter 6, 'Stress echocardiography').
- Generally: anterior wall, apex, and septum are supplied by the left anterior descending artery; lateral and posterior (inferolateral) walls by the circumflex artery; and inferior wall by the right coronary artery. However, basal septum in an apical 4-chamber view is right coronary artery territory and supply of the apex and posterior wall varies slightly depending on which coronary system is dominant (left or right).
- In each loop look at each segment and score as normal, hypokinetic (endocardial excursion <5mm), akinetic (endocardial excursion <2mm), or dyskinetic (endocardium moves out in systole).
- As movement may be passive, look for thickening in segments you are unsure about. Normal segments will thicken by >50% between diastole and systole. If present, report as normal or hypokinetic.
- Present the findings as a diagram.

Wall motion scores

Wall motion scoring permits semi-quantitative evaluation of the regional function assessment.

- Score normal regions as 1; hypokinetic as 2; akinetic as 3; and dyskinetic as 4. Score aneurysms as 5, and thinning with akinesis as 6 or thinning with dyskinesis as 7.
- Calculate (or let the software calculate) a *wall motion score index* by averaging scores of all individual segments. This is a semi-quantitative index of global systolic function analogous to ejection fraction.

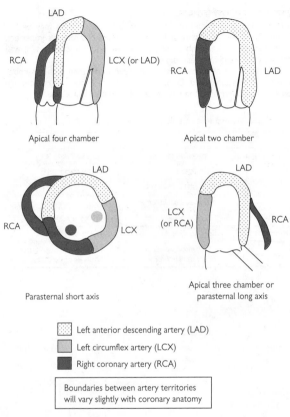

Fig. 3.55 Coronary artery supply to walls of left and right ventricle.

Quantitative assessment

Concordance of wall motion assessment between centres may be improved with the use of standard reading criteria, but remains imperfect. The benefit of a suitable objective measure would be to supplement wall motion scoring and help less expert readers.

Quantitation of regional function has been performed with a number of echocardiographic and Doppler modalities (Table 3.15). Although some are encouraging, none have entered mainstream practice.

Table 3.15 Assessment techniques for regional function

	Radial	Longitudinal
Displacement & thickening	Centre-line (from 2D)	Annular M-mode
	Colour kinesis	Tissue tracking
	Anatomical M-mode	
	Integrated backscatter	
Velocity	Speckle strain	TDI or speckle strain
Deformation	Speckle strain	TDI or speckle strain
Timing	TDI (time to peak systole or onset of diastole)	TDI (time to peak systole or onset of diastole)

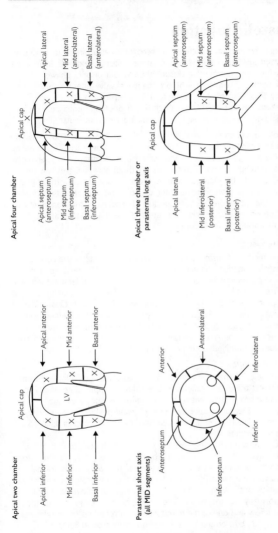

Fig. 3.56 17-segment model (16-segment is the same without the apical cap). Note that some segments are seen in multiple views. The posterior wall can also be referred to as the inferolateral wall. 'X's mark the 17 different segments of the ventricle, some of which are seen in the other views (unmarked segments).

Diastolic function

Diastolic dysfunction is increasingly recognized as an important influence on symptoms and haemodynamic status. Diastole extends from aortic valve closure to mitral valve closure and has four distinct phases:

• isovolumetric relaxation—before the mitral valve opens.
• early filling—accounting for up to 80% of ventricular filling.
• diastasis—as left atrial and left ventricular pressures equalize.
• atrial systole—accounting for the remainder of ventricular filling.

Diastolic dysfunction during the early phases is due to problems with active myocardial relaxation. This is usually present early in disease development (e.g. ischaemia, aortic stenosis, hypertension, hypertrophy) and is termed *abnormal relaxation*. With disease progression fibrosis develops and chamber compliance reduces (also seen with infiltrative disease). These changes affect later diastole and lead to *restrictive filling*. During the transition there is a period of apparently *pseudonormal filling* on some echocardiographic parameters at the mitral valve, although diastolic function remains impaired.

Assessment

Measurement of *transmitral flow* (left ventricular filling) is the cornerstone of diastolic function evaluation (i.e. E/A ratio). This measure is refined with: (1) *pulmonary vein flow* and *left atrial size* (to understand left atrial pressure) and (2) *tissue Doppler imaging* of the mitral annulus to study changes in myocardial movement (see Fig. 3.58 p. 201). *Colour M-mode propagation* has also been used. The report should comment on the presence and pattern of diastolic dysfunction (*abnormal relaxation*, *pseudonormal filling*, or *restrictive filling*). Also comment on likely underlying pathology, if identified, during the examination.

Mitral valve inflow

• In the apical 4-chamber view position the pulsed wave Doppler sample volume at the mitral leaflet tips. Use colour Doppler if necessary to optimize beam alignment with mitral inflow. Record a tracing.
• E/A ratio. Measure peak E-wave velocity and peak A-wave velocity. Normal filling is generally characterized by an E/A ratio of 0.75–1.5.
• Other measures.
  • *Deceleration time.* Measure the distance from peak to end of the E-wave. If the end is obscured by the A-wave extrapolate the slope to the baseline. A deceleration time of 160–260msec is normal.
  • *Isovolumetric relaxation time.* Measure the time from the end of the aortic outflow trace to the start of the mitral inflow trace. This normally requires two different Doppler recordings (one of aortic outflow and one of the mitral inflow) with timings taken relative to a fixed point on the ECG. This is normally around 80msec.
  • *Valsalva manoeuvre.* The mitral inflow pattern can be recorded again with the patient performing a Valsalva. If there is *pseudonormal* or *reversible restrictive filling* the trace will revert to an *abnormal relaxation* pattern. Failure to revert may reflect the presence of normal filling or simply be due to inadequate inspiratory effort.

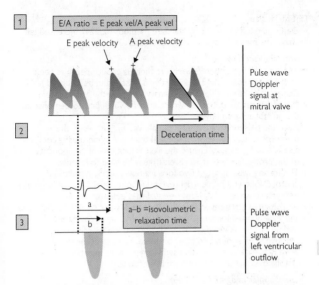

Fig. 3.57 Doppler measures of diastolic function. 1. E/A ratio uses peak of E and A wave velocities from pulsed wave Doppler at mitral valve tips. 2. Deceleration time is time from peak of E wave to baseline. 3. Isovolumetric relaxation time: a = time from R wave on ECG to start of mitral valve inflow; b = time from R wave to end of aortic outflow.

Left atrial size
- Determine left atrial size by standard methods (p. 224). Increased left atrial size implies raised left atrial pressure.

Pulmonary vein flow
- In the apical 4-chamber view ensure there is enough depth to see the pulmonary vein inflow. The easiest vein to see (and best aligned for Doppler) is the right upper pulmonary vein near the atrial septum. Placement can be optimized with colour flow mapping to demonstrate the pulmonary vein flow.
- Place the pulsed wave Doppler sample volume just inside the pulmonary vein and record a spectral tracing. A good tracing confirms a satisfactory position. Ensure the filter is kept low or components of the profile (such as atrial reversal) may be hard to identify.
- The tracing will consist of two forward flow phases, systolic and diastolic, followed by an atrial reversal (due to atrial systole). Normally the systolic wave is dominant or equal to the diastolic wave.
- A prominent atrial reversal (>30cm/sec peak velocity of the atrial wave and >20–30msec longer duration of the atrial wave compared to the duration of the A wave on the mitral inflow) is a specific but not very sensitive marker of raised filling pressure. Blunting of the systolic flow wave is a reliable marker of raised filling pressure in patients with systolic dysfunction, but not normal function.

Tissue Doppler imaging (see p. 46)
- In apical 4-chamber views place the pulsed wave tissue Doppler on the septal or lateral annulus of the mitral valve (there is no clear consensus about which is optimal). The tissue Doppler spectrum can be optimized by decreasing the sample volume and optimizing gain settings (excessive gain causes spectral broadening). Ensure it is aligned with the long axis of the ventricle.
- The Doppler pattern should be the same as the mitral valve inflow with an E wave and A wave (but below the baseline away from the probe). Measure the peak velocity of both. They are usually referred to as E' and A'.
- E/E' can also be calculated and relates to left atrial pressure. E/E' <8 suggests normal left atrial pressure and E/E' >15 suggests elevated left atrial pressure.

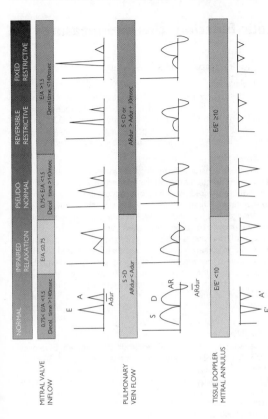

Fig. 3.58 Doppler patterns to characterize diastolic function. Mitral inflow can be repeated with a Valsalva manoeuvre and, if there is pseudonormal filling, the mitral inflow will change to an impaired relaxation pattern. Reversible restrictive describes a restrictive pattern that changes to an impaired relaxation pattern on Valsalva.

MITRAL VALVE INFLOW

PULMONARY VEIN FLOW

TISSUE DOPPLER MITRAL ANNULUS

NORMAL

IMPAIRED RELAXATION

PSEUDO NORMAL

REVERSIBLE RESTRICTIVE

FIXED RESTRICTIVE

0.75< E/A <1.5
Decel: time >140msec

E/A ≤0.75

0.75< E/A <1.5
Decel. time <140msec

E/A >1.5
Decel.time <140msec

S >D
ARdur < Adur

S<D or
ARdur > Adur+ 30msec

E/E' <10

E/E' ≥10

Diastolic function: tips and measures

Transmitral flow categorization (see Fig. 3.58, p. 201)

1. Impaired relaxation (see Table 3.16)

This is characterized by reduction of the peak transmitral pressure gradient (hence lower E velocity and E/A ratio [<1 in young, <0.5 in elderly]) and prolongation of the E deceleration slope (>220msec in young, >280msec in elderly). Cardiac pacing, left bundle branch block, and right ventricular overload may provoke the same changes.

2. Pseudonormal filling

As left atrial pressure increases with progressive left ventricular disease, E velocity and deceleration time return to normal. With exception of patients with more marked elevations of filling pressure and low heart rate, who may show a mid-diastolic('L') wave, transmitral flow patterns cannot be distinguished from normal without the performance of other steps. The first step is to suspect the condition—'normal' transmitral flow in the setting of left ventricular enlargement, hypertrophy, or systolic dysfunction is likely to be pseudonormal. The second step is to assess left atrial size, followed by estimation of filling pressure (as E/E′) and tissue Doppler of the mitral annulus. Note that, when left ventricular ejection fraction is preserved, E deceleration time, the Valsalva response, blunting of the pulmonary venous S wave (and S/D ratio), and flow propagation velocity may be unreliable indicators of diastolic dysfunction.

3. Restrictive filling

Continued elevation of filling pressure leads to increased E velocity (increase in E/A ratio >2) and shorter E deceleration time (<150msec). This finding is unusual with normal ejection fraction (indicating a restrictive cardiomyopathy (e.g. amyloidosis), and is more commonly associated with left ventricular dilatation and severe systolic dysfunction. The presence of reversibility (i.e. normalization with Valsalva or after diuresis) is prognostically very important.

Table 3.16 Age-adjusted normal cut-offs for selected diastolic parameters

	Age (years)		
	<40	**40–60**	**>60**
E deceleration time (msec)	<220	140–250	140–275
Septal E' velocity (cm/sec)	>9	>7	>6
Lateral E' velocity (cm/sec)	>11	>10	>7

Table 3.17 Useful criteria for differentiating normal from pseudonormal filling in adult subjects with normal left ventricular systolic function

	Normal	Pseudonormal
Lateral E' velocity (depending on age), cm/sec	>7–11	<7–11
Lateral E/ E'	<10	>10
PV A velocity, cm/sec	<35	>35
PV A duration—transmitral A duration, msec	<30	>30
Valsalva manoeuvre	No significant change in E/A ratio	E/A <1 or E/A decrease by >50%

PV, Pulmonary venous.

Left ventricular synchrony

The current selection criteria for cardiac resynchronization therapy include NYHA class III or IV heart failure symptoms and left ventricular ejection fraction <35% on maximal medical therapy, in the setting of a widened QRS (the relevant QRS width varies between trials, but usually is >120msec (usually left bundle branch block)). Despite using these criteria, 20–30% do not respond and it may be that others with heart failure would benefit.

Markers of dyssynchrony

Echocardiographic assessment of synchrony can be used for patient selection, pacing site selection, or both. Synchrony can be assessed between right ventricle and left ventricle (interventricular dyssynchrony—electromechanical delay in right ventricular and left ventricular outflow tracts) or within the left ventricle (intraventricular dyssynchrony—M-mode, tissue Doppler, strain, 3D). There are few comparisons between the markers and centres often offer a 'menu' of measurements. Below is a list, with findings that would suggest dyssynchrony.

- M-mode septum to posterior delay >130msec.
- Interventricular delay >40msec.
- Systolic strain (% delayed contraction >30).
- Septal to posterior wall delay >65msec by tissue Doppler imaging.
- Dyssynchrony index >32.6msec.
- Parametric markers—tissue strain index, tissue tracking.

Interventricular dyssynchrony

Interventricular dyssynchrony is the difference in time between onset of pulmonary flow and onset of aortic flow (≥ 40msec suggests dyssynchrony). Because separate views are needed for each measurement the onset of flow in each view is timed relative to the ECG trace.

- Obtain a parasternal short axis view (aortic valve level). Record a pulsed wave Doppler tracing through the pulmonary valve. Ensure there is a surface ECG recording.
- In an apical 4-chamber view place a pulsed wave Doppler in the outflow tract and record a tracing. Ensure there is surface ECG trace.
- Measure the distance from the start of the QRS to the start of the pulmonary valve flow on the first view; then measure the distance from the start of the QRS to the start of the aortic valve flow on the second view. The difference is the interventricular delay.

Intraventricular dyssynchrony (septal to posterior wall delay)

Intraventricular dyssynchrony is the delay between the septal and posterior wall peak contraction (≥ 130msec suggests dyssynchrony), i.e. the delay between the opposite walls of the left ventricle being fully contracted.

- In a parasternal long axis view drop the M-mode cursor perpendicular to the septal and posterior wall. On the tracing identify the peak of septal and posterior wall systolic motion. Measure the time difference between the two walls and this is the intraventricular delay.

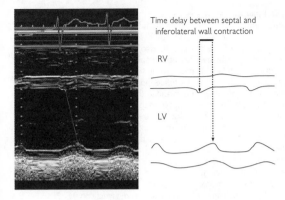

Time delay between septal and inferolateral wall contraction

RV

LV

Intraventricular delay = Delay between septum and inferolateral wall

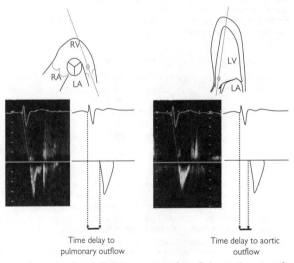

Time delay to pulmonary outflow

Time delay to aortic outflow

Interventricular delay = Delay to aortic outflow – Delay to pulmonary outflow

Fig. 3.59 Measurement of inter- and intraventricular dyssynchrony.

Tissue Doppler measures

Differences in movement of the mid- and basal segments of each wall of the left ventricle can be assessed by tissue Doppler imaging to provide some impression of the co-ordination of the ventricle. The assessment can be based on eight measures from apical 4- and 2-chamber views, or 12 measures, which include measures in the apical 3-chamber view.

- In apical 4-chamber place the tissue Doppler sample volume on each side of the mitral valve annulus and in the mid-segments of the septum and lateral wall. Record tracings in each position.
- Repeat the process in the apical 2-chamber view on each side of the annulus and the mid-segments of the inferior and anterior walls.
- This can then be repeated in the apical 3-chamber view in all four basal and mid-segments.
- Measure the time from the start of the QRS to the systolic phase of motion on each tracing (p. 46).
- The standard deviation of the eight (or 12) measures provides a global index of dyssynchrony (>33msec suggests dyssynchrony).
- An alternative measure is the delay between the basal septum and basal lateral wall in the apical 4-chamber view (>60msec suggests dyssynchrony).
- Finally if any of the eight (or 12) measures are >100msec different then this suggests dyssynchrony.

Use in follow-up: how to define success?

The most widely used markers include clinical improvement (formalized as improvement in heart failure class or quality of life score) and improved exercise capacity (e.g. lengthening of a 6 minute walk). Echocardiographic markers include ≥15% decrease in left ventricle volumes, ≥5% increase in ejection fraction, any decrease in left ventricle mass, or a decrease in mitral regurgitation severity.

Unresolved issues

A number of potential contributions from echocardiography remain unresolved.

- What is the optimal synchrony marker to predict recovery? There are several novel markers being developed.
- Should echocardiography be used to assess ischaemia/viability?
- Is guidance regarding optimal pacing site useful?
- Should echocardiography be used to make adjustments to pacing parameters over time as cardiac function varies?

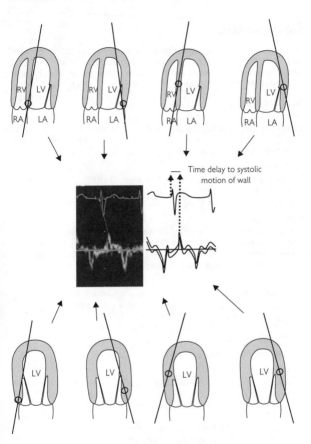

Fig. 3.60 Tissue Doppler imaging in basal and mid-segments of left ventricle walls from apical 4- and 2-chamber views. For a 12-segment model the apical 3-chamber view is used as well.

Optimization

Two key elements need optimization after resynchronization therapy: ventricular filling and left ventricular cardiac output. This can be done with two pacing parameters: delay between pacing atrium and ventricle (AV delay) and delay between pacing left and right ventricle (VV delay).

Assessment

Start

Ensure you have the appropriate pacemaker programmer and a technician. Start by collecting the standard baseline dyssynchrony measures (p. 204) and record the current programmed AV and VV delay.

AV delay

The aim is to choose the shortest AV delay that still allows complete ventricular filling. There are two approaches. Both use apical 4-chamber view with a pulsed wave Doppler profile of mitral valve inflow.

Iterative method
- Program a long AV delay (e.g. 150msec) on the pacemaker. Look at the A-wave and decrease the delay in 20msec steps until the A-wave starts to be truncated. Then gradually extend the delay by 10msec steps until the A-wave is just complete (Fig. 3.61).

Ritter method
- Program a short AV delay (e.g. *short delay* = 50msec) and measure distance from start of QRS to end of A wave (*QAshort*).
- Program a long AV delay (e.g. *long delay* = 150msec) and measure distance from start of QRS to end of A wave (*QA long*).
- Calculate optimal delay as:

    optimal delay = long delay + QAlong − QAshort

VV delay

In an apical 5-chamber view place pulsed wave Doppler in left ventricular outflow tract. Keep it in the same position throughout the study.
- Start the VV delay with left ventricle paced 80msec before the right ventricle.
- Record a spectral profile and annotate with the VV delay.
- Calculate the vti by tracing the spectral profile.
- Reduce the delay by 20msec to 60msec and record another vti.
- Repeat, reducing delay by 20msec until there is no delay (0msec). Then start pacing RV first, increasing in 20msec increments up to 80msec.
- Also, try left and right ventricle pacing alone.
- Look at results and identify parameter with maximal vti. There should be a graded pattern away from the optimal delay. Choose this as the new VV delay.
- If decision is to pace right ventricle first AV delay should be reset.

    new optimal AV delay = previous optimal AV delay − VV delay

Finish

Program new AV and VV delay. Finish study with full re-evaluation of synchrony to ensure improvement following reprogramming.

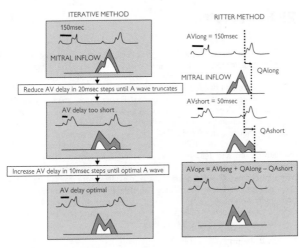

Fig. 3.61 Two methods to measure AV delay.

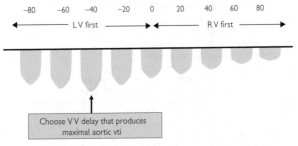

Fig. 3.62 VV delay assessed from recordings of aortic vti at different programmed delays. The VV delay with maximal aortic vti is selected.

Right ventricle

Normal anatomy

The right ventricle is formed by a free wall, divided into anterior and posterior portions, and the interventricular septum. The inflow area (tricuspid valve, chordae tendinae, papillary muscles, and chamber walls) is trabeculated and divided from the non-trabeculated outflow tract by a muscle bundle (crista supraventricularis). Towards the apex a muscular moderator band connects the free wall and septum. The combination of a thin free wall and thick septum leads to an irregular crescent shape with asymmetric contraction. The right ventricle maintains blood flow from the venous system to the pulmonary vasculature and from there to the left atrium and left ventricle. Size and function can therefore be affected by pulmonary problems (e.g. pulmonary hypertension, pulmonary embolism), left-sided heart disease (e.g. left ventricular failure, mitral valve disease), and right ventricular disorders (e.g. right ventricular infarction, right ventricular dysplasia, right ventricular hypertrophy). Septal defects have important effects on right ventricle function because they expose the right heart to systemic pressures.

Normal findings

Views

- The key views are: parasternal long axis; parasternal right ventricular inflow and outflow; parasternal short axis (aortic valve, mitral valve, and mid-papillary levels); apical 4- and 3-chamber; subcostal.

Findings

- Parasternal long axis. The right ventricle lies nearest the probe and this view can be used for M-mode measures.
- Parasternal right ventricular inflow and outflow. These can give excellent views of the tricuspid and pulmonary valves.
- Parasternal short axis (aortic valve, mitral valve, and mid-papillary levels). The right ventricle wraps around the left ventricle and therefore can be scanned through at multiple levels (as for the left ventricle). At the aortic valve it can be seen with both tricuspid and pulmonary valves and Doppler measures can be performed. As the plane moves towards the apex, the right ventricle is seen as a crescent to the left of the left ventricle. These views can give an impression of size and, in combination with septal appearance, of right ventricular pressure.
- Apical views. In the 4-chamber view the right ventricle lies on the left with the right atrium behind. This is a standard view for measures of cavity size and can give some impression of function based on movement of the tricuspid annulus.
- Subcostal view. The right ventricle lies nearest the probe with the ventricular septum horizontal. This is the best view to look for septal defects with colour flow and Doppler.

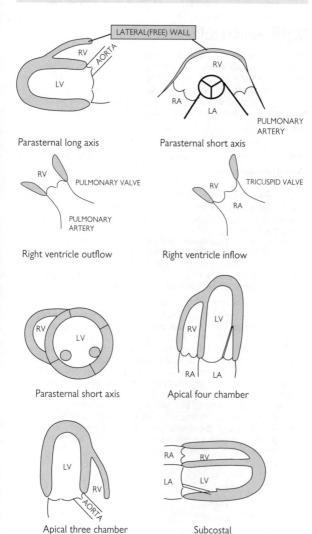

Fig. 3.63 Key views to assess the right ventricle.

Right ventricular size

The right ventricle has a complex shape so assessment of size is often performed qualitatively. However, the right ventricle has significant clinical relevance and a more thorough assessment is usually warranted. Both right ventricular wall thickness and cavity size can be quantified but, unlike other right-sided echocardiography measures, e.g. pulmonary valve function, techniques cannot be borrowed directly from the left heart.

Assessment

Assess the right ventricle in several views. If it does not appear normal comment on cavity size, as well as wall thickness and outflow tract size.

Right ventricular cavity size

Qualitative assessment

- In the apical 4-chamber view look at right ventricular area and mid-cavity diameter. Both should be smaller than the same left ventricular measures (assuming normal left ventricular size). Normally two-thirds the size.
- If left and right are similar in size then the right ventricle is *moderately dilated.* If larger than left then *severely dilated* and the right ventricle may form the apex: if so this can be reported as *apex forming.*
- Ensure apical views are not foreshortened. It is easy artificially to make the right ventricle form the apex and be bigger than the left ventricle.

Quantitative assessment

- A parasternal long axis view can be used with M-mode at the mitral valve tip level to measure cavity size but this should be supported by measurements from apical views.
- To assess right ventricular size quantitatively acquire a standard apical 4-chamber view. The three basic measures are taken in end-diastole: *right ventricular length*; *mid-cavity diameter*; and *diameter at the tricuspid annulus.* Right ventricular area can also be traced in systole and diastole.
- Other measures relate to the right ventricular outflow measured in the parasternal short axis (aortic valve) view at end-diastole. Again there are three measures: the vertical diameter from *aortic valve to free wall*; the diameter of the *pulmonary valve annulus*; and a diameter a few centimetres into the *pulmonary artery.*

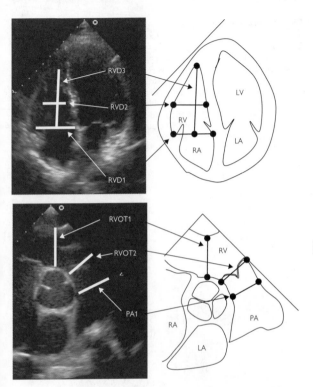

Fig. 3.64 Six standard measures of right ventricular size from apical 4-chamber (top) and parasternal short axis (bottom) views. Apical 4-chamber view: RVD1, basal RV; RVD2, mid RV; RVD3, base–apex. Parasternal short axis view: RVOT1, mid-ventricle (aortic valve to free wall); RVOT2, pulmonary valve level; PA1, pulmonary artery.

Right ventricular wall thickness

This can be assessed in parasternal long axis and apical 4-chamber views but the most consistent measures are from the subcostal view.

- In the parasternal view use a 2D image or M-mode trace with cursor perpendicular to the ventricular wall at the mitral valve tip level. Measure wall thickness at end-diastole. Normal is less than 0.5cm.
- In the subcostal view use a clear 2D image frozen in end-diastole (or perpendicular M-mode trace). Measure from edge-to-edge of the free wall at the level of the tricuspid valve chordae tendinae.
- In either view take care not to include epicardial fat or coarse trabeculations in the measurement.

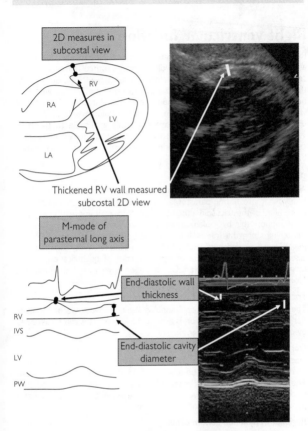

Fig. 3.65 Measurement of right ventricular wall thickness from a 2D subcostal view (top) and M-mode in parasternal long axis view (bottom).

Right ventricular function

Right ventricular function is traditionally assessed qualitatively. The key to assessment is to study movement of the right ventricular free wall (the septum largely contributes to left ventricular function). The movement of the right ventricular free wall differs from movement of the left ventricle, being predominantly towards the apex rather than into the middle of the ventricle. The techniques based on changes in volume or area that are used to assess the left ventricle are not easily applicable to the right ventricle. The complex geometry makes it difficult to measure accurate volumes. However, with advances in 3D imaging these approaches may become possible.

Assessment

Assess right ventricular function from the apical 4-chamber view. Confirm your impression in parasternal and subcostal views. Concentrate on movement of the tricuspid annulus to get an overall impression of function. Support this by looking at regional wall motion abnormalities and thickening along the free wall to the apex; note whether areas are *normal*, *akinetic*, or *dyskinetic* (use same criteria as in left ventricular regional assessment, p. 194). Because of the difficulties of quantification, report function as *normal* or *impaired*. Comment on any regional abnormalities. Normal values are in Table 3.18, p. 218.

Tricuspid annulus movement

The lateral side of the tricuspid annulus should move towards the apex during systole. Normal motion is around 1.5–2.0cm. This can be assessed by eye or with tissue Doppler imaging.

Fractional area change

Ejection fraction is difficult to measure because of complex geometry but fractional area change can be assessed from an apical 4-chamber view. The area of the right ventricle should be traced in end-diastole and end-systole. The difference between the two measures can be reported as a percentage relative to the end-diastolic area.

Regional wall motion abnormalities

The right ventricle free wall is predominantly supplied by the right coronary artery. The septum, apex, and, in some patients, the distal free wall are supplied by the left anterior descending artery.

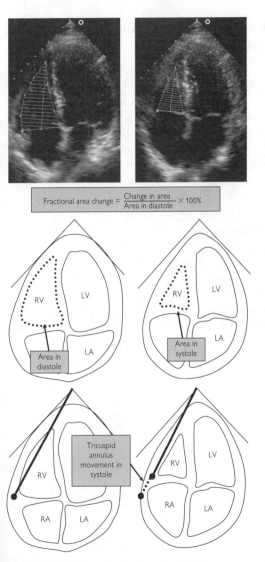

$$\text{Fractional area change} = \frac{\text{Change in area}}{\text{Area in diastole}} \times 100\%$$

Fig. 3.66 Right ventricular function assessed by fractional area change or (more commonly) movement of tricuspid annulus.

Right ventricular size and function: normal ranges

Table 3.18 Parameters to assess right ventricle size and function

	NORMAL	MILD	MODERATE	SEVERE
RV dimensions (apical 4-chamber)				
Basal RV diameter, cm	2.0–2.8	2.9–3.3	3.4–3.8	>3.8
Mid RV diameter, cm	2.7–3.3	3.4–3.7	3.8–4.1	>4.1
Base–apex length, cm	7.1–7.9	8.0–8.5	8.6–9.1	>9.1
RVOT diameter (parasternal short axis)				
Mid-ventricle, cm	2.5–2.9	3.0–3.2	3.3–3.5	>3.5
Pulmonary valve level, cm	1.7–2.3	2.4–2.7	2.8–3.1	>3.1
PA diameter (parasternal short axis)				
Pulmonary artery, cm	1.5–2.1	2.2–2.5	2.6–2.9	>2.9
RV area and fractional area change (apical 4-chamber)				
RV diastolic area, cm^2	11–28	29–32	33–37	>37
RV systolic area, cm^2	7.5–16	17–19	20–22	>22
Fractional area change, %	32–60	25–31	18–24	<18

In relation to Fig. 3.64 apical 4-chamber view: basal RV = RVD1; mid RV = RVD2; base–apex = RVD3.
In relation to Fig. 3.64 parasternal short axis view: aortic valve to free wall = RVOT1; level of pulmonary valve = RVOT2; pulmonary artery = PA1.

Right ventricular overload

Identifying volume or pressure overload in the right ventricle can aid clinical assessment of right heart function. Although often considered together they usually represent two different initial pathologies. Right *volume overload* suggests a left-to-right shunt or right-sided valvular regurgitation. *Pressure overload* suggests pulmonary hypertension or pulmonary stenosis. Pressure overload can develop from volume overload, and occasionally vice versa, in which cases features of both will be present.

Assessment

The key points to look at when evaluating the two situations are the following.

- What happens to right ventricle size and thickness (pp 212–5)?
  - *Volume overload* leads to increased cavity size and *pressure overload* leads to increased wall thickness. However, one can lead to the other and the two findings will coexist.
- How does the interventricular septum behave during the cardiac cycle?
  - Simply, *volume overload* is related to a flattened septum in *diastole*, whereas *pressure overload* is associated with a flattened septum in both *diastole* and *systole*.

Assess right ventricular systolic pressure (p. 148) to help support your impression of right ventricular pressure or volume overload.

Volume overload

- Obtain a clear parasternal short axis (mid-papillary level) view.
- *Ventricular size and wall thickness.* In volume overload the right ventricle should be *dilated* (the same size or bigger than the left ventricle) so comment on size. In chronic overload the right ventricle may start to hypertrophy but this will be *eccentric* as there will still be dilatation.
- *Septum.* The septum will flatten in *diastole* due to the large right ventricular volume and create a D-shaped ventricle (as volume overload worsens it will start to bow into the left ventricle). But then in *systole* the left ventricle reverts to a circular shape. This creates abnormal septal motion towards the left ventricle in diastole and towards the right ventricle in systole.

Pressure overload

- Use the same parasternal short axis (mid-papillary level) view.
- *Ventricular size and wall thickness.* In chronic pressure overload the right ventricular free wall thickens (normally half left ventricular thickness) but the cavity will remain the same until the right ventricle starts to fail.
- *Septum.* As pressure increases the septum will flatten out towards the left ventricle through both *diastole* and *systole*. With chronic pressure overload and increase in wall thickness the right ventricle will start to behave more like a left ventricle and the septum will bow into the left ventricle and contract towards the right ventricle during systole. This also creates *paradoxical septal motion* (but for a different reason from volume overload).

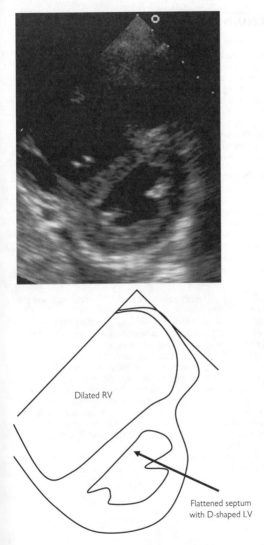

Fig. 3.67 Example of right ventricular volume overload in a parasternal short axis view. Note dilated right ventricle and flattened septum in diastole.

Left atrium

Normal anatomy

The left atrium receives blood from the four pulmonary veins. It acts as a reservoir and as a conduit to transport blood to the left ventricle. It has contractile function and atrial systole contributes approximately 25% of left ventricular filling. Morphologically, the atrium can be considered as having a body and an appendage. The common anatomical variations related to the atrium are those associated with the atrial septum, such as aneurysm, patent formanen ovale, atrial septal defect, or lipomatous hypertrophy. Rare anatomical variants can occur within the atrium such as cor triatriatum, in which the left atrium is separated into a superior and an inferior chamber.

Normal findings

Views

- The key views for the left atrium are: parasternal long axis, and apical 4- and 2-chamber. The apical views are the most useful to assess left atrial volume and left atrial haemodynamics.
- The parasternal short axis (aortic valve level) includes the left atrium and can be useful to look at the septum. The subcostal view aligns the left and right atrium perpendicular to the probe so can be useful for Doppler assessment of the septum.

Findings

- Parasternal long axis. The left atrium lies below the aortic root and the view is used for simple linear measures of left atrial size.
- Parasternal short axis (aortic valve level). The left atrium lies below the aortic valve. The interatrial septum is seen on the left and the left atrial appendage can occasionally be seen on the right.
- Apical 4- and 2-chamber. The left atrium lies at the bottom of the images and the views allow assessment of left atrial volume. The septum can also be studied. However, it lies vertically in the image and it is difficult to identify defects or do Doppler measures. Pulmonary veins are seen at the back of the atrium in the apical 4-chamber (particularly the right upper vein that lies by the septum). In the apical 2-chamber the left atrial appendage can sometimes be seen pointing out to the right. Generally, the left atrial appendage is only rarely visualized by transthoracic imaging.
- Subcostal view. The septum lies horizontal in the image and this is the best view to look for septal defects with colour flow and Doppler.

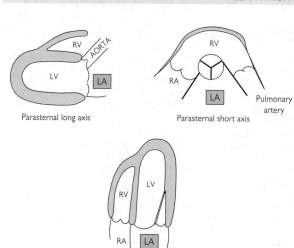

Parasternal long axis

Parasternal short axis

Apical four chamber

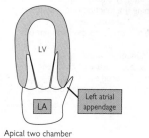

Apical two chamber

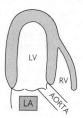

Apical three chamber

Fig. 3.68 Key views to assess left atrium.

Left atrial size

Left atrial enlargement is of clinical importance as it is associated with adverse cardiovascular outcome from a range of pathologies including myocardial infarction, stroke, dilated cardiomyopathy, and diastolic left ventricular failure with increased filling pressure. Atrial enlargement is also associated with atrial fibrillation.

Assessment

Preferred assessment is with volumes measured in apical views. Historically, linear measures in parasternal views are quoted. This is the antero-posterior diameter. If the atrium has enlarged along the long axis of the heart this may be missed with single anteroposterior linear measures.

Volumetric measures

Volume measures use the same principles and equations as for left ventricular volume assessment (p. 166). The left atrium can be modelled with the area–length formula, Simpson's method (which cuts the atrium into a series of discs and adds up the volumes of each disc), and the ellipsoid method. All calculations are usually done automatically by the machine software but require measurement of atrial length and diameters or planimetry of cross-sectional area. If measures are done in the 4-chamber view it is assumed that the atrium is spherical. Use of both 4- and 2-chamber views allows 3D assessment.

- Obtain a clear apical 4-chamber view with enough depth to include the whole of the left atrium.
- Record a loop and scroll through to identify end-systole.
- Planimeter around left atrium excluding the junction of the pulmonary veins and left atrial appendage (if visible). Record the area.
- Measure the length from back of the left atrium to the midpoint of a line across the mitral annulus.
- Repeat the process in the apical 2-chamber view.
- Use the shorter of the two lengths as the measure of atrial length.
- The machine will calculate volumes by Simpson's method.
- The *area–length formula* for left atrial volume is calculated as:

$$\frac{8 \times \text{area in 4-chamber} \times \text{area in 2-chamber}}{3 \times \pi \times \text{atrial length}}$$

- The *ellipsoid fomula* is:

$$\frac{4\pi \times (\text{length}/2) \times (\text{anteroposterior diameter}/2) \times (\text{apical view diameter}/2)}{3}$$

Linear measures

- In a parasternal long axis view, record a 2D loop and identify end-systole. Measure perpendicularly across the atrium from edge to edge.
- Alternatively, drop the M-mode cursor across the atrium at the level of the aortic valve tips, perpendicular to the walls. Measure left atrial size at end-systole (maximal size).

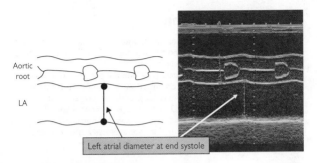

Fig. 3.69 M-mode measures of anteroposterior left atrial size in parasternal long axis view.

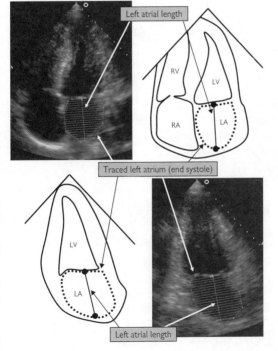

Fig. 3.70 Area tracing of left atrium in apical views to provide a more accurate assessment of left atrial size.

Left atrial function

Indices of left atrial function that incorporate left atrial ejection fraction corrected for cardiac output and body surface area have been reported in the literature, but are not in clinical use.

Indirect measures of atrial function include the presence of P waves on the ECG, a transmitral A wave on pulsed wave Doppler (the best way to demonstrate normal atrial contraction), and the presence of an atrial reversal wave on pulsed wave Doppler of the pulmonary vein. The presence of a P-wave on ECG but absent A-wave on mitral inflow suggests atrial dysfunction. This can occur, for example, early after cardioversion from atrial fibrillation.

Left and right atria: normal ranges

Table 3.19 Parameters to assess left and right atria

	WOMEN			
	NORMAL	**MILD**	**MODERATE**	**SEVERE**
Atrial dimension				
LA diameter, cm	2.7–3.8	3.9–4.2	4.3–4.6	>4.6
LA diameter/BSA, cm/m²	1.5–2.3	2.4–2.6	2.7–2.9	>2.9
RA minor axis, cm	2.9–4.5	4.6–4.9	5.0–5.4	>5.4
RA minor axis/BSA, cm/m²	1.7–2.5	2.6–2.8	2.9–3.1	>3.1
Atrial area				
LA area, cm²	<20	20–30	31–40	>40
Atrial volume				
LA volume, mL	22–52	53–62	63–72	>72
LA volume/BSA, mL/m²	**<29**	**29–33**	**34–39**	**>39**
	MEN			
	NORMAL	**MILD**	**MODERATE**	**SEVERE**
Atrial dimension				
LA diameter, cm	3.0–4.0	4.1–4.6	4.7–5.2	>5.2
LA diameter/BSA, cm/m²	1.5–2.3	2.4–2.6	2.7–2.9	>2.9
RA minor axis, cm	2.9–4.5	4.6–4.9	5.0–5.4	>5.4
RA minor axis/BSA, cm/m²	1.7–2.5	2.6–2.8	2.9–3.1	>3.1
Atrial area				
LA area, cm²	<20	20–30	31–40	>40
Atrial volume				
LA volume, mL	18–58	59–68	69–78	>78
LA volume/BSA, mL/m²	**<29**	**29–33**	**34–39**	**>39**

BSA, Body surface area
Bold rows identify best validated measures

Right atrium

The right atrium acts as reservoir for blood from the coronary sinus and inferior and superior vena cavae. It has some unique anatomical features that can be mistaken for pathology. These include the Eustachian valve, which *in utero* directs blood from the inferior vena cava through the foramen ovale but becomes redundant after birth. If it does not regress it is seen attached to the right atrial wall between the inferior vena cava and border of the fossa ovalis. A Chiari network is a remnant from the embryological stage before the Eustachian valve forms and is a thin membrane, typically fenestrated, near the orifice of the inferior vena cava and extending further across the right atrium than the Eustachian valve.

Normal views and findings
- The right atrium can be seen in a modified right ventricular inflow view and parasternal short axis view (aortic valve level).
- The apical 4-chamber view is useful for volume measurements and Doppler interrogation of tricuspid valve inflow.
- The subcostal view often provides excellent views of the right atrium and right atrial inflow from the inferior vena cava.

Right atrial size

Techniques to measure right atrial size are borrowed from those for the left atrium but assessment is less clinically relevant. Right atrial size measurements are most often used in assessment of right ventricular systolic pressure (p. 148). There is little research or clinical data so normal ranges are fairly simplistic without reference to sex or body size.

Qualitative measures
The simplest assessment is to compare the left and right atria in an apical 4-chamber view. If the right atrium appears larger than the left it is dilated.

Quantitative measures
- *Minor axis* is a simple linear measure. On an apical 4-chamber view measure across the middle of the atrium from lateral wall to septum. Ranges are in Table 3.19 (p. 227).
- Area can be reported. Trace around the right atrium joining the lateral and septal sides of the tricuspid annulus with a straight line.
- A volume can be calculated using the area–length equation (p. 170) with measures from an apical 4-chamber view. Right atrial length is required and can be measured from the back of the atrium to the middle of the annulus.

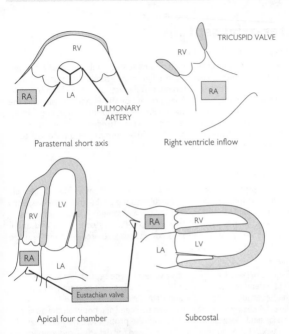

Fig. 3.71 Key views to assess right atrium.

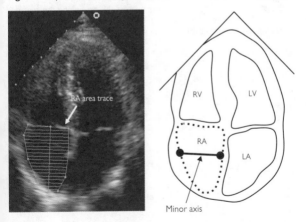

Fig. 3.72 Assessment of right atrial size from area measures in apical views.

Interatrial septum

Normal anatomy

The atrial septum divides the left and right atria. Embryologically it develops as two distinct sheets, the primum and secundum septum. In utero the septum, specifically the foramen ovale, acts as a portal for blood to pass from the inferior vena cava, directed by the Eustachian valve, to the left side of the heart, bypassing the lungs. After birth the foramen closes. In around 80% of people it seals but remains evident as a depression in the septum called the fossa ovalis. In 20% it remains as a potential communication between right and left heart.

Normal findings

Views

The atrial septum is best assessed in a subcostal view. This is the only view that has the septum perpendicular to the probe and therefore aligns the septum for Doppler or colour flow assessment. The atrium can also be assessed in the parasternal short axis (aortic valve level) and apical 4-chamber views. Agitated saline contrast can be used to investigate the possibility of a patent foramen ovale.

Findings

- Parasternal short axis (aortic valve level). The septum lies in the far field extending from the aortic ring (usually at the bottom left) with the left atrium on the right and right atrium on the left.
- Apical 4-chamber. The septum can be seen lying between the atria in the far field. Because it is in line with the probe there may be areas of ultrasound dropout that can be confused for defects. Colour flow mapping in this view can be tried.
- Subcostal view. The right atrium lies nearest the probe and the septum lies across the screen. This view can be used for colour flow mapping and Doppler alignment through the septum.

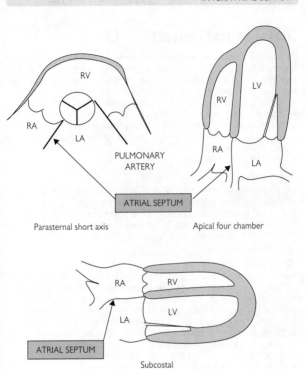

Parasternal short axis   Apical four chamber

Subcostal

Fig. 3.73 Key views to assess the atrial septum.

Atrial septal defects

Atrial septal defects are the commonest congenital heart defects. Although they can occur on their own they are frequently associated with other defects and a full echocardiographic assessment should be performed. They can also be iatrogenic (e.g. after cardiac surgery and transeptal puncture) or accidental (e.g. after pacing). There are four types of congenital defect.

- Secundum atrial septal defect (65%)—fossa ovalis/central septum.
- Primum atrial septal defect (15%)—more muscular septum by valves.
- Sinus venosus defect (10%)—near the superior vena cava/posterior and superior septum.
- Coronary sinus defects are much rarer.

Assessment

Initial assessment should be with 2D imaging, followed by colour flow mapping to study direction of flow and then Doppler to quantify the size of the shunt. Where suspicion of a defect remains high a contrast study can be performed with Valsalva to identify a left to right shunt (p. 234). Full assessment may require a transoesophageal study (see Chapters 4 and 5).

2D and colour flow mapping

Study the septum in all the standard views and look for gaps in the septum. To avoid overcalling septal dropout the defect should be apparent in different planes. There may be indirect evidence of a problem that prompts more careful study, in particular: right atrial and right ventricular enlargement without other cause; an abnormally directed colour flow jet in the right atrium on colour flow mapping; abnormal septal motion; or an aneurysmal septum. Comment on:

- the position of the defect and, therefore, likely classification;
- any associated defects (particularly relevant for primum defects);
- the size of the defect in two directions if possible (this can be done in subcostal views with long axis and sagittal planes through the defect);
- direction and timing of flow from colour flow mapping. Usually predominantly left to right during systole but with chronic right ventricular overload flow starts to occur right to left.

Doppler quantification of shunt

The principle of shunt quantification is comparison of right and left ventricle stroke volumes. Their ratio (called Qp/Qs) should be 1 but with shunting to the right the ratio increases and to the left the ratio declines. Accuracy depends on accurate measures of outflow tract diameter.

- Obtain left ventricular outflow tract pulsed wave Doppler vti from apical 5-chamber view and diameter from parasternal long axis.

$$Qs = \pi \times (LVOTdiameter/2)^2 \times aortic\ vti.$$

- Measure right ventricular outflow tract pulsed wave Doppler vti and diameter from a parasternal short axis (aortic valve level) view.

$$Qp = \pi \times (RVOT\ diameter/2)^2 \times pulmonary\ vti.$$

- Report the ratio Qp/Qs.

Primum atrial septal defects and associated defects

Primum defects occur when there is failed development of the primum septum. To make the diagnosis there must be no atrial septal tissue extending from the base of the atrio-ventricular valves.

The atrial septal defect on its own is a *partial atrio-ventricular canal* defect. If extending to involve the ventricular septum and atrio-ventricular valves it forms a *complete atrio-ventricular canal* or *endocardial cushion defect*. The valves often have abnormal atrio-ventricular valve rings and lie in the same plane in apical views (instead of the usual apical displacement of the tricuspid valve).

If there is a primum septal defect look for and comment on:
• inlet ventricular septal defect;
• cleft mitral valve leaflet—generally involving the anterior mitral valve leaflet at around '12 o'clock' in the parasternal short axis (mitral valve level) view. Invariably associated with regurgitation, often eccentric;
• mitral and tricuspid regurgitation;
• partial attachment of the anterior mitral valve leaflet to the ventricular septum—best seen from the parasternal long axis view after forward and backward displacement of the probe.

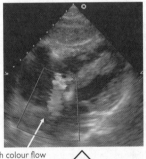

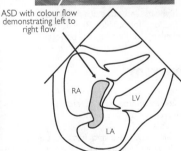

ASD with colour flow demonstrating left to right flow

RA

LV

LA

Fig. 3.74 Colour flow mapping of atrial septum in subcostal view.

Patent foramen ovale

If the foramen ovale fails to seal after birth (~20–30% of the population) it remains possible for pressure changes in the left and right atria to reopen the hole. This is of clinical interest because patent foramen ovale are relatively easy to close percutaneously and their presence raise the possibility that emboli, e.g. clots or fat, could pass from the right heart to the systemic circulation and cause strokes. Furthermore, foramen ovale are associated with decompression illness and, possibly, migraines.

To identify a patent foramen ovale right to left flow needs to be identified for a short period during the cardiac cycle (flow throughout the cardiac cycle identifies a septal defect). Sometimes this can be done with colour flow but usually contrast is needed.

Contrast study for atrial shunts and patent foramen ovale

There are three elements to a good contrast study for an atrial shunt.

- *A stable image*—use apical 4-chamber view (or subcostal view) optimized so that all four chambers are seen. Try the view with the patient doing a Valsalva to ensure you can keep all chambers in view.
- *Good quality contrast*—draw up a mixture of 8mL saline, 1mL of air, and (ideally) 1mL of blood (from the patient!) into a syringe. Attach with a second syringe to a 3-way tap (use syringes with Luer locks to avoid the syringes bursting off). Force the mixture back and forth until frothy. Inject rapidly through a venflon inserted into an antecubital vein. It must completely and rapidly opacify the right atrium.
- *A good Valsalva*—shunting may be evident at rest so the first contrast injection should be without Valsalva. If no bubbles appear in the left heart repeat the injection with a Valsalva manoeuvre. The critical time of a Valsalva is when the patient relaxes. It is then that right-sided pressures transiently elevate relative to the left and contrast shunts. Get the patient to take a breath and bear down hard. Inject the contrast and when it has filled the right atrium tell them to relax. If there is a shunt a few bubbles will appear in the left atrium and left ventricle within 5 beats of the patient relaxing. If bubbles appear later this is more consistent with a pulmonary arteriovenous malformation.

Set the system to capture 10 beats and start acquisition on contrast injection. Look back through the loop for bubbles. Repeat the study with more contrast until all three elements of the study are perfect.

Atrial septal aneurysm

Atrial septal aneurysms are an area of excessive mobility of the atrial septum and in 75% of cases are associated with patent foramen ovale. The technical definition is movement of the septum (at least 10mm in width) away from the normal plane of the septum (to left or right) by ≥10mm. Usually the septum will move back and forth as the relative pressure gradient between atria varies, but may be fixed. Comment on presence and look for underlying reasons.

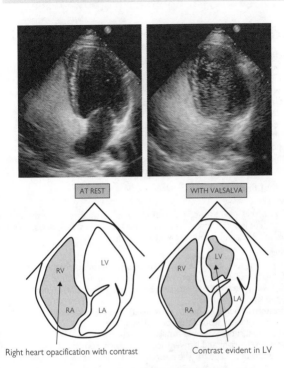

| AT REST | WITH VALSALVA |

Right heart opacification with contrast

Contrast evident in LV

Fig. 3.75 Contrast injection: left-sided bubbles with Valsalva (on right) demonstrating a patent foramen ovale. Also note septal aneurysm.

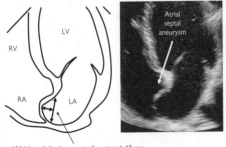

Width and displacement of septum > 10 mm

Fig. 3.76 Demonstration of septal aneurysm. At least 10mm wide with at least 10mm movement.

Ventricular septum

Normal anatomy

The ventricular septum divides the left and right ventricle. The ventricular septum can be divided simply into (1) a small membranous portion below the aortic valve and forming part of the left ventricular outflow tract and (2) a muscular septum, spreading inferiorly, anteriorly, and apically. These have separate embryological origins.

The muscular septum can be subdivided into three areas: the *inlet* septum between the mitral and tricuspid valves; the *trabecular* septum extending to the apex and forming the bulk of the septum on echocardiographic views; and the *outlet* septum close to the aortic and pulmonary valves. These subdivisions are used to classify ventricular septal defects.

Normal findings

Views

Any view that studies the ventricles can also be used to study the ventricular septum. Therefore, parasternal long and short axis views, apical 4-, 5-, and 3-chamber, and subcostal are all useful.

Findings

- Parasternal long axis. The membranous septum (or sometimes part of the muscular outlet septum) is seen in the left ventricular outflow tract, with the mid-segments of the trabecular (muscular) septum lying to the left.
- Parasternal short axis (aortic valve level). The membranous and outlet septum are seen around the aortic ring.
- Parasternal short axis (mid-papillary muscle level). The septum lies between the right and left ventricles and mainly consists of the muscular (trabecular) septum. The muscular inlet septum may be seen at the bottom of the septum.
- Apical 4- and 5-chamber: The trabeculated (muscular) septum can be viewed right up to the apex. In a 4-chamber view the muscular inlet septum is seen between mitral and tricuspid valves. In the 5-chamber view the membranous septum by the aortic valve comes into view.
- Subcostal view. The septum lies perpendicular to the probe and this view provides an opportunity for aligning colour flow mapping and Doppler through the septum.

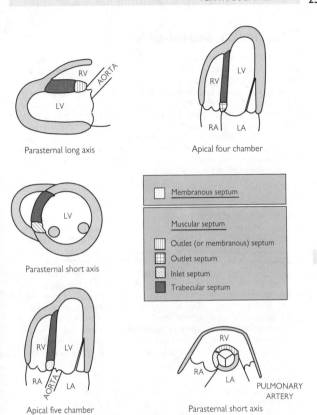

Parasternal long axis

Apical four chamber

Parasternal short axis

Membranous septum

Muscular septum
Outlet (or membranous) septum
Outlet septum
Inlet septum
Trabecular septum

Apical five chamber

Parasternal short axis

Fig. 3.77 Key views to assess the ventricular septum.

Ventricular septal defects

Ventricular septal defects are one of the common congenital heart defects. They can occur anywhere within the septum and are named according to their location—*membranous* or *muscular* (inlet, outlet, or trabeculated). If they involve both the membranous and muscular septum they are called *peri-membranous*. *Gerbode defects* are a specific type from left ventricle to right atrium. As well as being congenital they can occur due to ischaemia (post-infarction, often quite apical in trabecular septum with multiple holes) or be iatrogenic following cardiac surgery or pacing. Membranous (and peri-membranous) are easiest to identify, with muscular defects the most often missed because the defect is small or altered in shape by ventricular contraction.

Assessment Initial assessment should be with 2D imaging, followed by colour flow. Doppler can quantify the size of any shunt (p. 232).

2D and colour flow imaging

- Study the septum in all views and look for gaps. To avoid overcalling septal dropout the defect should be apparent in different planes.
- Colour flow imaging over the septum, particularly in the subcostal and parasternal views, is essential to scan for abnormal colour flow jets appearing in the right ventricle and originating from the septum.
- The septum is curved and cannot be seen entirely in one plane. Peri-membranous defects are easiest to see in parasternal long axis and short axis (aortic valve level) views with tilting to scan through the septum. These views also identify outlet defects, which can be differentiated from peri-membranous defects because they lie nearer the pulmonary valve. The inlet and trabecular defects are better seen in apical and subcostal views but may need probe tilting to scan the septum.

Comment on

- Position of the defect and, therefore, likely classification.
- Characteristics of the defect, e.g. multiple small defects.
- Size of the defect (in two directions if possible, e.g. subcostal views with long axis and sagittal planes through the defect). Measure size from 2D images or colour flow jet.
- Direction and timing of flow from colour flow mapping. With large chronic defects right ventricular pressure will increase and the left to right flow will reduce. Colour flow may be less evident.
- If possible, use pulsed or continuous Doppler aligned across the defect to measure the pressure gradient between ventricles using the Bernoulli equation (= $4 \times \text{velocity}^2$). Right ventricular pressure can be measured from the pressure gradient. If the aortic valve is normal then systolic blood pressure will equal left ventricular systolic pressure.

  RV systolic pressure = systolic blood pressure – gradient across the defect

- Left and right ventricular size and function, as well as evidence of right ventricular pressure or volume overload (p. 220).
- Associated problems, e.g. aortic valve dysfunction and regurgitation.

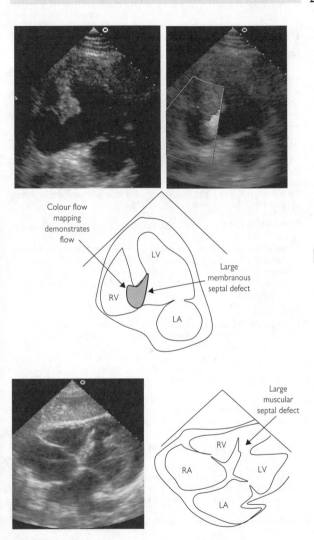

Fig. 3.78 Examples of ventricular septal defects. The top figure shows a large congenital peri-membranous defect in an apical view. The lower figure demonstrates a trabecular muscular defect secondary to ischaemia seen in a subcostal view.

Pericardium

Normal anatomy

The pericardium surrounds the heart. An outer, supportive, fibrous pericardium blends superiorly into the aorta and pulmonary arteries and inferiorly attaches by ligaments to the diaphragm, sternum, and vertebrae. On the inside of the fibrous layer and the outer surface of the heart are two serous membranes that allow the heart to move. There are two irregular holes through the membranes: one around the aorta and pulmonary arteries and the other around the pulmonary veins and vena cavae. The membranes join around the edges of the holes to create an enclosed, 'deflated' sac that can fill with fluid. Because they wrap round the blood vessels two pockets (or sinuses) are created: the transverse sinus between aorta and pulmonary artery and the oblique sinus between the pulmonary veins on the back of the left atrium. These are important because localized collections can form in the pockets.

Normal findings

Views

- Part of the pericardium can be seen in all views and should be studied in all scan planes—only part of the pericardium may be affected in disease or there may be a localized collection.
- The best views are parasternal long and short axis, apical 4-chamber, and subcostal.

Pericardium

- The *pericardial surfaces* are difficult to see because they adhere to surrounding structures but may appear as a thin, slightly brighter line around the heart.
- Measures of pericardial thickness do not correlate well with pathology specimens but the pericardium is normally 1–2mm thick. CT or magnetic resonance imaging should be used to measure thickness.

Pericardial space

- The *pericardial space* is seen as a black line around the heart. It is normal to have a few millimetres of fluid.

Distinguishing pericardial from pleural fluid

In the parasternal long axis view use the descending aorta as a landmark. The pericardial sac tucks in between the aorta and left atrium, so pericardial fluid will extend up to the gap and lie in front of the aorta. Pleural fluid will track behind the aorta and over the left atrium.

If both pericardial and pleural fluid are suspected look for the pericardium lying as a continuous dividing line within the fluid in an apical view.

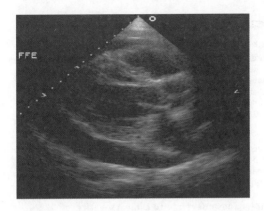

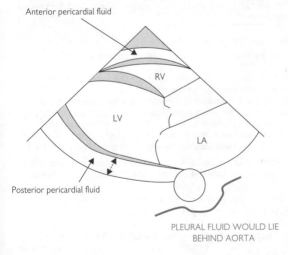

Fig. 3.79 Parasternal long axis view showing heart lying in global pericardial effusion. Measure depth on 2D (double-ended arrow) or M-mode and report measurement site.

Pericardial effusion

Amount of pericardial fluid

- Measure fluid thickness using 2D or M-mode in several places and views. Report the depth and where the measurement was made.
- For global effusions, grade as *mild*, *moderate*, or *large* based on depth (depth also approximates to volume of fluid).

<0.5cm	Minimal	50–100mL
0.5–1cm	Mild	100–250mL
1–2cm	Moderate	250–500mL
>2cm	Large	>500mL

- More accurate volume measures can be made with planimetry from traced pericardial and heart borders in apical views. It is possible to produce even more accurate measures with 3D echocardiography, although there is not usually any clinical indication.

> **Thickness does not relate to clinical severity**
> Rapid accumulation of a small quantity can have as severe a haemody-namic effect as slow accumulation of a large quantity. Look for features of tamponade.

Appearance of pericardial space

- Fluid is the black echolucent area and will be serous, blood, or pus. It is difficult to differentiate with echocardiography.
- Strands (fibrin) can occur in any condition that causes inflammation (infection, haemorrhage, or uraemia).
- Masses are more unusual and could be haematoma, tumour, cyst, or related to infection, e.g. fungus. Comment on size, shape, appearance, movement, attachments to surfaces, e.g. pericardium, ventricle. Haematoma is usually the same echocardiographic density as myocar-dium—so may be difficult to see—but suggests a haemopericardium.

Localization Look at effusion in all views and comment whether global (most common) or localized. Specify where the effusion is localized.

> **Problems with localized effusions**
> Suspect localized effusions after cardiac surgery (blood) or infections (loculation). Localized effusions may only be evident because of res-tricted pulmonary vein flow (oblique sinus) or unusual compression of a cardiac chamber. Consider transoesophageal echocardiography in patients with haemodynamic problems after cardiac surgery to look for localized effusions.
> - Apparent posterior localization may be because a small effusion has shifted posteriorly due to gravity in a supine patient.
> - A localized anterior space in parasternal views may actually be mediastinal (e.g. fat, fibrosis, thymus).

Evidence of cardiac tamponade See p. 244.

Best site for pericardiocentesis See p. 252.

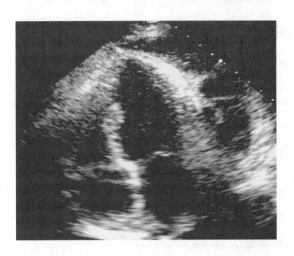

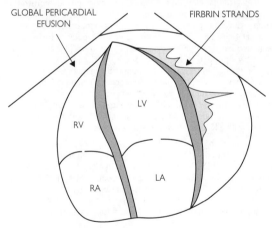

GLOBAL PERICARDIAL EFUSION

FIRBRIN STRANDS

LV

RV

LA

RA

Fig. 3.80 Apical 4-chamber view with global pericardial effusion and fibrin strands.

Cardiac tamponade

Cardiac tamponade is a clinical diagnosis based on tachycardia (>100bpm), hypotension (<100mmHg systolic), pulsus paradoxus (>10mmHg drop in blood pressure on inspiration), raised JVP with prominent × descent. Echocardiography provides supporting evidence.

2D findings suggestive of tamponade As intra-pericardial pressure rises and begins to exceed right heart pressure, parts of the cardiac chambers collapse during the cardiac cycle. Clinical signs usually appear before the left heart is affected.

- Right atrium appears to collapse faster than usual in atrial systole.
- Parts of right ventricle start to collapse during ventricular diastole. First the right ventricular outflow during early diastole (at lowest pressure); then, as intra-pericardial pressure increases, collapse extends to involve whole of right ventricle and whole of diastole.
- Combination of rapid atrial collapse in atrial systole followed by rapid ventricular collapse in ventricular diastole creates the appearance of a 'swinging right atrium and ventricle'.

Doppler findings suggestive of tamponade

Doppler findings in tamponade are the echocardiographic demonstration of the exaggerated variation in right and left ventricular inflow during respiration—clinically demonstrated as pulsus paradoxus.

- In an apical 4-chamber view place pulsed wave Doppler at tricuspid valve inflow. Switch on physiological respiration trace (if available) and slow sweep speed to 25cm/sec. (See Fig. 3.82, p. 249.)
- Acquire a tracing and measure maximum and minimum E-wave velocities (these correspond with respiration: maximum in inspiration).
- Do the same at the mitral valve (E-wave maximum in expiration).
- Normal variation is <15% at mitral valve and <25% at tricuspid valve. Greater than this supports tamponade but clinical signs are usually associated with ~40% variation at the mitral valve.

Exaggerated flow changes through the heart during respiration can also be demonstrated in the left and right ventricular outflow tracts (increased flow in inspiration on the right and in expiration on the left).

- Use pulsed wave Doppler in right ventricular outflow tract in parasternal short axis. Record vti and peak velocity in inspiration and expiration.
- Do the same at the left ventricular outflow tract in apical 5-chamber.
- Normally vti and peak velocity vary <10% during respiration.

Problems with assessment of tamponade

2D and Doppler measures are only accurate with 'normal' relations between intra-pericardial, intrathoracic, and intraventricular pressures. Increased ventricular 'stiffness' (ventricular hypertrophy, intraventricular haematoma) or increased right ventricular pressure (pulmonary hypertension) makes the ventricle less likely to collapse. Low volume states mean the change in ventricular inflow on Doppler is less pronounced. Doppler indices are not validated in ventilated patients.

Pulsus paradoxus

There is normally a swing of 5mmH$_2$0 in intrathoracic pressure with respiration. Inspiration leads to an increase in blood flow into the lungs and therefore an increase in flow into the right heart and reduced flow into the left heart. Expiration forces blood out of the lungs and increases flow into the left heart and reduces flow into the right heart. This accounts for the normal variation in blood pressure ('left-sided pressures') with respiration. Increased pericardial fluid increases intrapericardial pressure. Left and right ventricular filling is impaired and this filling is exacerbated on the left on inspiration leading to an exaggerated drop in blood pressure on inspiration.

Changes in 2D and Doppler with increasing tamponade

1 Tricuspid valve inflow pattern
2 Mitral valve inflow pattern
3 Abnormal right atrial collapse in atrial systole
4 Right ventricular outflow collapse in ventricular diastole
5 Left ventricular outflow collapse in ventricular diastole

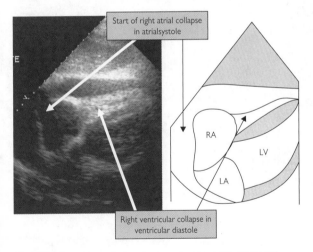

Fig. 3.81 Subcostal long axis view showing early atrial systolic collapse and ventricular diastolic collapse.

Constrictive pericarditis

Constrictive pericarditis is uncommon and often has vague signs and symptoms with a long history. It can be due to chronic inflammation as a result of infection (classically tuberculosis), cardiothoracic surgery, radiation, or connective tissue disease. It can be transient with pericardial inflammation. Diagnosis is clinical. Echocardiography can be supportive and differentiate from restrictive cardiomyopathy. Magnetic resonance imaging or CT are also usually required to assess the pericardium.

2D findings suggestive of constriction

- Look for the pericardium. May appear normal thickness (1–2mm) or thickened (up to 10mm) (measurements are inaccurate so use other modalities for actual measures). May appear bright or there may be shadowing from calcium (a marker of chronic inflammation).
- Assess the left ventricle. Usually normal systolic function: consider other causes if not. Assess septal motion in parasternal views with 2D and M-mode. Classically, septum appears to 'flutter' as left and right ventricle fill during diastole. Probably due to waves of competitive filling of the 2 ventricles. Seen as early diastolic notching on M-mode, or paradoxical and then normal motion on 2D.

Differentation from restrictive cardiomyopathy

Clinical features of constrictive pericarditis and restrictive cardiomyopathy are similar. Echocardiography is useful to differentiate.

	Restrictive cardiomyopathy	Constrictive pericarditis
Similarities between conditions		
E/A ratio	Increased	Increased
Deceleration time	Decreased	Decreased
Differences between conditions		
LV function	May be abnormal	Usually normal
Pericardium	Normal	May be bright or thick
Septal motion	Usually normal	May be abnormal
Atria ·	Biatrial enlargement	Usually normal size
Mitral annulus velocity	Decreased	Normal
Ventricular inflow on respiration	Normal variation	Increased variation

Doppler findings suggestive of constriction

- Assess mitral and tricuspid inflow during respiration just as for tamponade (p. 244). Constrictive pericarditis causes the same changes as tamponade (>25% variation at tricuspid and >15% at mitral). As the ventricles are supported by 'stiff' pericardium no ventricular collapse.
- Look for features of diastolic dysfunction (p. 198). Exaggerated E/A ratio on mitral inflow and shortened deceleration time (time from peak to end of E-wave; normal >160msec).
- Use tissue Doppler (if available). In apical 4-chamber place cursor on lateral mitral annulus. In constrictive pericarditis myocardial function is normal and peak mitral annulus velocity is therefore normal (>10mm/sec). If reduced, consider restrictive cardiomyopathy.

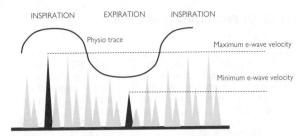

Fig. 3.82 Diagram representing PW Doppler trace at tricuspid valve. There is significant variation in tricuspid valve inflow (>25%) consistent with cardiac tamponade or constrictive pericarditis. The same recording can be done at mitral valve but maximum E-wave velocity will be in expiration and normal variation is <15%.

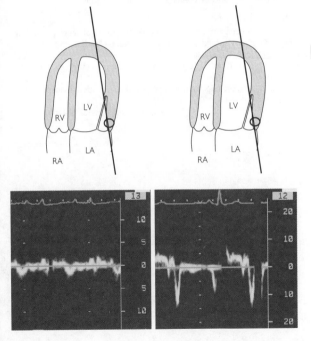

Fig. 3.83 Tissue Doppler imaging of lateral mitral annulus showing reduced movement in restrictive cardiomyopathy (left) compared to normal myocardial function (right). Normal motion is >10cm/sec.

Other pericardial diseases

Congenital pericardial disease

Congenital absence of pericardium is rare. Usually suspected in 2D because of an obvious gap or herniation of part of the heart (often left or right atrial appendage or parts of ventricle). The heart may be abnormally positioned with right atrial or ventricular dilatation and paradoxical septal motion. Record where the pericardium is missing and any functional effects of herniation.

Congenital pericardial cysts are more common. Usually benign. Comment on size, mobility, position, attachment, appearance (fluid, masses).

Pericardial tumours

Primary cardiac tumours or *metastatic tumours* can involve the pericardium. Comment on any masses, reporting the position, size, appearance, attachments, and functional effects on cardiac function.

Acute pericarditis

There are no echocardiographic features diagnostic of acute pericarditis. Echocardiography should be used in suspected pericarditis to look for:
• complications (e.g. effusions);
• left ventricular function (e.g. abnormal function may suggest myocarditis);
• underlying causes (e.g. tumour or regional wall motion abnormalities suggestive of myocardial infarction);
• other causes for clinical signs (e.g. endocarditis, pericardial effusion).

Pericardiocentesis

Echocardiography is very useful during pericardiocentesis. Pericardiocentesis is usually done from subcostal or apical positions so assess pericardial fluid in both views.

Before the procedure record:
- depth of fluid in each position;
- depth from skin to the outer boundary of fluid (a guide as to how far to introduce the needle).
- Angle of the echo probe to achieve images can be a guide to the angle to be used for the needle.

During the procedure record the following.
- The needle can sometimes be seen advancing into pericardial space.
- If unclear whether needle is in pericardial space, inject agitated saline contrast down needle. Contrast should be seen clearly filling the pericardial space if needle is correctly positioned… or filling another cardiac chamber if not!

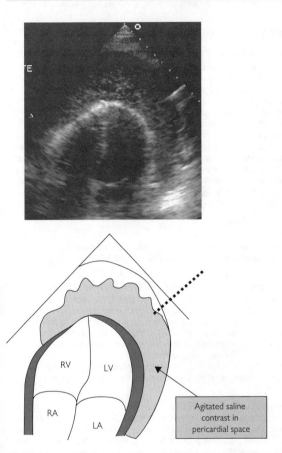

Fig. 3.84 Pericardiocentesis from subcostal position monitored by echocardiography from apex. Agitated saline contrast has been injected down the pericardiocentesis needle and is seen circulating in the pericardial space. This confirms the correct location of the needle.

Aorta

Normal anatomy

The aorta is the main conductance artery of the body, carrying blood from the heart to all major branch vessels. It has a functional role, distending during systole and recoiling in diastole, to propel blood. The aortic wall has three layers: tunica intima, a thin inner layer, lined by endothelium; tunica media, a thicker middle layer of elastic tissue for tensile strength and elasticity; tunica adventitia, a thin outer layer, predominantly collagen, housing the vasa vasorum and lymphatics.

There are four major sections: (1) ascending aorta from aortic valve annulus including sinuses of Valsalva, sinotubular junction (the narrowest point), and up to right brachio-cephalic artery; (2) aortic arch from brachio-cephalic to aortic isthmus (just distal to left subclavian artery); (3) descending aorta from isthmus to diaphragm; (4) abdominal aorta from diaphragm to aortic bifurcation and origin of iliac arteries.

Normal findings

Views

Parts of the aorta can be seen in all windows. Full evaluation requires a combination of views and additional, non-standard transducer positions.

Proximal ascending aorta

- Proximal ascending aorta is best seen in the parasternal long axis view. Additional views include, particularly if dilated, the right parasternal views or left parasternal views from higher intercostal spaces for ascending aorta (particularly with patient in extreme left lateral position to bring aorta more anterior). Doppler interrogation is limited to qualitative assessment of flow and aortic regurgitation severity.
- Apical views. The ascending aorta can also be visualized in apical 5- and 3-chamber views. 2D image quality is limited at this depth but orientation is optimal for Doppler to assess aortic regurgitation.

Aortic arch

Suprasternal views (and supraclavicular views) allow assessment of aortic arch and brachiocephalic vessels. Both transverse and longitudinal views are possible but the latter is most useful to identify head and neck vessels. Descending aorta is only partially in plane and, artefactually, appears to taper. Descending aorta blood flow can be used to assess aortic regurgitation severity and aortic coarctation.

Descending thoracic aorta

Descending thoracic aorta is seen in cross-section posterior to the left atrium in the parasternal views. The proximal segment of descending aorta is seen in the suprasternal view. Additional views of the longitudinal section of the descending thoracic aorta can normally be visualized from an apical 2-chamber view with lateral angulation and clockwise rotation of probe. The distal thoracic aorta and proximal abdominal aorta can be visualized from the subcostal view.

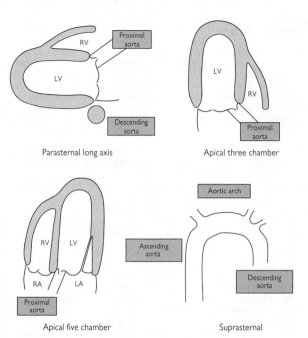

Fig. 3.85 Key views to assess the aorta.

The pathological significance of the isthmus

The isthmus is the point where the relatively mobile ascending aorta and arch become fixed to the thorax and thus the aorta is vulnerable to trauma at this point. Coarctations also commonly develop here.

Aortic size

The terms *proximal aorta* or *aortic root* refer to the aortic annulus, sinuses of Valsalva, sinotubular junction, and proximal ascending aorta. Measurement of the aortic root is of crucial importance in the diagnosis of Marfan syndrome, and in the serial monitoring of patients with, or at risk of, progressive dilation of the ascending aorta. While a single measurement of the proximal aorta may suffice in the normal examination, a minimum of four measurements should be routinely made and recorded from the parasternal long axis view when monitoring aortic disease.

Assessment

- Make measurements from a parasternal long axis view in systole (with valve leaflet tips open to their maximum).
- They can be made from 2D images frozen in systole or from M-mode aligned at different positions through the proximal aorta.
- A complete assessment includes measurement of:
  - annulus (normal 2.3 ± 0.3cm);
  - sinus of Valsalva, at aortic leaflet tip level (normal 3.4 ± 0.3cm; <2.1cm/m^2);
  - sinotubular junction;
  - proximal ascending aorta (normal 2.6 ± 0.3cm).
- 2D measurement at the sinuses gives higher values than M-mode measurements. Comment on how the measurements were made and use the appropriate normal values. In a normal study a single aortic diameter may be sufficient. When possible report size relative to body surface area.
- Where needed, continue the assessment by providing measurements of the arch from suprasternal views, descending aorta from parasternal views, and, for completeness, abdominal aorta from subcostal views.
  - Aortic arch.
  - Descending thoracic aorta (normal <1.6cm/m^2).
  - Abdominal aorta (normal <3cm; <1.6cm/m^2).

Serial measurements and identification of dilatation

- In serial measurements the annulus is not prone to dilatation. Any significant change should raise suspicion of methodological error and caution over interpreting measurements elsewhere. In effect, the annulus acts as a control for serial studies.
- Measurements at the sinus of Valsalva are the key. They tend to be the site of initial ectasia when the aortic root does dilate in Marfan syndrome. In the normal adult it measures less than 3.7cm but can vary with body surface area. Normograms that adjust for body surface area maximize sensitivity for the detection of aortic dilatation in adults, but for practical purposes the upper normal limit in the adult is 2.1cm/m^2 and anything below this can be reported as normal.

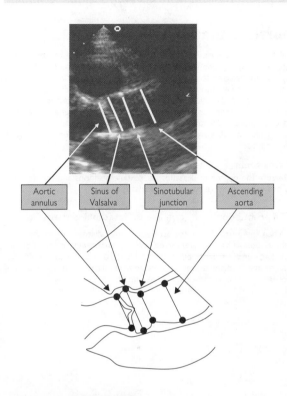

| Aortic annulus | Sinus of Valsalva | Sinotubular junction | Ascending aorta |

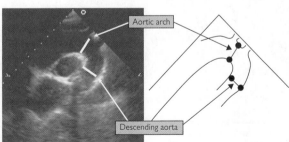

Aortic arch

Descending aorta

Fig. 3.86 Measurement of aortic size at key locations from parasternal long axis (top) and suprasternal (bottom) views.

Aortic dilatation

Dilatation of the aorta is an increase in diameter more than expected for age and body size and is the most commonly identified aortic abnormality. When localized to the sinus of Valsalva the risk of complications is significantly lower than when there is generalized aortic dilatation but still higher than no dilatation! Causes include: degenerative disease (hypertension, atherosclerosis, cystic medial necrosis, post-stenotic); collagen vascular disease (Marfan syndrome, Ehlers–Danlos); inflammatory disorders (rheumatoid, systemic lupus erythematosus, ankylosing spondylitis, Reiter syndrome, syphilis, aortic arteritis); trauma (blunt or penetrating).

Assessment

Measure the degree of dilatation at multiple positions and report where and how the measurements were made.

Differentiation of degenerative dilatation from Marfan

When the aorta dilates due to degenerative disease, the contours of the sinuses of Valsalva and the normal slight narrowing at the sinotubular junction are maintained. In contrast, dilatation of the aorta in Marfan syndrome is characterized by enlargement of the sinuses of Valsalva, resulting in loss of narrowing at the sinotubular junction.

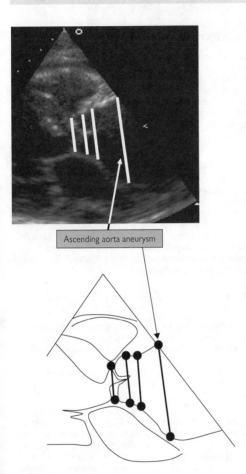

Ascending aorta aneurysm

Fig. 3.87 Example of dilatation of the proximal ascending aorta seen in a parasternal long axis view.

Marfan syndrome

Marfan syndrome is an autosomal dominant connective tissue disorder due to mutation in the fibrillin 1 gene. It is a multisystem disorder that affects both locomotor and cardiovascular systems, and the eyes. The incidence is approximately 1 in 10,000 births of whom approximately 26% are a spontaneous mutation, i.e. have no family history. Many individuals have some of the skeletal features of Marfan syndrome without the actual condition and the diagnosis is dependent on diagnostic criteria (Ghent criteria).

Assessment

Echocardiography is key for the criteria and should report on the presence of the following.

- Major criteria: (1) dilatation of the ascending aorta—with or without aortic regurgitation—involving at least the sinuses of Valsalva; (2) dissection of the ascending aorta.
- Minor criteria: (1) mitral valve prolapse, with or without mitral regurgitation; (2) main pulmonary artery dilatation in the absence of stenosis under 40 years of age; (3) calcification of the mitral annulus under 40 years of age; (5) dilatation or dissection of the descending thoracic or abdominal aorta under 50 years of age.

Indications for considering elective aortic root replacement

Prophylactic surgery is indicated for progressive aortic root dilatation:

- aortic diameter >55mm in adults with connective tissue disease;
- aortic diameter >50mm in children and adults with a family history of dissection;
- rapid change in the aortic root size—more than 2mm per year;
- aortic diameter >60mm in adults without connective tissue (atherosclerotic aneurysm).

There is an increased risk in pregnancy. If the aortic diameter is >40mm, monitoring with echocardiography and clinical examination should be considered monthly. Progressive root dilatation should lead to consideration of surgery prior to, or contemporaneous with, delivery of the child. Special precautions would also be required at the time of delivery which should take place under the care of a specialist team managing complex pregnancy with cardiac disease.

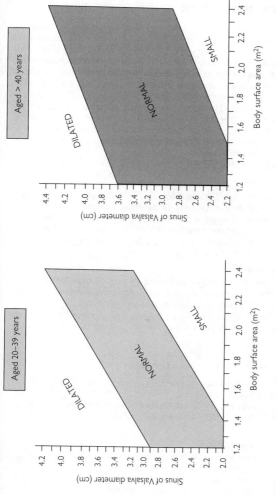

Table 3.20 Ranges of normal sinus of Valsalva size according to age

Aortic dissection

Aortic dissection originates from an intimal tear, leading to sub-intimal haemorrhage, which can extend within a false lumen back to the aortic valve or forwards, throughout the aorta. Aortic dissection is life-threatening, with an early mortality of 1% per hour. Presentation is usually with severe chest pain. The differential includes other causes of chest pain such as acute myocardial infarction or chest wall pain, and aortic intramural haemorrhage or expanding thoracic aneurysm. Risk factors for dissection include: Marfan syndrome, aortic dilatation/aneurysm, hypertension, aortic valve disease—particularly bicuspid valve (risk 5× normal).

The Stanford classification is the simplest and most pragmatic.
- Type A: involvement of the ascending aorta irrespective of involvement elsewhere.
- Type B: limited to the arch and/or descending thoracic aorta.

Assessment

Prompt diagnosis is crucial and transthoracic echocardiography is of value in initial management. Examine for diagnostic features and for secondary complications. A negative transthoracic study does not exclude aortic dissection and, where there is a high index of suspicion, further imaging with transoesophageal echocardiography, CT, or magnetic resonance imaging will be required.

Diagnostic features
- Look for the presence or absence of any possible *dissection flap* in *all* aortic views (parasternal, suprasternal, subcostal). A flap will appear as a linear mobile structure with motion independent of the aortic wall.
- Look for a *false lumen* using colour flow Doppler placed over the aorta in all aortic views. There will be different patterns of flow in the true and false lumen.

Beam-width artefact and reverberation
- Beam-width artefact and reverberation can mimic a dissection flap.
- M-mode of aortic wall motion and a suspected flap will demonstrate flap motion that is different from aortic wall movement. Whereas a reverberation artfact will move with the wall.

Secondary complications
- Measure aortic root size from parasternal views, size of arch and descending aorta from suprasternal views, and size of descending thoracic and abdominal aorta from subcostal views.
- Comment on and quantify aortic regurgitation.
- Comment on pericardial fluid and perform Doppler analysis of trans-mitral and trans-tricuspid blood flow to diagnose tamponade. A small acute collection can cause tamponade without obvious pericardial fluid.
- Assess left ventricular systolic function, and comment on any regional wall motion abnormalities that might suggest coronary artery involvement.

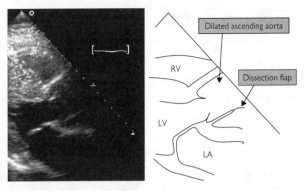

Parasternal long axis view

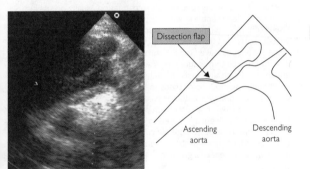

Suprasternal view

Fig. 3.88 Examples of aortic dissection flap seen in parasternal long axis and suprasternal views.

Aortic coarctation

Aortic coarctation is a congenital narrowing in the proximal descending thoracic aorta, usually located immediately proximal to the entry site of the *ductus arteriosus*. It may be suspected in a patient with hypertension and a weak femoral pulse, radiofemoral delay, or systolic murmur. Aortic coarctation first diagnosed in adulthood is usually asymptomatic as the stenosis is not usually severe and collaterals are present. 50–80% will have a bicuspid aortic valve and other cardiac abnormalities (e.g. sub-aortic membrane, supravalvular aortic stenosis).

Assessment

Echocardiography is required in diagnosis and follow-up. Aortic coarctation can be relatively complex and further imaging (usually magnetic resonance imaging) is performed if intervention is being considered.

Diagnosis

The suprasternal view is the most useful.

- Identify the brachiocephalic vessels—coarctation usually occurs just distal to the left subclavian with post-stenotic dilatation common.
- Use colour flow mapping of the descending aorta to identify a high velocity narrowed flow stream with turbulence (even if 2D poor).
- Place continuous wave Doppler through the point of maximum colour flow turbulence to measure a typical systolic velocity gradient. The gradient will typically persist to end-diastole ('diastolic tail').
- Continuous wave Doppler tends to overestimate the gradient and better correlation with catheter gradients can be obtained if the proximal velocity is measured with pulsed wave Doppler and the modified Bernoulli equation used to calculate flow.
- If coarctation is suspected but difficult to image, continuous wave Doppler using a pencil probe in the suprasternal postion will often allow measurement of a gradient in the descending aorta.

Follow-up

All patients with previous repair of coarctation of the aorta should be followed up throughout adult life. Echocardiography should be repeated annually. Where visualization is inadequate alternative imaging such as CT or magnetic resonance imaging may be needed.

- Examine and report the residual gradient.
- Look for abnormalities in the aorta and comment on development of any aneurysm at the site of previous repair.

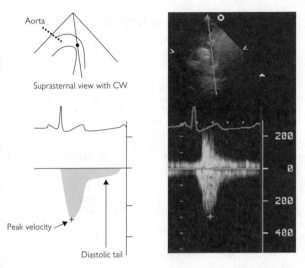

Fig. 3.89 Doppler profile in coarctation of the aorta from a suprasternal view. Note the increased peak velocity and prolonged flow throughout diastole ('diastolic tail').

Sinus of Valsalva aneurysm

Sinus of Valsalva aneurysms can be congenital resulting from incomplete fusion of the distal bulbar septum that divides the aorta and pulmonary arteries. They tend to have a long sac of mobile tissue projecting into adjacent structures, forming a 'wind sock' appearance. Acquired aneurysms, usually due to endocarditis, lead to more symmetrical dilatation, with no excess tissue. If rupture occurs, a fistula develops between aorta and adjacent chamber, with left to right shunting and clinical features that can vary in severity from acute haemodynamic compromise to a new continuous murmur. 85% affect right coronary sinus and project/rupture into the right ventricle; 10% affect non-coronary sinus and project/rupture into the right atrium; 5% affect left coronary sinus and project/rupture into the left atrium.

Assessment

- Use parasternal long and short axis views to diagnose and measure.
- If rupture suspected, use parasternal short axis view at and above the aortic valve. Colour flow mapping will usually confirm site of communication and continuous flow. If possible the coronary artery should be visualized to exclude coronary artery fistulae.
- Continuous wave Doppler will show a high velocity systolic and diastolic signal.
- Comment on the size of the right atrium (which reflects acute right atrial overload) and left atrial and left ventricular size (which will reflect the extent of chronic volume overload).

Aortic atherosclerosis

Atherosclerosis of the aorta can result in dilatation, aneurysm, or dissection and is a risk factor for coexisting coronary artery disease and cerebrovascular disease.

Assessment

Aortic atheroma can be visualized with transthoracic echocardiography (although transoesophageal is more appropriate) in either the proximal ascending aorta or, more commonly, in the descending abdominal aorta.

Atherosclerotic thoracic aortic aneurysm may also be detected by transthoracic imaging, either at the aortic root or behind the left atrium in the descending thoracic aorta (parasternal long axis view). More rarely, descending abdominal aortic aneurysm may be picked up in subcostal views. The extent of the aneurysm cannot usually be accurately quantified, but the extent of dilatation and presence or absence of laminar thrombus can be commented upon. Further imaging will frequently be required.

Modified subcostal view

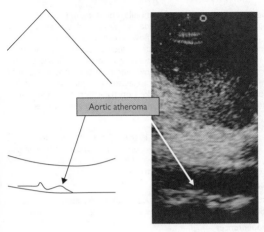

Aortic atheroma

Fig. 3.90 A subcostal view aligned to view the abdominal aorta. Note the thickening of the wall and irregular appearance consistent with an atherosclerotic plaque.

Mechanical prosthetic valves

All mechanical valves consist of a mobile component (occluder), the restraining system (to restrict occluder motion), and the sewing ring (attaches prosthesis to vessel). Blood flow is restricted through these and normal pressure gradients are therefore higher across mechanical, compared to native, valves. Valve components are metallic or plastic coated, with a carbon layer. These cause shadows and reverberations so scanning from different positions is required to assess the valve. In particular, mitral prosthesis regurgitation is masked on transthoracic images and if valve dysfunction is suspected transoesophageal imaging may be required.

Ball and cage (Starr Edwards)

The ball and cage valve consists of a sewing ring attached to a cage made of 3 or 4 struts. The blood flows on all sides around a Silastic ball occluder, which moves within the cage. Blood flow is directed laterally within the valve and converges downstream.

Assessment

Use all standard imaging planes adjusted where necessary with slight rotation or tilting to minimize shadows.

Normal appearances

Whether valve is open or closed there will be significant shadows from the sewing ring and reverberation from the ball. Structures and flows behind the valve are masked. Physiological regurgitation is trivial central jet.

Tilting disc (e.g. Medtronic-Hall, Omniscience)

A single circular disc suspended within a frame, with an off-centre hinge point. Opening therefore creates two orifices, one large (major) and one small (minor).

Assessment

Use standard imaging planes with slight rotation or tilting as necessary. Images are usually best when through the central hinge point or perpendicular to the closed disc. For mitral prostheses use apical windows for assessment. For aortic prostheses use apical windows for Doppler and parasternal to differentiate valvular from perivalvular regurgitation.

Normal appearances

There are shadows from the sewing ring and reverbations from the disc throughout the cardiac cycle.

- *Valve closed*. Structures and flow behind the valve are masked. Physiological regurgitation is two small jets between disc and ring. Some may have a jet associated with the central strut and some a very long central jet.
- *Valve open*. Disc opens to 55–75°. The major orifice may leave a sector to display deeper structures. The strut can be seen in a central position underneath the sewing ring. Two colour jets can be displayed. Continuous wave Doppler velocities are similar through minor and major orifice.

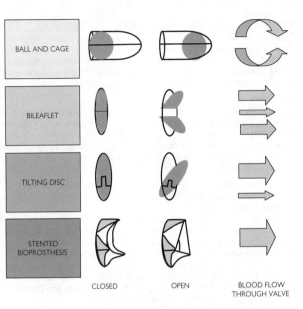

	CLOSED	OPEN	BLOOD FLOW THROUGH VALVE
BALL AND CAGE			
BILEAFLET			
TILTING DISC			
STENTED BIOPROSTHESIS			

Fig. 3.91 Diagram of mechanical prosthesis design and blood flow.

When to use transoesophageal echocardiography?

Transthoracic echocardiography usually provides good alignment with the transprosthestic flow. Therefore detection of prosthesis stenosis is not a problem. However, transthoracic assessment of regurgitation is limited by shadowing and distance to the transducer. Aortic valve prosthesis haemodynamic assessment is usually better by the transthoracic approach. Indications for transoesophageal imaging are these.

- Transthoracic imaging is inconclusive or non-diagnostic.
- Transthoracic findings not in agreement with clinical findings.
- Suspected problems of mitral mechanical valve prosthesis.
- Suspected prosthetic valve endocarditis.
- Suspected prosthetic valve thrombosis.
- Intraoperative use (to guide repair, assess success, complications).

Bileaflet (e.g. Carbomedics, St. Jude)

These consist of two leaflets, separately hinged in the centre of the prosthesis. Three orifices are created in the open position: two large lateral orifices and one small central orifice. In aortic valve replacement supra-annular placement is possible and may be used in double valve replacement in order to get a greater separation of the valves.

Assessment

As for single tilting disc, use standard imaging planes, mainly apical for mitral prostheses and both apical and parasternal for aortic valves. Before making diagnosis of impaired motion of one or both discs, ensure transducer has been rotated thoroughly to obtain a position in which the cursor (ultrasound beam) is aligned perpendicularly to the central line of the disc coaptation.

Normal appearances

There will be shadows from the sewing ring and reverberation from discs throughout the cardiac cycle.

- *Valve close.* Discs close at about 25° and mask structures and flow behind the valve. Physiological regurgitation is up to four jets originating at pivot points near the edge of the valve.
- *Valve open.* Discs open to 55–75° and two separate discs are often seen. There is more flow acceleration through the narrow central orifice. Therefore continuous wave measures through the centre may overestimate the overall pressure gradient, especially for small aortic prosthetic valves. Use mean rather than peak gradient.

Physiological regurgitation

Physiological regurgitation is normal with tilting disc and bileaflet prostheses. There are two components: (1) an initial backward flow during valve closure; (2) holosystolic flow designed to 'wash' the valves and reduce risk of valve thrombosis. These are referred to as 'wash' or 'closing' jets.

Differentiation of closing jets from pathological regurgitation?

Physiological jets

- Flow is contained within the sewing ring.
- Colour flow pattern is usually thin and laminar.
- Jet length usually less, <2–3cm.

Pathological jets

- Any perivalvular jets (outside the sewing ring).
- Different from the expected signature of the physiological pattern for the valve.

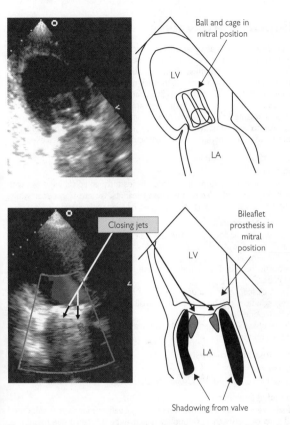

Fig. 3.92 Examples of apical views of mitral mechanical prostheses. The top figure demonstrates a ball and cage valve and the lower figure a bileaflet prosthesis with two closing jets. Note shadows behind the sewing ring.

Bioprosthetic valves

Bioprosthetic valves are made from porcine aortic valve or bovine peri-cardium. The leaflets are stiffer than native valve leaflets. Bioprostheses may be stented or stentless. Stents or struts support the cusps and pro-trude downstream (into the aorta with aortic bioprostheses or left ven-tricle with mitral bioprostheses). Struts and the ring are metallic so cause shadowing (although less than mechanical prostheses). Some models can be implanted in a supravalvular position. Although their flow profile is similar to that of native valves, there is still an increased pressure gra-dient across the prosthetic valves, particularly stented bioprostheses.

Stented bioprosthesis
Assessment
Use standard scan planes. Image prostheses through apical windows with the beam perpendicular to the closed leaflets. Rotate transducer whilst using colour flow mapping to assess perivalvular regurgitation

Normal appearance
There will be shadows from the sewing ring and stents protruding down-stream throughout the cardiac cycle. In the apical view usually two struts are displayed and, in the short axis, the ring and three struts are visible. If the aortic root is dilated there may be free space between sewing ring and root.
- *Valve closed.* Leaflets appear thin like a native valve. Physiological regurgitation may be present as a small central jet (usually early post-operatively)
- *Valve open.* Valve opens widely with leaflets parallel to the stent (2–4mm distance).

Stentless bioprosthesis
Assessment
Use standard scan planes. Usually no shadowing.

Normal appearance
Usually very similar to native aortic valve. Leaflets may appear thickened and junction between valve and annulus may be thickened due to sutures. Pulmonary valve homografts may have supravalvular thickening and ste-nosis. Ideally, no regurgitant jet but sometimes minor distortion during implantation or due to mismatch of prosthesis causes mild central regur-gitation. Jet may be eccentric if due to distortion.

Homografts and autografts
May be used in endocarditis or as an autograft in young patients in aortic valve disease (Ross procedure: native pulmonary valve is used for aortic valve replacement and a bioprosthesis is implanted as pulmonary valve). Scan planes and appearances are as for stentless bioprosthesis.

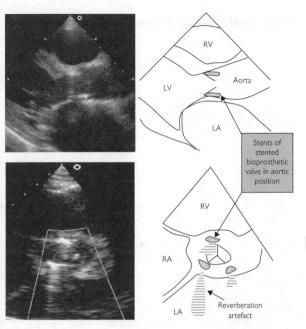

Fig. 3.93 Examples of stented bioprosthetic valves. The top figure shows a parasternal long axis view of an aortic prosthesis and the lower figure a parasternal short axis view. Note the bright struts with artefacts extending away.

Prosthetic valve abnormalities

Vegetation, thrombus, pannus Extended masses on prostheses. Pannus is excessive endothelial proliferation causing obstruction and/ or failure in complete valve closure. Pannus is sometimes difficult to distinguish from thrombus. Both may be present. No specific texture differentiates masses so to differentiate use:

- appearance—thrombi usually larger, protrude from the sewing ring, and less echocardiographically dense;
- clinical information—suboptimal anticoagulation makes thrombus more likely; bacteraemia makes vegetation more likely;
- associated abnormalities—vegetations may be associated with paravalvular abscesses, leaks.

Bioprosthetic valve degeneration Observed in most prostheses after several years. Infrequent in first 3 years. Leaflet calcification results in irregular thickening (usually >3mm in thickness). Rigid leaflets have decreased cusp motion, cause stenoses, and may rupture resulting in prolapse (or flail cusp) and valvular regurgitation.

Prosthetic valve dehiscence—'rocking' valve Exaggerated mobility of valve ring indicates dehiscence. Assess with 2D. Usually associated with severe paravalvular regurgitation. Valve dehiscence is usually preceded by paravalvular leaks.

Valve prolapse In bioprostheses, prolapse of leaflet tissue is possible and is seen in standard views. Usually leaflets are degenerated (irregular thickening and calcification) and valvular regurgitation will be present.

Structural damage For example, broken occluder or restraining system; will be combined with intravalvular regurgitation.

Sutures Seen as immobile, dense structures within the ring. Can be difficult to differentiate from focal fibrosis. They will be mobile if dehisced.

Strands Mobile, filamentous strands on normal and abnormal valves (rarely seen adjacent to native valve). Thought to be fibrin strands (they can disappear after thrombolysis of thrombosed prostheses). Poor reproducibility in imaging these structures as visualization is highly dependent on machine settings.

Pseudo-microbubbles Look like single contrast microbubbles. Probably due to microcavitation. Found with normal valves but more often if valve dysfunction. Appear as dots, moving away from prosthesis; visible only shortly after valve closure (unless valvular or paravalvular leak).

In contrast, spontaneous echo contrast is seen only in areas of low blood velocity (therefore not at orifices or leakages of prosthetic valves) and is smoke-like in appearance with swirling patterns.

Diastole   Systole

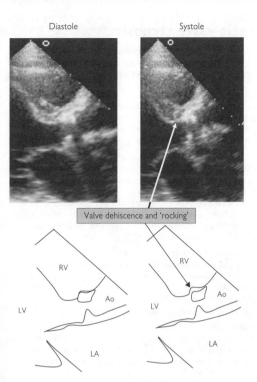

Valve dehiscence and 'rocking'

Fig. 3.94 Example of aortic prosthesis rocking.

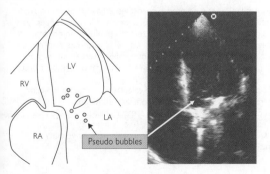

Pseudo bubbles

Fig. 3.95 Microbubbles associated with closure of a mitral prosthesis.

Prosthestic valve stenosis

Prosthetic valve stenosis suggests an acceleration of blood through the prosthetic valve because of some pathology. Pressure gradients may go up with thrombus/pannus and, rarely, vegetations or degeneration.

Assessment

If stenosis is suspected initial assessment should be to look for pathology that might explain stenosis (thrombus, vegetation, valve dysfunction) and check the level of any obstruction (outflow tract, valve level). Then gather supportive information about severity of any stenosis.

Grading severity

Pressure gradient and velocity

Techniques are as for native valves (continuous wave Doppler) but mechanical prostheses can have 2 or 3 different-sized orifices so application of Bernoulli equation is not straightforward and calculations can vary depending on Doppler alignment. With cage-and-ball prostheses it is almost impossible to get optimal Doppler alignment. In clinical practice calculation of effective orifice area is useful.

Orifice area—aortic valve prostheses

Use same technique as for native valve (continuous wave, pulsed wave, and left ventricular outflow tract diameter). Reporting orifice area also avoids problems with variation in cardiac output. For St Jude bileaflet aortic prosthesis a Doppler velocity index has been validated:

• vti across LVOT/vti across aortic valve <0.23 suggests severe stenosis

Orifice area—mitral valve prostheses

Use techniques as for native valves. The pressure half-time tends to underestimate effective orifice area but can be used. Width of the forward flow may be an alternative, if measured in two orthogonal planes.

What is abnormal for prosthetic valves?

Normal mechanical and stented bioprostheses have a pressure gradient equivalent to mild or moderate stenosis. Normal ranges vary between manufacturers and valves so refer to published information to give clinical advice. Pressure gradients also vary with haemodynamics, such as cardiac output, so there is considerable interpatient variability. General principles about what might need investigation are best based on calculated orifice area.

• Aortic prostheses may be stenotic if calculated valve area is <1cm^2 or there has been a >30% change from last follow-up.
• Mitral prostheses may be stenotic if pressure half-time >200msec and peak diastolic velocity >2.5m/sec (if only mild regurgitation).
• Tricuspid prostheses may be stenotic if peak diastolic velocity >2.5msec (if only mild regurgitation).

Prosthetic valve regurgitation

- *Transvalvular regurgitation* describes regurgitation within the sewing ring. This can be caused by leaflet prolapse (bioprostheses), incomplete disc closure due to clot, pannus (mechanical prostheses), or structural damage (broken retainment system, dislodged disc).
- *Paravalvular regurgitation* has its origin outside the sewing ring. This can occur immediately after surgery (usually trivial and resolves after protamine or with endothelialization during first few post-operative weeks). It can be due to dehiscence of the sewing ring, or secondary to endocarditis.

Assessment Decide if regurgitation is *transvalvular* or *paravalvular*. When jet is easily displayed it is often *paravalvular*, as physiological and *transvalvular* regurgitation is shadowed by valve. If difficult to be sure, comment.

Use multiple views and look at jet position with colour flow (use systematic approach similar to identification of mitral leaflet scallop prolapse). Short axis views of rings are very useful to position jets. 3D echocardiography may give further information. If *paravalvular*, report extent and localization with figure or reference to 'clock face' in parasternal short axis view (for mitral valve, area adjacent to aortic valve is 12 o'clock).

Transoesophageal echocardiography provides a comprehensive assessment of severity and cause. It should always be performed if transthoracic screening suggests there may be clinically significant regurgitation.

Grading severity

Pathological regurgitant jets are usually eccentric and often multiple. Shadowing from sewing ring, struts, or disc limits field of view. Therefore, colour flow area, PISA, and vena contracta are not reliable. Assessment of severity is often qualitative, in which case indirect supportive measures should also be provided and transoesophageal echocardiography advised.

Supportive measures
- Increase in cavity diameters compared to previous studies.
- If no prosthetic stenosis, an increase in forward flow velocity (due to volume overload). For mitral protheses moderate to severe regurgitation is suggested by a peak velocity >1.9m/sec and mean gradient >5mmHg. If no aortic stenosis and only mild regurgitation then a ratio of vti mitral prothesis/vti aortic valve >2.5 suggests moderate to severe regurgitation.
- Pulmonary venous flow for mitral regurgitation (systolic flow reversal). If left ventricular function is impaired a blunted pulmonary vein flow pattern is 'normal' after mitral valve replacement.
- Aortic flow pattern for aortic regurgitation (diastolic flow reversal).

Other techniques With *transvalvular* regurgitation (both mitral and aortic) one option is to measure the proportional area of the sewing ring occupied by the jet in a short axis view: <10% is mild; 10–25% is moderate; and >25% is severe.

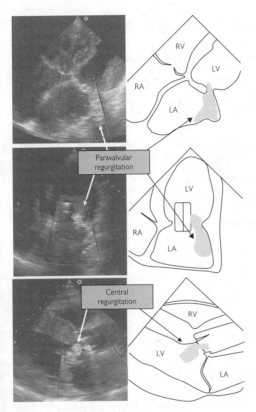

Fig. 3.96 Examples of paravalvular and transvalvular regurgitation.

Endocarditis

Diagnosis of endocarditis is based on clinical factors (positive blood cultures with appropriate organisms, predisposing factors, new valve dysfunction, peripheral stigmata) supported by echocardiographic abnormalities (Duke's criteria are widely used). A normal echocardiogram never excludes endocarditis and, if clinical suspicion is high, transoesophageal echocardiography should always be performed. If normal, repeat imaging can be considered to monitor for developing pathology.

Assessment

For diagnosis use a full systematic examination with focus on valves (main site). Bear in mind clinical situation: right-sided valves if intravenous infection (drugs, lines), known abnormal valves (prosthetic or degenerative), previous endocarditis (old vegetations). For monitoring use full examination and make sure you comment on change from previous findings.

For all studies report on: vegetations (location, number, size); abscess (particularly valve rings); fistulae (e.g. aorta to right heart); valve dysfunction (including severity, dehiscence, rupture); pericardial effusion.

Vegetation

Key features to help diagnose: (1) attachment to upstream-side valve; (2) irregular shape; (3) oscillating motion distinct from valve; (4) related valve dysfunction. Comment on number of vegetations, attachments, size (measure in at least two directions and provide overall assessment—small, moderate, large).

Abscess

Abscesses can be peri-valvular or valvular. Appearances initially are often of a thickening and 'spongy' appearance to valve ring (particularly aortic root) or valve leaflet. An echo-free, fluid-filled centre may develop. Abscesses may open into adjacent cardiac chambers (technically the space is then no longer an abscess).

For each abscess comment on location with reference to position around valve (e.g. annulus right coronary cusp). Measure size in different planes and judge as small, moderate, or large. Comment on functional effects of abscess (e.g. outflow tract or valve distortion).

Fistula

Fistulae usually develop following an abscess and describe an abnormal connection between two cardiac chambers. Use colour flow mapping to track fistulae and identify jets in cardiac chambers. If aligned, use Doppler to quantify flow direction and size.

Comment on physical size (length and width) and which chambers are connected. Give an estimate of haemodynamic significance (e.g. size of shunt left to right heart, change in ventricular size and function, degree of regurgitation if fistula across valve).

Severity of valvular lesion See valve sections.

Pericardial effusion See pericardial section (p. 242).

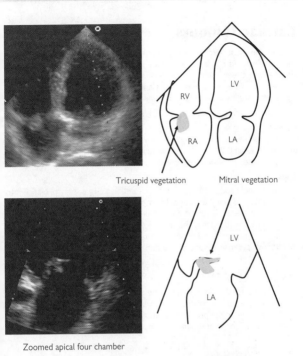

Tricuspid vegetation   Mitral vegetation

Zoomed apical four chamber

Fig. 3.97 Apical 4-chamber views of tricuspid (top) and mitral (bottom) vegetations. Note irregular appearance and valve leaflet attachment.

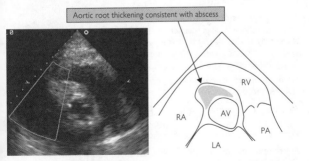

Aortic root thickening consistent with abscess

Fig. 3.98 Parasternal short axis view that demonstrates thickening of aortic root in 10 o'clock position consistent with an aortic root abscess.

Cardiac tumours

One of the most 'exciting' things to see in echocardiography is a cardiac mass that should not be there. Once seen it is easy to forget about continuing with the systematic collection of information but this is essential in order to understand what effect any mass may be having. Masses will be vegetations, cysts, tumours (benign and malignant), or thrombus.

Primary tumours—benign (80%)

Myxoma

Myxoma is the most common primary tumour (30% of tumours: 74% left atrium; 18% right atrium; 4% left ventricular free wall). 10% are familial so family counselling should be considered if other familial cases.

Appearances and assessment
Globular, finely speckled mass with well defined edges. May prolapse into left ventricle. Usually attached to interatrial septum (fossa ovalis 90%). Attachment best visualized in apical and subcostal 4-chamber views. Tumour calcification may be seen infrequently. Determine length and diameter of myxoma. Quantify severity of coexisting mitral regurgitation or effective stenosis caused by myxoma.

Myxoma or thrombus?

No specific finding differentiates the two but thrombus is more often irregular, layered, immobile, broad-based (myxoma typically has a stalk), and located near the posterior wall of the left atrium. The left atrium is more likely to be dilated with an abnormal mitral valve.

Papillary fibroelastoma

10% of primary tumours. Found attached most commonly to mitral and aortic valves with small pedicles. Rarely attach to left ventricular outflow tract or papillary muscles.

Appearances and assessment
Small (rarely >1cm in diameter), mobile, pedunculated, echocardiographically dense mass. May mimic vegetation or Lambl's excrescences. Usually no other valve abnormalities. Comment on size, location, and functional effects.

Other tumours Lipoma (10%), fibroma (4%), rhabdomyoma (9%—children more common).

Primary tumours—malignant (20%)

Typical tumours are sarcomas, angiosarcomas, and rhabdomyosarcomas. Primary lymphomas also reported. Final diagnosis often requires biopsy.

Appearances and assessment
Often irregular and invade into myocardium. Can be recognized as unusual, localized myocardial thickening. Report location, extent, and functional effects (valvular or ventricular dysfunction, restrictive or constrictive physiology, pericardial fluid). Comment on concerns about cause.

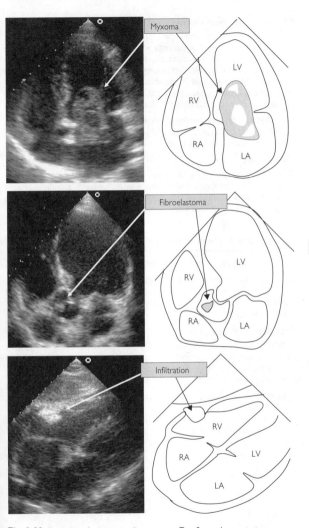

Fig. 3.99 Examples of primary cardiac tumours. Top figure demonstrates a myxoma prolapsing through the mitral valve. The middle figure is an apical 5-chamber view that demonstrates a fibroelastoma on the aortic valve. The bottom figure is a subcostal view of an infiltrative mass, probably malignant tumour.

Secondary tumours—metastases

Forty times more common than primary malignant tumours. Cardiac metastases occur in 5% of patients who die of malignant tumours. Most common tumours to metastasize to heart are: melanoma, bronchogenic carcinoma, breast cancer, lymphoma, gastrointestinal adenocarcinoma, laryngeal carcinoma, pancreatic cancer, mucinous adenocarcinoma of cervix/ovary. Often clinical presentation is with tachycardia, arrhythmias, or heart failure and most common finding is a pericardial effusion.

Appearances and assessment Usually seen as wall thickening and there may be an associated pericardial effusion. Tumour mass may protrude into a cardiac chamber. Comment on size, location, and functional effects.

Valve cysts

Fluid-filled cysts can be found on valves often due to myxomatous degeneration. They appear as round structures, often with a pedicle attachment. The cyst has a fluid-filled appearance and there may be floating structures inside. Comment on location, size, and functional effects.

Pericardial cyst

Cysts can form in pleura or pericardium. Most commonly cysts are seen around the right costophrenic location (70%), then left costophrenic angle (30%), and rarely in upper mediastinum, hila, or left cardiac border.

Appearances and assessment Pericardial cysts appear as an ovoid space adjacent to a cardiac chamber. The differential is between cyst and loculated pericardial effusion, dilated coronary sinus or ventricular pseudo-aneurysm.

Extra-cardiac tumours

Tumours within the thorax, but separate from the heart, can be incidentally picked up during echocardiography. Parasternal views identify mediastinal cysts or thymomas. Other extra-cardiac tumours include haematoma, teratoma, diaphragmatic hernia, and pancreatic cysts.

Appearances and assessment Comment on location, suspected cause, and functional effects. Key effects are displacement of the heart, compression of cardiac chambers, evidence of superior vena cava obstruction, cardiac tamponade, constrictive pericarditis, pulmonary or tricuspid stenosis.

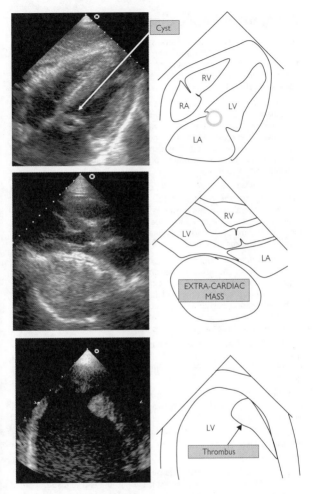

Fig. 3.100 Examples of tumours. Top figure is a subcostal view of a mitral valve cyst. The middle figure demonstrates a large extra-cardiac mass causing chamber compression. The bottom figure shows an apical left ventricle thrombus.

Congenital heart disease

Common congenital heart defects, such as atrial and ventricular septal defects (pp 232 and 238) and coarctation of the aorta (p. 264), have distinct methods of assessment using standard techniques. More complex congenital disease is dealt with in specialist texts. Some of the disorders that may be seen during routine echocardiography are included here.

Patent ductus arteriosus Patent ductus arteriosus connects aorta to pulmonary artery. Identify the aortic end in descending aorta (suprasternal view) just distal to left subclavian. Pulmonary end empties into left pulmonary artery just to left of pulmonary trunk (use modified parasternal short axis views). Colour flow demonstrates a jet directed the wrong way in pulmonary trunk towards pulmonary artery. Report functional effects of left to right shunt.

Persistent left superior vena cava Persistent left superior vena cava drains into the coronary sinus. An apical 4-chamber view cutting below the mitral valve demonstrates the sinus. It is usually dilated. Agitated saline contrast injected into the left arm opacifies the sinus before the right atrium. Usually no significant haemodynamic effects but it complicates pacemaker placement.

Anomalous pulmonary drainage This describes drainage of pulmonary veins into right atrium. Total drainage requires a septal defect for oxygenated blood to reach systemic circulation. In partial drainage one or two pulmonary veins still drain to left. Most easily assessed with transoesophageal echocardiography. Right upper pulmonary vein may drain to right atrium or superior vena cava; left pulmonary veins may connect to innominate vein; right pulmonary veins may connect to inferior vena cava.

Tetralogy of Fallot Combination of right ventricular outflow obstruction, ventricular septal defect, right ventricular hypertrophy, and aorta overriding the septum. Assessment pre-operatively should focus on, and quantify, each aspect.

Double outlet right ventricle Both aorta and pulmonary artery arise from right ventricle. Ventricular septal defect allows oxygenated blood to reach systemic circulation.

Persistent truncus arteriosus Single trunk divides into systemic and pulmonary arteries. Associated with ventricular septal defect and single valve in trunk.

Hypoplastic left ventricle Usually involves whole of left heart with disordered valve development and small left atrium and ventricle.

Single ventricle Single ventricle with mitral, tricuspid, aortic, and pulmonary valves connected. Chamber can be of left or right origin with remnants of other ventricle seen.

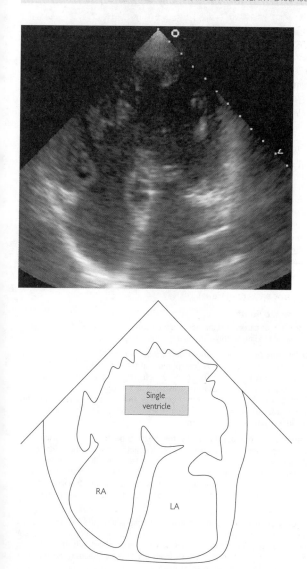

Fig. 3.101 Apical 4-chamber view of a single ventricle.

Obstructive congenital disorders

Many congenital defects can be organized, and assessed, according to their restriction or obstruction to blood flow. They can be demonstrated using standard 2D imaging and Doppler quantifications.

Right ventricular inflow
- Ebstein anomaly and tricuspid atresia (p. 138).

Right ventricular outflow
- Subvalvular—outflow tract (use short axis views).
- Pulmonary valve—pulmonary stenosis (p. 144).
- Supravalvular—pulmonary artery (use short axis views).

Left ventricular inflow
- Pulmonary veins—stenosis or obstruction. Usually requires transoesophageal echocardiography to document.
- Atrium—atrial membranes (either across the middle of atrium—cor triatriatum—or supravalvular).
- Mitral valve—congenital stenosis (p. 94), double inlet valve.

Left ventricular outflow
- Subvalvular—fibromuscular (wall thickening) or membranous (discrete membrane present) (use parasternal and apical views).
- Aortic valve— bicuspid valve (p. 126).
  - Supravalvular level—membranous or fibromuscular thickening (use parasternal views).

Cardiac orientation

Disorders of cardiac orientation are a fundamental congenital abnormality. Assess according to three independent developmental aspects.

Atrial situs (atrial orientation) and venous inflow Normal is *situs solitus* and abnormal *situs inversus* (morphological left atrium on right). Abdominal organs usually match atria (liver on left suggests *inversus*). Use subcostal views. Left atrium has long, thin atrial appendage and rounded shape. Right atrium has broad, short appendage and Eustachian valve. Identify where inferior vena cava and pulmonary vein connect (vein inflow does not identify atria as connections vary).

Ventricle morphology Normally the heart tube folds to the right and heart lies in left chest with right ventricle anteriorly. If tube folds to the left the right ventricle lies on other side of left ventricle. Atrio-ventricular valves stay with ventricles. Identify right ventricle from trabeculations, 3 papillary muscles, tri-leaflet valve, moderator band, and triangular cavity. Left ventricle has smooth surface, 2 papillary muscles, bileaflet valve, and bullet shape.

Arterial connections Identifies arterial transposition and occurs if valves are in 'right' position but folding rotates ventricles, or if ventricles are 'right' but arteries are switched. Use parasternal short axis and long axis views. Identify pulmonary artery from orientation (heading posteriorly) and bifurcation. Ascending aorta heads superiorly. Use suprasternal views to see if the arch goes to the left (normal) or right.

Surgical correction of congenital heart disease

Complete repairs

With effective correction there may be little echocardiographic evidence of repair. A full systematic study should be used and reports made of any residual functional effects on valve function, as well as disorders of left or right ventricle appearance or function. Residual shunts or abnormal vascular connections should be commented upon.

Shunts

These are designed to increase blood flow into the pulmonary artery to improve oxygenation.

Blalock–Taussig shunt

This shunt connects the subclavian or innominate artery to a branch of the pulmonary artery. The shunt can be made on the left or right. It can be seen in suprasternal views and both colour flow mapping and Doppler assessment can be attempted to identify stenosis or changes in flow.

Glenn shunt

The Glenn shunt anastomizes the superior vena cava to the pulmonary artery.

Fontan procedure

This is used to bypass an abnormal right ventricle by directing venous flow to the pulmonary circulation. There are a range of Fontan procedures and it can be difficult to evaluate with echocardiography without knowing the surgical details.

Transoesophageal: examination

Introduction

Transoesophageal echocardiography has emerged over only the last 30 years. The first M-mode transoesophageal images were published in the 1970s by Dr Frazin, a cardiologist in Chicago, who attached a traditional probe on to the end of an endoscope. It did not catch on as a technique because the patient found it difficult to swallow the probe.

By the early 1980s 2D imaging with superior, smaller probe technology had become realistic, significantly advanced by the introduction of the electronic, phased-array probe. The early probes were single plane and it was not until the 1990s that biplane probes became a reality. These were finally superseded by multiplane imaging, a move that provided the leap in functionality that we take for granted today.

Transoesophageal echocardiography uses all the same technology as transthoracic imaging. 2D echocardiography and colour and spectral Doppler can all be performed as well as tissue Doppler imaging and 3D reconstructions. However, transoesophageal imaging possesses a major advantage in that there is little tissue between the probe and the heart to degrade the image and the ultrasound beam does not need to penetrate as far. Higher ultrasound frequencies can therefore be used (typically 5–7.5MHz) which enhances spatial resolution.

A lot of the clinical applications have been driven by interest in intra-operative monitoring and this remains a key application of the technique. However, real-time imaging with unparalleled spatial and temporal resolution makes the image quality superior to all other modalities within the imaging window provided by the oesophagus. As the procedure is well tolerated, transoesophageal echocardiography has guaranteed usefulness for cardiology studies, particularly where detailed anatomical and functional imaging is needed.

Performing the study

There are many different patients in whom transoesophageal echocar-diography is requested, ranging from patients who require elective monitoring of stable clinical problems such as aortic dissection to those with emergency haemodynamic problems. The background to each study will therefore vary considerably. This section is written to provide a framework to perform a structured and compre-hensive, transoesophageal echocardiogram in any situation.

For intraoperative studies or those on intensive care units the patient is already sedated or anaesthetized and, unless planned before an operation, may not have given consent. However, even in these situa-tions the majority of the framework for performing a study is still relevant. All aspects of assessing indications and contraindications should be carried out, as well as preparation of machine, probe, and monitoring. The only real differences from elective studies in awake patients are usually the patient position (lying on their back), the presence of other things in the mouth (tracheal tubes), and depth of sedation (general anaesthetic or deep sedation).

Indications

There are generally accepted, evidence-based uses of transoesophageal echocardiography that have evolved in clinical situations where there is a need for high spatial and temporal resolution to assess pathology.

- *Evaluation of valve pathology.*
  - Pre-surgical evaluation for repair of mitral or aortic valves.
  - Evaluation of cause of dysfunction.
- *Intracardiac shunts.*
- *Cardiac embolic source.*
  - Intracardiac shunts.
  - Left-sided thrombus—ventricle, left atrial appendage.
  - Left-sided valve abnormalities/masses/vegetations.
  - Aortic atheroma.
- *Endocarditis.*
  - Diagnosis.
  - Monitoring.
- *Evaluation of prosthetic valve dysfunction.*
- *Congenital heart disease.*
- *Aortic dissection and aortic pathology.*
- *Cardiac masses (where transthoracic imaging inadequate).*
- *Imaging during procedures.*
  - Percutaneous procedures—ASD/PFO closure, mitral balloon valvotomy.
  - Electrophysiology and pacing—transseptal puncture, lead placement.
  - Cardiothoracic surgery.[1]
- *Haemodynamic monitoring in anaesthetized patient.*
  - Peri-operative monitoring.
  - Intensive care monitoring.
- Poor transthoracic windows or inadequate image quality.

---

1 American Society of Anesthesiologists. Practice guidelines for perioperative transesophageal echocardiography. *Anesthesiology* 1996; **84**: 986–1006.

Contraindications and complications

Consider contraindications before starting. Absolute contraindications tend to be oesophageal problems that make the procedure technically impossible and increase the risk of traumatic injury. The decision to go ahead despite relative contraindications depends on the importance of the clinical information to be gathered, whether there are alternative ways to gather the data, and operator experience. During and after the procedure be vigilant for possible complications and ensure the patient is fully informed of these risks when taking consent.

Absolute contraindications
- Oesophageal tumors causing obstruction of the lumen.
- Oesophageal strictures.
- Oesophageal diverticula.
- Patient not co-operative.

Relative contraindications
- Oesophageal reflux refractory to medical therapy.
- Hiatal hernia.
- Odynophagia or dysphagia.
- Previous oesophageal or gastric surgery.
- Previous oesophageal or gastric bleed.
- Oesophageal varices: using a sheath is said to reduce the risk as the gel reduces the pressure of the probe tip. However, transgastric views are not advised and there must not have been a bleed in the preceding 4 weeks.
- Severe cervical arthritis.
- Profound oesophageal distortion.
- Recent radiation to head and neck.
- Significant dental pathology.

Complications
A study of complications in around 10,000 patients showed a very low incidence.[1] Failed intubation occurred in around 2%. All other complications had an incidence of less than 1%.
- Intubation problems—termination because of choking.
- Pulmonary problems—bronchospasm, hypoxia.
- Cardiac problems—ventricular extrasystole, tachycardia, atrial fibrillation, AV block, angina.
- Bleeding—from pharynx, related to vomiting, from oesophagus.
- Perforation—risk of perforation increases in small patients and in all conditions that make the oesophagus friable, e.g. prior radiation to head, neck, or oesophagus, steroid treatment, gastro-oesophageal reflux disease, prolonged duration of probe in patient.
- Probe failure.

1 Daniel, W.G. et al. Safety of transoesophageal echocardiography. A multicenter survey of 10,419 examinations. *Circulation* 1991; **83**: 817–21.

Antibiotic prophylaxis for transoesophageal echocardiography?

Antibiotic prophylaxis is not recommended for any indication under current guidelines. It remains reasonable to consider antibiotics in occasional cases, for example a patient with a prosthetic heart valve and evidence of poor oral hygiene, in whom the study is being performed for an indication other than suspected endocarditis. In these individual cases, practice is governed by clinical common sense rather than evidence.

Information for the patient

For elective or planned studies patients should be provided with information or have a detailed verbal explanation. Informed consent is essential as it is a semi-invasive procedure and sedation is used.

Example of an information sheet

You have been asked to attend for transoesophageal echocardiography (TOE). A TOE is a test that allows the doctor to look closely at the heart without other organs obscuring the view. In order to carry out the procedure, the scope, which is a long flexible tube, is passed through the mouth and down the gullet.

Before the procedure? You should not have anything to eat or drink for at least 6 hours before the procedure. When you arrive you will be seen by a doctor who will take a medical history and after explaining the procedure, ask you to sign a consent form. If you have any concerns, please do not hesitate to ask, as we would like you to be as relaxed as possible. We will be pleased to answer any queries.

What happens during the procedure? A blood pressure cuff will be attached to your arm and a small monitor placed on your finger to monitor the oxygen levels in the blood. The doctor will spray your throat with some local anaesthetic. A mouth guard is placed between your teeth to protect the tube and your teeth. You will be asked to turn on to your left side and the room's main lights will be turned off. Your sedation is then given through a small tube (cannula) which will be inserted into your arm. When you are sleepy the procedure will start. There will be several people looking after you including the doctor, a nurse and a technician. The procedure takes 10–20 minutes to examine all areas carefully.

Benefits? The benefits from transoesophageal echocardiography are that it can: define the nature of cardiac symptoms; decide which further therapeutic and diagnostic procedures you may have to undergo.

Risks? Risks from transoesophageal echocardiography are tiny. Usually the investigation is tolerated well; some patients may have some mild symptoms during the test (mostly coughing). Serious risks are very rare and include palpitations 0.75% (7 patients in every 1000), angina 0.1% (1 patient in every 1000), bronchospasm/hypoxia 0.8% (8 patients in every 1000), bleeding 0.2% (2 patients in every 1000), oesophagus perforation, extremely rare less than 0.01% (1 in every 10000 patients). Your doctor would not recommend that you have a transoesophageal echocardiogram unless they felt that the benefits of the procedure outweighed these small risks.

After the procedure? The sedation may last up to an hour. Your blood pressure and respiration will be checked and you may have an oxygen mask on while you are awake. The sedation has an amnesic effect so you should remember little of the procedure when you wake up.

Preparing for the study

Setting up the environment

- With the patient on their bed, ensure there is a blood pressure cuff on the arm and set to automatic monitoring every 5 to 10 minutes. Check a baseline blood pressure.
- Set up stable ECG monitor on the machine.
- Monitor oxygen saturations and check a baseline saturation level.
- Provide supplemental oxygen, usually via nasal specs at 2L/min.
- Ensure suction is available and working.
- Check bed height and position so operator and nursing staff are not bending over the patient but standing upright during the procedure.
- Check relative position of machine, patient, and operator to ensure operator has a clear view of images.

Nursing

- The nurse should talk to the patient and check identity and consent.
- The nurse stands behind the patient or at the head of the bed to reassure the patient and support the head and mouthguard.
- During the procedure the nurse should monitor haemodynamics and saturations and inform the operator if they change.
- They should monitor for secretions and give suction as required.
- After the procedure they should stay with the patient to ensure adequate recovery from the sedation.

Operator

- Check notes for indications and purpose of study. Check past medical history, allergies, and any contraindications.
- Make sure patient has been starved for at least 6 hours and has taken out any false teeth/loose bridges/loose teeth.
- Ensure the apparatus is ready: probe prepared, attached, and selected; probe steering works; transoesophageal machine presets selected; ECG tracing and patient details on machine.
- Sedation drawn up, local anaesthetic spray available, and IV cannula in arm ready for sedation.
- Ensure gel ready to be applied to probe.
- Then, give local anaesthetic spray.
- For the awake patient, ask them to roll on to their left side and ensure a stable position—often achieved if the patient brings their right leg over their left in a 'recovery position' arrangement. If in an ITU setting, ask if the patient is able to be rolled on to their left side.
- Ensure the head of the bed is flat, the patient has their head on a pillow, and there is a mat under the head to absorb any secretions.
- For the awake patient, ask them to drop their chin on to their chest.
- Place the mouth guard between their teeth.
- Give sedation and start the intubation.

Preparing for transoesophageal echocardiography— a 10 point plan

1 Put sheath on the probe.
2 Review referral form/notes for indication, contraindications.
3 Ask patient when was last meal (should be >6 hours before), previous problems with swallowing, known oesophageal disease, allergies.
4 Insert patient name and hospital number on scanner and ask patient to confirm.
5 Insert IV cannula.
6 Attach probe to the scanner, test steering, and whether probe is accepted by the scanner.
7 Start blood pressure monitoring and pulse oximetry, nasal specs for oxygen supply (2L/min).
8 Apply local anaesthesia to patient's throat; then rotate patient into a left lateral decubitus position.
9 Put in mouth guard.
10 Give sedation.

Preparing and cleaning the probe

The probe can easily be damaged either externally (by chemicals or misuse) or by the patient (beware teeth!). There are also important health and safety issues about protecting the patient from the probe.

Checking the probe

Check over the probe at the start of the procedure. Look for evidence of damage to the coating and layers. There may be breaks or 'bubbling' in the coating. In extreme situations the underlying wire shielding may be exposed with a risk of current leak or heating to the patient. If you are concerned about the integrity of the probe use a different probe and contact the manufacturer.

Preparing and cleaning

There are two options for probe preparation and cleaning.

The probe is used without a cover

- In this case it is essential it is sterilized between cases. After the investigation the probe should be washed down with water and then immersed in a tube containing glutaraldehyde solution (licensed for endoscope disinfection) for a fixed period of time according to manufacturer guidelines.
- Glutaraldehyde can cause allergies or breathing problems. Therefore ensure regular fresh air in the room where the probe is cleaned. Furthermore, the probe needs to be rewashed with water to ensure the solution is removed before the probe is used on the next patient.
- The handgrips and controls of the probe should be wiped with an alcohol-based agent. Alcohol should not normally be used to clean the transducer face at the tip of the probe.

The probe is used with a purpose-designed sheath

- Sheaths protect the probe from infection and provide electrical isolation from the patient.
- There are both latex and latex-free versions.
- To prepare, fill the sheath tip with the supplied gel using a syringe.
- Then feed the probe all the way into the sheath and fix the upper end with the supplied plastic clip.
- Avoid air bubbles in the gel around the transducer as these degrade image quality. Press them further up the sheath or pull and release the sheath tip to expel them away from the transducer.
- When performing a series of studies there is no need to carry out a complete disinfection between patients. After each investigation remove the sheath and wipe off any gel left on the probe. Then clean the probe with water and an alcohol-based agent.
- If the sheath breaks during the procedure or a perforation is seen afterwards, immerse the probe in disinfectant solution as above.
- In patients with a high infection risk (HIV, hepatitis B, etc.) disinfect the probe with a commercial solution after sheath removal (as above) and sterilize the controls with alcohol-based solutions.

Probe movements

A combination of probe movements is required to gather all the images. For many of the views, changes in sector angle are the primary control, with physical movements used to optimize the image.

Withdrawal and advance Moving the probe forward and backwards in the oesophagus is the simplest manoeuvre. The depth of the probe is best controlled with the hand nearest the patient's mouth. This hand can also judge the size of small movements forward and back relative to the mouth guard. The depth of probe insertion is marked on the probe in centimetres. This number should be used when images need to be annotated to record probe depth. It measures the distance from probe tip to front incisors.

Rotation (or turning) The probe can be rotated clockwise or anti-clockwise within the oesophagus. This is achieved by twisting the hand-held control section with one hand, and the probe near the mouthguard with your other hand. This movement is usually used to orientate the heart in the image plane and to look at the descending aorta.

Sector angle On the controls there are usually two buttons side by side. These rotate the angle of the imaging plane forward and backward between 0° and 180°. The angle plane can also sometimes be changed directly from the ultrasound machine. The current angle plane is displayed on the screen.

Angulation (or retro-/anteflexion) The large wheel on the control panel moves a few centimetres of the transducer tip forward and backward. Angulation forward is usually used to press the transducer against the oesophagus wall or stomach to improve contact and image quality. Angulation backwards can be effective at lengthening out the left ventricle.

Lateral motion The small wheel on the control panel causes movement of the transducer tip from side-to-side. This is very rarely used and for the most part can be ignored. Occasionally, with difficult images or abnormally positioned hearts, small lateral motions may be helpful.

Position lock Most probes have a lever behind the control wheels that locks the probe in position. For most studies this is not required and can be ignored. For long periods of monitoring—particularly in transgastric views intraoperatively—the lock can be used. However, there is an increased risk of traumatic injury with movement of the probe with the lock on. Care must be taken to remove the lock before the probe is repositioned.

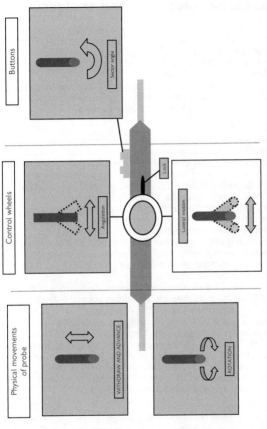

Fig. 4.1 Probe movements and the controls on the handset that allow motion. The main controls are the large wheel (angulation) and the buttons (sector angle). The small wheel and lock are rarely needed.

Anaesthetic, sedation, and analgesia

Local anaesthetic

- Start with a local anaesthetic, Xylocaine® (lignocaine) spray.
- With the patient sitting up, spray several times on to the back of their throat. Ask them to hold the liquid for a few seconds and then swallow.
- Warn the patient that the spray has an unusual taste, their mouth and throat will feel numb, and their swallow may feel strange or difficult.
- The spray will need 2 to 3 minutes to have an effect.

Sedation and analgesia

There are no standard guidelines for transoesophageal echocardiography and it is possible to perform the study with no sedation. However, the following routines can be used (borrowed from other endoscopic procedures). A benzodiazepine provides sedation and amnesia, and an opioid analgesia. Remember that '*the difference between good and bad sedation is around three minutes*', i.e. wait for the sedation to work.

- Ensure reversal agents are available and accessible (flumazenil for midazolam and naloxone for pethidine or fentanyl). Life support equipment should be accessible and the operator ALS trained.
- Start with 2mg IV midazolam and 25mg IV pethidine—this is usually sufficient for most patients. Aim for the patient to be '*drowsy but rousable*'. In certain patients and situations lower starting doses are advisable (see below).
- Wait 3–5 minutes then assess level of sedation (patient response, haemodynamics). If not adequate, give further bolus of 1–2mg IV midazolam and consider further 25mg IV pethidine.
- Repeat the '*wait and bolus*' regime until adequate sedation.
- Total sedation should not exceed 10mg midazolam and/or 75mg pethidine. Stop and consider a general anaesthetic at a later date.
- Once sedation is appropriate start intubation. If intubation is difficult because the patient is awake return to the sedation routine.
- During the procedure (after intubation) if the patient becomes distressed consider giving further boluses of sedation.

Specific situations

- In younger patients (and some older patients) increasing doses of midazolam can increase agitation and be counterproductive. Consider using more analgesia and less sedation from the outset.
- In older patients (particularly >80 years) oversedation is a problem so start with 1mg IV midazolam, withhold the opioid, and wait longer between boluses as the sedation may be slower to circulate.
- Use lower starting doses for those with significant left ventricular failure or respiratory disease, hypotension, or neurological impairment.

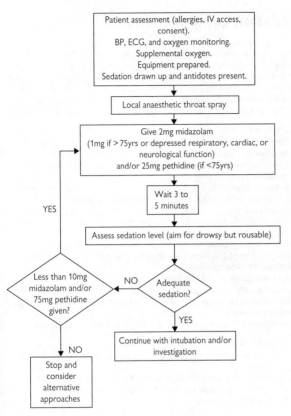

Fig. 4.2 Flow chart for sedation protocol.

Sedation complications

Although by using low dose conscious sedation with up-titration complications are relatively infrequent, it is always essential to be vigilant. Monitoring of the patient during the procedure is mandatory. Several expert bodies have produced guidelines for how to give sedation if you are not an anaesthetist. It is advisable to have a local policy for how to use sedation for transoesophageal echocardiography and an audit process so that problems or adverse events associated with the procedure are identified.

Peri-procedure

- Monitor for drops in blood pressure and saturations throughout the procedure. These are the commonest side-effects of sedation.
- If hypotensive, patients may be mildly dehydrated as they are nil by mouth so consider IV fluids.
- Drops in saturations may be temporary at the start of sedation and can be corrected with increased supplemental oxygen.
- If there are ever any concerns about the level of sedation or degree of haemodynamic or respiratory changes reverse the sedation and stop the procedure (if still ongoing).
- To reverse the midazolam give flumazenil. This is relatively short-acting so after a period of time, if the sedative effects return, consider further boluses or even an infusion.
- To reverse the opioid give naloxone.
- In those with left ventricular failure, lying flat with sedation can precipitate acute failure so be alert for clinical signs and treat with diuretics, etc. if necessary.
- Allergic reactions can occur with sedation so treat as appropriate.

Post-procedure

- After the procedure, the patient should be monitored until they are fully awake.
- If the procedure has been elective and the patient is going home afterwards they should be advised not to drive or operate heavy machinery for 24 hours.

Intubation

Intubation is a key skill to learn. Unless you intubate successfully the procedure cannot start! The skills needed to perform successful intubation in elective studies with light sedation are broadly similar to those skills needed for intubation in intraoperative or intensive care settings. Everyone develops their own techniques but a standard procedure is as follows.

Intubation with light sedation

- Ideally have two people, one to hold the controls and the other to hold the end of the probe and intubate. If on your own, lie the probe along the bed and concentrate on intubation. Some people can hold the controls in one hand and feed the probe with the other, but this requires an uncomplicated passage of the probe.
- Talk confidently and calmly to the patient. Guide them through the procedure and the swallows. After intubation reassure them and tell them to take gentle breaths through the nose. The attitude of the operator and how they relate to—and relax—the patient often determines the success of the procedure.

The routine

- The patient should be lying on their left side with their chin towards their chest. This encourages the probe to pass into the oesophagus (exactly what you try to avoid with chin-lift during resuscitation).
- Check the mouth guard is in position between the teeth.
- Wipe gel over the probe tip to about 40cm. Too much increases the risk of aspiration and too little makes probe movement difficult and uncomfortable for the patient.
- Check probe controls and put a curve on the end of the probe.
- Ensure the curve on the tip lines up with the expected curve into the back of the mouth; then pass the probe through the mouth guard and on to the tongue.
- Ask the patient to swallow once to get the probe to the back of the mouth and then a second time to pass it into the oesophagus.
  The second step should be timed to coincide with the swallow.
- To direct the probe a finger can be placed in the mouth beside the mouth guard. This guides the probe into the back of the mouth.
  It is especially useful when learning, when the probe is not passing smoothly, or in the anaesthetized patient.
- When the probe is in the oesophagus stop and do not move anything for a few minutes while the patient settles.
- The operator should then remove one glove and get into position.
  One gloved hand controls the probe at the mouth guard and the other holds the controls. The operator usually stands facing the patient with their right hand at the patient's mouth and looks over their shoulder at the images. An alternative arrangement is to stand at right angles, with the left hand at the patient's mouth, facing the machine.

Intubation in the anaesthetized patient

- Use the same probe preparation and use a mouth guard.
- Ensure there is a curve on the probe; then use a finger to guide the tip into the back of the mouth.
- If the patient is on their back get someone to lift the chin towards the chest.
- The probe may pass smoothly into the oesophagus with light pressure. If there is resistance induce a reflex swallow with some forward pressure on the back of the tongue.
- If a tracheal tube is in place, passage of the probe into the oesophagus may be restricted by the tracheal tube. To overcome this, ask for the assistance of the anaesthetist, either to temporarily deflate the cuff or to manipulate the tracheal tube.

What to do if the probe does not pass or patient is agitated?

You should not need to give more than a gentle steady force to the probe. If resistance is felt assume it has gone the wrong way.

- If you are not already using your finger to guide the probe, do so.
- Feel where the tip of the probe has gone. It may have doubled back on itself in the mouth or you may feel it heading up or down. Withdraw slightly, adjust the rotation, and then try to advance again, with a swallow.
- If it is not clear where the probe has gone, withdraw entirely, check the curve on the probe and its direction, then restart.
- If the patient cannot swallow because they are too sedated use a finger to direct the probe.
- If the patient starts coughing think whether you may have passed the probe into the trachea. Withdraw the probe and start again.
- If the patient becomes very agitated, stop and consider whether to try again after more sedation and/or analgesia.
- In around 2% of cases intubation fails. Know when to stop. After two or three attempts have been unsuccessful consider getting help from a more experienced operator, if available. If the patient is becoming very agitated despite adequate sedation and analgesia, stop. If the investigation is essential, the study can always be rearranged with a general anaesthetic to ensure patient compliance and/or an anaesthetist to aid intubation.

Image acquisition

Standard acquisition

Acquisition of transoesophageal images should always be performed in a standardized way—with a set sequence of views. Virtually all the views have corresponding transthoracic views and therefore, if you have prior training in transthoracic imaging, think about these views to identify structures. As with performing a transthoracic study, all the views should be recorded for comprehensive data collection. Even when there is a specific question (e.g. exclusion of atrial clots before cardioversion) a full dataset should be acquired to ensure nothing is missed.

The 'screenwiper' principle

The best initial sequence of views (scan planes) is summarized by the *screenwiper principle*. The following pages go through how to collect transoesophageal data following the screenwiper principle.

• Starting from 0° the sector is moved across in steps to around 135° and then back again in a series of steps.
• At each step the view needs only minor modifications of probe position to optimize the image. This reduces major probe movements and minimizes patient discomfort.

Each view is examined in:
• 2D imaging;
• then colour flow Doppler recordings;
• and, if needed, spectral Doppler recordings (PW and/or CW).

After the *screen wiper* is complete additional views can then be used, as required, to look at pulmonary veins, transgastric views, the aorta, or any abnormal findings.

Optimize the views using small changes in transducer position
Adjust by angulation, moving the transducer up and down, and rotating the sector (tips will be given for each of the views). Don't move too fast and too much. Slight changes have a big impact on the image!

Most scan planes have several different structures
All structures cannot always be viewed in a single recorded loop. Slight adjustments of the probe position and/or sector may be needed and loops recorded for each structure.

If you get lost
If during a transoesophageal investigation you become disoriented find the 4-chamber view again. Reset the rotation to 0° and then try some rotation and repositioning of the probe until the four chambers come back into view.

Basic screenwiper study

1 Four chamber view
2 Five chamber view
3 Short axis aortic view (± right ventricle inflow/outflow)
4 Long axis aortic view
5 Interatrial septal view (bicaval view)
6 Two chamber view (left atrial appendage view)

Then further views

7 Left pulmonary venous view
8 Right pulmonary venous view
9 Pulmonary artery view
10 Transgastric views*
11 Descending aorta view
12 Aortic arch view

* Not necessary in all patients.

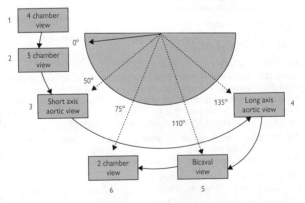

Fig. 4.3 'Screen wiper' principle showing sequence of sector angles for first 6 views. Once in position, the image can be optimized with slight variation in sector angle (usually <5°) followed by slight adjustments in depth and tilting as necessary.

Four chamber view

This is the first view to acquire and is similar to the transthoracic 4-chamber view (but upside down). After intubation, advance the probe to around 35cm from the teeth.

Finding the view
- Rotation should be set at 0°.
- The atria will probably be the first feature you see.
- Turn the probe to swing all four chambers into view.
- Withdraw and advance the probe slightly to avoid the left ventricular outflow tract but keep a clear view of the mitral valve.
- If the left ventricular outflow tract is still seen, try adding up to 15°.
- If necessary, improve contact by probe angulation.

What do you see?
Use this view to assess
- Global and regional left ventricular function and wall thickness.
- Right ventricular size and function.
- Mitral valve morphology (orifice, prolapse).
- Tricuspid valve morphology.

Use this view to measure
- Right and left ventricular size (although beware foreshortening).
- Mitral Doppler measurements.

Key features of view
Mitral valve Key view for mitral valve to assess morphology and haemo-dynamics. A2 segment of anterior mitral leaflet (aML) and P2 segment of the posterior mitral leaflet (pML) often seen. Colour flow mapping will show stenosis and/or regurgitation. Supplement with continuous or pulsed wave Doppler as for transthoracic echocardiography.

Tricuspid valve Lateral leaflet is better displayed than septal. To get a better view of the tricuspid valve advance the probe slightly deeper into the oesophagus. Supplement with Doppler as required.

Left and right atria The main cavity of both atria and the interatrial septum can be seen. However, fossa ovalis is not usually seen. Turn the probe slightly left and right to scan through the atria.

Left ventricle Parts of the interventricular septum and the lateral wall are displayed. Often left ventricle is foreshortened and measurement of end-diastolic and end-systolic volumes may be inaccurate. Retroflex the probe to lengthen out the left ventricle but beware contact may be lost.

Right ventricle An impression of size and function of the right ventricle relative to the left is obtained, although there is a risk of foreshortening, as with the left ventricle.

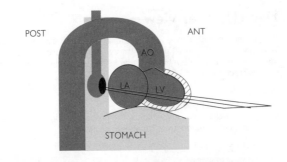

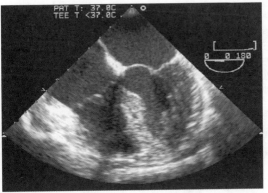

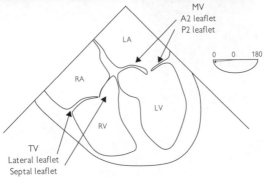

Fig. 4.4 Position of probe and classical image for a 4-chamber view. Without ante- or retro-angulation of the probe the left ventricle is usually foreshortened.

Five chamber view

This is the second view and it is similar to the transthoracic apical 5-chamber view. The main purpose is to get to the appropriate level for the aortic short axis view. However, an initial view of the left ventricular outflow tract is provided.

Finding the view
- Rotation should be set at 0°.
- From the 4-chamber view withdraw the probe very slightly until the left ventricular outflow tract comes into plane.

What do you see?

Use this view to assess
- Left ventricular outflow tract obstruction.
- Aortic regurgitation.

Use this view to measure
- No specific measurements.

Key features of view
Most of the features are as for the 4-chamber view.

Left ventricular outflow tract Look at the size of the outflow tract and use colour flow mapping within the tract to look for aortic regurgitation or flow turbulence due to obstruction.

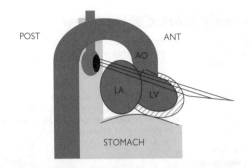

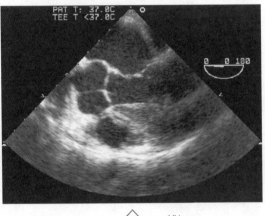

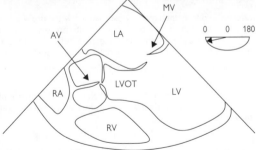

Fig. 4.5 Probe position for 5-chamber view with classic image.

Short axis (aortic valve) view

The perfect short axis view of the aortic valve, it can also provide information on the right heart and interatrial septum. It is equivalent to the parasternal short axis.

Finding the view
- From the apical 5-chamber view rotate the sector to around 50°.
- Optimize further with slight clockwise rotation of the probe.
- The probe may need to be withdrawn or advanced slightly to get the right scan plane. Focus on a clear view of the aortic valve.

What do you see?
Use this view to assess
- Aortic valve morphology and pathology.
- Perivalvular processes.
- Sometimes, tricuspid and pulmonary valves.
- Coronary artery origins can also be seen.
- Interatrial septum for patent foramen ovale.

Use this view to measure
- Left atrial diameter.
- Aortic valve orifice area and aortic root diameter.

Key features of view
Aortic valve The valve lies in the centre: left coronary cusp on the right; right coronary cusp at the bottom; and non-coronary on the left. Colour flow identifies regurgitation and, by adjusting the image to go through the tips of valve, planimetry can be used to measure aortic valve orifice area.

Aortic root Around the valve is the aortic root. Infection or aortic surgery can make this thickened or 'boggy'. Abscesses may also be seen.

Transverse sinus Between the aortic root and the left atrium is the transverse sinus (part of the pericardial space). This is only visible if it contains fluid.

Coronary arteries To display the coronary ostia withdraw the probe a few millimetres. Left main stem is at 2 o'clock and right coronary artery at 6 o'clock. The left coronary system can sometimes be tracked to, and beyond, the bifurcation. Colour flow and Doppler demonstrate flow.

Left atrium Lying between the probe and the aortic valve, this is a standard view for linear measures of left atrial size.

Tricuspid valve This can sometimes be seen below and to the left of the aortic valve. Better views are obtained from the right ventricular inflow/outflow view.

Pulmonary valve This lies below and to the right of the aortic valve

Interatrial septum The interatrial septum abuts the aortic root in the 10 o'clock position. The fossa ovalis is not usually seen but sometimes a patent foramen ovale or shunt can be demonstrated using colour flow or contrast.

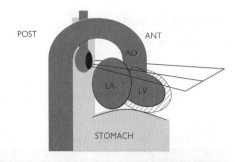

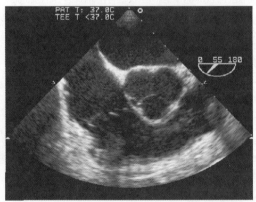

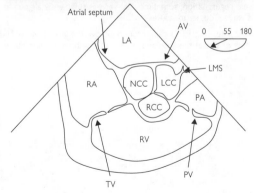

Fig. 4.6 Short axis view of aortic valve. LMS, Left main stem.

Short axis (right ventricular inflow/outflow) view

This view may be included for better display of the pulmonary valve and tricuspid valves.

It is very similar to the aortic view and can be skipped if the valves have already been adequately displayed. It is equivalent to the parasternal short axis transthoracic view.

Finding the view

- From the short axis aortic view rotate the sector to around 70–80°.
- The probe may need to be withdrawn or advanced slightly to get the right scan plane. Focus on a clear view of the pulmonary and tricuspid valves.
- The optimal view will include the tricuspid and pulmonary valve with the right ventricle wrapped around the aortic valve—a right ventricular inflow–outflow view.

What do you see?

Use this view to assess

- Pulmonary valve morphology and pathology.
- Tricuspid valve morphology and pathology.
- Base of right ventricle.

Use this view to measure

- Right ventricle and outflow tract size.

Key features of view

Pulmonary valve This lies below and to the right of the aortic valve. Use colour flow to assess for regurgitation.

Tricuspid valve Lies below and to the left of the aortic valve. Use colour flow to assess regurgitation; sometimes the valve is sufficiently aligned for continuous wave Doppler measures.

Right ventricle The ventricle wraps around below the aortic valve and measurements of size at the base and in the outflow tract are sometimes possible.

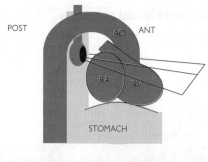

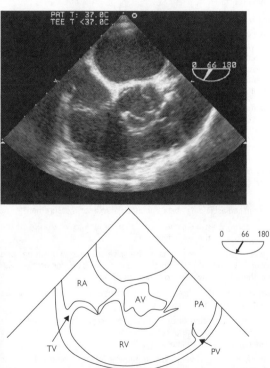

Fig. 4.7 Short axis view focused on right heart with change in sector.

Long axis (aortic valve) view

This view is equivalent to a transthoracic apical 3-chamber view or parasternal long axis view. It is used to assess the aortic and mitral valves as well as left ventricle, outflow tract, and left atrium. In some people the mitral valve is not seen well as it lies more inferiorly. An adjusted long axis view will then be needed to assess the mitral valve.

Finding the view

- From the short axis views rotate the sector to around 135°.
- Withdraw, advance, and turn the probe slightly to get the scan plane.
- Focus on a clear view of the aortic valve and ascending aorta.
- The optimal view will include two clear valve leaflets and a straight ascending aorta.

What do you see?

Use this view to assess

- Aortic valve morphology and pathology.
- Mitral valve morphology and pathology.
- Perivalvular processes.
- Left ventricular outflow tract and membranous septum.
- Ascending aorta.

Use this view to measure

- Aortic root, sinuses, and ascending aorta.
- Left atrial size.

Key features of view

Aortic valve The right coronary cusp is seen at the bottom and non-coronary cusp at the top. Colour flow will demonstrate regurgitation and this can be a good view for identifying vegetations or masses.

Aortic root The entire aortic root, including sinuses of Valsalva, sinotubular junction, and ascending aorta, should be visible for measurement.

Ascending aorta Slight adjustment can often bring into view a lot of the proximal portion of the ascending aorta.

Mitral valve A2 and P2 segments of the valve are seen and can be used for colour flow and other Doppler measures. However, for proper visualization the probe may need to be advanced slightly.

Left atrium The atrium lies nearest the probe and linear size can be measured from probe to aortic root.

Left ventricle The septum (including the membranous septum below the aortic valve) and inferolateral (or posterior) wall can usually be seen to assess wall motion abnormalities.

Right ventricle The right ventricular outflow is just seen below the aortic valve and sometimes the pulmonary valve is partially visible

Transverse sinus This lies between aortic root and left atrium and is visible if it contains fluid.

LONG AXIS (AORTIC VALVE) VIEW

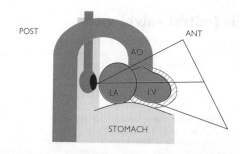

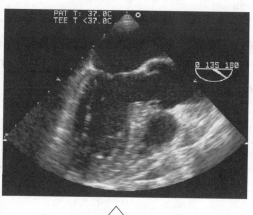

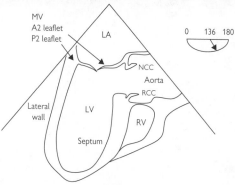

Fig. 4.8 Long axis view demonstrates aortic valve and left ventricle.

Long axis (mitral valve) view

This view is a slight adjustment of the long axis aortic view but focused on the mitral valve. If the views of the mitral valve were already optimal in the aortic long axis image this view can be skipped.

Finding the view
- From the long axis aortic view, at around 135°, advance the probe slightly.
- Focus on a clear view of the mitral valve and try and get an unforeshortened left ventricle.
- The optimal view will include two clear mitral valve leaflets.

What do you see?
Use this view to assess
- Mitral valve morphology and pathology.
- Left ventricular global and regional function.

Use view to measure
- Doppler measures of mitral regurgitation and stenosis.

Key features of view
The features are similar to those of the long axis aortic view (except the aortic valve may be less clear).

Mitral valve A2 and P2 segments of the valve are seen. Colour flow can map regurgitation and assess flow convergence and vena contracta. The valve is also usually aligned for Doppler measures.

Atrial septum (bicaval) view

This is a unique transoesophageal view with no equivalent transthoracic image. It is perfect for studying both atria and the septum.

Finding the view

- From the long axis views rotate the sector to around 110°.
- Turn the probe clockwise away from the left ventricle. You will see the septum come into view as a line across the screen.
- Withdraw, advance, and turn the probe. Focus on a clear view of the septum, with the 'dip' of the fossa ovalis in the centre.
- The optimal view includes inferior and superior vena cavae on either side with the right atrial appendage visible on the right.

What do you see?

Use this view to assess

- Drainage of superior and inferior vena cavae.
- Assessment for atrial septal defect and patent foramen ovale.
- Drainage of right upper pulmonary vein.
- Eustachian valve.

Use this view to measure

- The tricuspid regurgitation jet may be aligned for Doppler measures.
- A slightly adjusted view can be used to look at the right upper pulmonary vein flow.

Key features of view

Left and right atria The left atrium is nearest the probe.

Interatrial septum This is the most prominent feature and can be qualitatively assessed for thickness and atrial septal defects. Colour flow mapping and contrast provide more detailed information on interatrial shunts.

Inferior vena cava and Eustachian valve These lie on the left of the image and flow can be mapped with colour flow. The Eustachian valve is seen as a mobile strand originating from the orifice of the inferior vena cava.

Superior vena cava and christa terminalis These lie on the right of the image with the christa terminalis usually seen as a bright bar below the superior vena cava separating it from the right atrial appendage.

Right atrial appendage This is a wide-mouthed, shallow, trabeculated appendage lying on the right of the image below the superior vena cava. Atrial pacing wires may be seen hooking into the appendage.

Tricuspid valve The tricuspid valve may be seen in the far field. To optimize the valve image advance the probe. Colour flow can assess regurgitation and the valve is often aligned for Doppler measures.

Right upper pulmonary vein To see the vein the probe needs to be turned anticlockwise slightly to focus on the superior vena cava. The right upper pulmonary vein lies close to the superior vena cava. The vein is often aligned for Doppler measures. This view is used to look for abnormal pulmonary venous drainage.

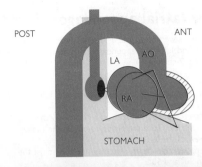

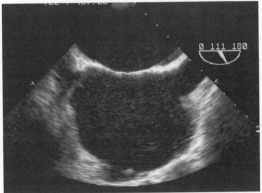

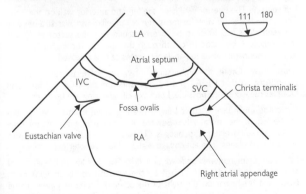

Fig. 4.9 Bicaval view.

Two chamber (atrial appendage) view

This view is important for several features of the left heart: mitral valve; left ventricular function; and left atrial appendage. The view is equivalent to the transthoracic apical 2-chamber view.

Finding the view

- Rotate back from the bicaval view to see mitral valve and left ventricle.
- Change the sector to around 75°.
- Withdraw and advance the probe to focus on a clear view of the mitral valve and left ventricle. Turn the probe to obtain the longest (unforeshortened) view of the left ventricle.
- To see the left atrial appendage clearly you may need to adjust the sector angle between 90° and 50°.
- The optimal view includes mitral valve, left atrial appendage, and an unforeshortened left ventricle. An unforeshortened left ventricle and left atrial appendage may not be visible in the same view and in this case separate images should be stored for each feature

What do you see?

Use this view to assess

- Global and regional left ventricle function, wall thickness.
- Mitral valve morphology (orifice, prolapse).
- Left atrial appendage.
- Left upper pulmonary vein.

Use this view to measure

- Left ventricle diastolic and systolic dimensions.
- Ejection fraction.
- Mitral valve.
- Left atrial appendage velocities.

Key features of view

Left ventricle The inferior wall is on the left and anterior wall on the right. This is the preferred view for measurement of left ventricular size because the ventricle is less likely to be foreshortened with the sector at 70–90° (the plane can be made to cut through the apex by turning the probe). Regional abnormalities and papillary muscles can be assessed.

Mitral valve Often a commissural view, i.e. valve is cut along its commisure so that P1, A2 and P3 segments are seen. Colour flow and Doppler measures are possible. Long axis of valve ring can be assessed.

Left atrial appendage A curved finger heading down from the left atrium to the left of the mitral valve. Beware of variation in anatomy, multiple lobes, or retroverted appendages. These will need assessment with atypical scan planes. The appendage is aligned for Doppler measures.

Left upper pulmonary vein and 'warfarin' ridge. This lies above the left atrial appendage and is divided from it by the warfarin (or coumadin) ridge (seen as a bright bar on the right of the screen). Probe may need to be withdrawn slightly to view vein. Vein is aligned for Doppler measures.

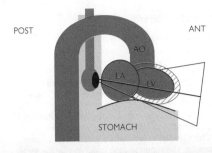

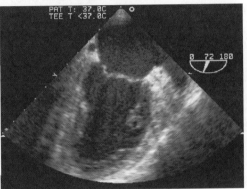

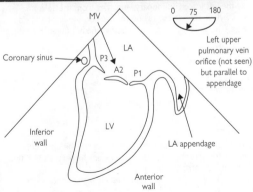

Fig. 4.10 2-chamber view cutting across mitral valve commissure.

Pulmonary vein views

Each pulmonary vein requires a separate view.

Finding the views

Right upper pulmonary vein
- The right upper pulmonary vein is best seen in the adjusted atrial septal (bicaval) view lying close to the superior vena cava. This view also allows Doppler alignment.
- The vein can also be identified starting from the apical 4-chamber 0° view. Rotate the probe to the right-hand side of the image and withdraw slightly. The right upper pulmonary vein is seen adjacent to, and wrapping around, the superior vena cava. Varying the sector angle between 0° and 20° can be useful to lengthen out the vein.

Right lower pulmonary vein
- The right lower pulmonary vein is best identified starting from the apical 4-chamber 0° view. Rotate the probe to focus on the right-hand side of the image (as when finding the right upper pulmonary vein) and then advance the probe slightly. The vein should be seen just below the right upper pulmonary vein.

Left upper pulmonary vein
- The left upper pulmonary vein is best seen in the adjusted 2-chamber view lying parallel to, and above, the left atrial appendage. This view also allows Doppler alignment.
- The vein is also seen with sector set to 0°. Rotate the probe to focus on the left-hand side of the image and withdraw slightly. Look for the vein orifice.

Left lower pulmonary vein
- To identify the left lower pulmonary vein start from the apical 4-chamber 0° view. Rotate the probe to focus on the left-hand side of the image. The vein should be seen below the left upper PV orifice.

What do you see?

Use these views to assess
- All four pulmonary veins.

Use these views to measure
- Pulmonary vein flow in upper pulmonary veins.

Identifying pulmonary veins

- At 0° the lower veins roughly lie perpendicular to the ultrasound beam (across the screen) while the upper veins lie parallel with the beam (pointing towards the probe).
- As the names suggest the lower veins lie below the upper veins. If an upper vein is identified then advance the probe slightly to see the lower vein and vice versa.
- Colour flow mapping is very useful to identify the veins. The colour flow will demonstrate blood flow out of the veins into the atrium.

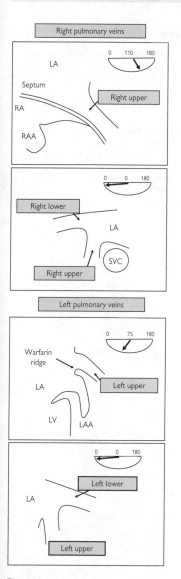

Fig. 4.11 Different viewing positions to identify pulmonary veins.

Coronary sinus view

Seeing the coronary sinus can be useful in some procedures such as electrophysiology studies or pacing device placement. It also allows assessment of congenital abnormalities such as a persistent left superior vena cava.

Finding the view
- Start from a 4-chamber view at 0°.
- The coronary sinus wraps around and below the mitral valve, opening into the right atrium. Therefore advance the probe so that the image plane cuts below the mitral valve. This may be helped by some retroflexion of the probe.
- The optimal view has the coronary sinus perpendicular across the screen opening into the right atrium.

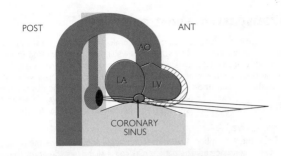

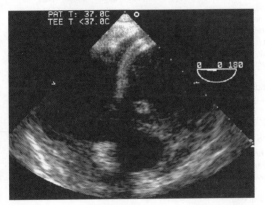

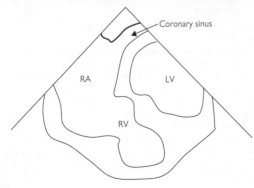

Fig. 4.12 Coronary sinus view.

Transgastric short axis views

Transgastric scanning can be quite uncomfortable to the conscious and mildly sedated patient. Transgastric views should be performed in well-sedated, compliant patients when further information is required. They can also be routinely performed intraoperatively. Short axis views are equivalent to transthoracic parasternal short axis views and can often be adjusted to create mid-papillary and mitral valve level views. They can be particularly useful intraoperatively to monitor left ventricular function.

Finding the view

- From the 4-chamber view, with sector angle at 0°, advance the probe several centimetres. The patient may rouse slightly as you enter the stomach.
- Angulate the probe forwards hard to try and get it at right angles.
- Withdraw the probe so the transducer tip presses on the upper stomach wall, against the diaphragm, underneath the heart.
- Make slight adjustments by turning the probe, as well as withdrawing and advancing until the left ventricle is seen in short axis.
- Keep the probe angulated forward.
- By withdrawing and advancing the probe along the bottom of the heart it is theoretically possible to see the left ventricle at several levels, e.g. mid-papillary, mitral valve.
- The optimal view is an on-axis cross-section through the left ventricle.

What do you see?

Use this view to assess

- Global and regional left ventricular function, wall thickness.
- Mitral valve morphology.
- Can provide information on right ventricular size and function.
- Pericardial effusions may be seen.

Use this view to measure

- Left ventricular size and wall thickness.

Key features of view

Left ventricle (mid-papillary level) With a clear short axis cut through the ventricle the septum, anterior, lateral, and inferior walls of the ventricle can be reviewed. This is an ideal view for measures of left ventricular size and thickness.

Mitral valve (mitral valve level) A slight withdrawal of the probe from the mid-papillary level should bring the image plane up to the mitral valve. You should be able to scan through the chordae up to the leaflet tips. Use colour flow to highlight regurgitation jets.

Right ventricle The right ventricle can be seen as a crescent around one side of the left ventricle. This view can give an impression of right ventricular size and function.

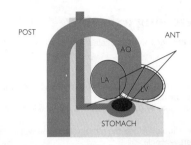

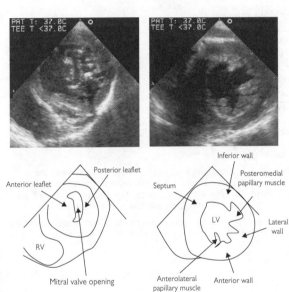

Fig. 4.13 Transgastric short axis views at mitral valve (left) and mid-ventricle (right) levels.

Transgastric long axis view

The long axis view provides an unparalleled view of the mitral subvalvular apparatus.

Finding the view
- From the short axis (mid ventricle) view rotate the sector angle to 90°.
- Keep hard probe angulation.
- Make slight adjustments by turning the probe until the left ventricle is seen in long axis.
- The optimal view should include the mitral valve, subvalvular apparatus, and left ventricle.

What do you see?
Use this view to assess
- Global and regional left ventricular function, wall thickness.
- Mitral valve morphology.
- Subvalvular mitral apparatus.

Use this view to measure
- Left ventricular size and wall thickness.

Key features of view

Left ventricle Similar to the 2-chamber view the inferior wall is nearest the probe and anterior walls in the far field. Foreshortening occurs easily. This can provide information on wall thickness as well as global and regional function.

Mitral valve and subvalvular apparatus A commissural view, the leaflet anatomy is not always clear but the subvalvular apparatus can be incredibly detailed. The different order chordae tendinae as well as both papillary muscles can be reviewed. Colour flow can map regurgitation.

Left atrium and left atrial appendage The left atrium is present but not usually in great detail. You may notice the left atrial appendage in the far field.

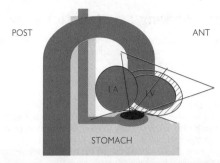

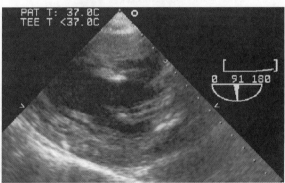

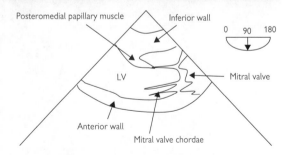

Fig. 4.14 Transgastric long axis view of left ventricle.

Transgastric long axis (aortic) view

The long axis view can be modified slightly to bring the left ventricular outflow tract into the image for Doppler measures across the aortic valve.

Finding the view
- From the long axis view rotate the sector angle to 110°.
- Keep hard probe angulation.
- Make slight adjustments by turning the probe until the left ventricular outflow tract is seen in the far field. Colour flow may help to identify flow through the aortic valve.
- The optimal view should include the left ventricular outflow tract aligned in the far field for Doppler measures.

What do you see?
Use this view to assess
- Doppler measures of aortic valve velocities.

Use this view to measure
- Aortic and left ventricular outflow tract velocities.

Key features of view
Aortic valve and left ventricular outflow tract. The aortic valve may be seen close to the mitral valve in the far field. Colour flow mapping may make this more apparent. The valve and outflow tract are aligned in this view for Doppler measures.

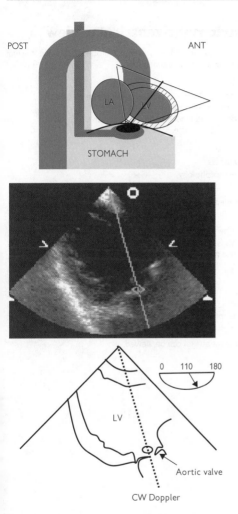

POST

ANT

LA

LV

STOMACH

0   110   180

LV

Aortic valve

CW Doppler

Fig. 4.15 Transgastric long axis view of left ventricle outflow tract.

Transgastric right ventricular view

This view can be difficult to find. However, if available, it can give a useful assessment of the right ventricle and inflow.

Finding the view
- From the transgastric long axis view turn the probe clockwise.
- The right ventricle should appear in long axis.
- The optimal view should include the tricuspid valve, subvalvular apparatus, and right ventricle.

What do you see?
Use this view to assess
- Tricuspid valve morphology.
- Subvalvular tricuspid apparatus.

Use this view to measure
- No specific measurements.

Key features of view

Right ventricle This is an unusual 2-chamber view of the right ventricle and atrium but can give an impression of right-sided chamber size.

Tricuspid valve and subvalvular apparatus As with the mitral views the subvalvular apparatus is usually detailed. Colour flow can map regurgitation and there can be a qualitative assessment of tricuspid valve function. As the right ventricle is relatively difficult to see with transoesophageal imaging this may provide a good window to look for tricuspid valve pathology, e.g. vegetations and masses.

Right atrium The right atrium can be viewed.

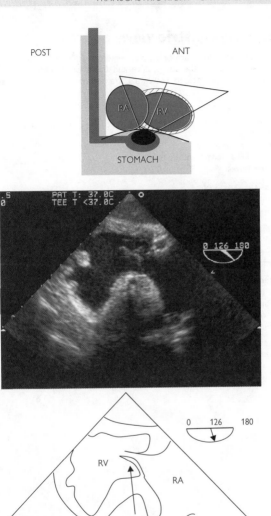

Fig. 4.16 Transgastric right ventricle view.

Deep transgastric view

Deep transgastric views are only really required when Doppler information is needed about the aortic valve and transthoracic imaging is not possible. The view tries to recreate a transthoracic apical 5-chamber view.

Finding the view
- From the transgastric long axis view advance the probe further into the stomach.
- Set the sector to 0°.
- Ensure full angulation of the probe and good contact with the stomach wall.

What do you see?
Use this view to assess
- Left ventricular outflow tract and aortic valve.

Use this view to measure
- Left ventricular function.
- Aortic and left ventricle outflow tract velocities (if seen—may need some sector angle adjustment).

Key features of view
Aortic valve and left ventricular outflow tract The aortic valve lies in the far field and may be highlighted by colour flow mapping. The primary purpose of this view is to align the valve and outflow tract for Doppler measures.

Left ventricle Similar to the 5-chamber view. The septum and lateral wall are seen.

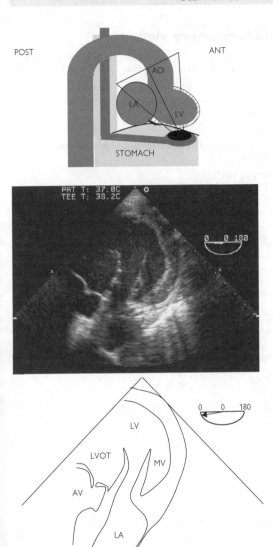

Fig. 4.17 Deep transgastric view.

Pulmonary artery view

A view to study the pulmonary arteries. Can be useful to assess size of artery or to look for large pulmonary emboli.

Finding the view
- Start from the short axis aortic view. The sector may need to be reduced slightly to 40°.
- Withdraw the probe slowly until you have a short axis view of the ascending aorta.
- The probe may need to be angulated forward gently to demonstrate the pulmonary artery.

What do you see?
Use this view to assess
- Ascending aorta for dissection or dilatation.
- Pulmonary artery.

Use this view to measure
- Aortic and pulmonary artery size.

Key features of view

Pulmonary arteries The right pulmonary artery is seen wrapping around the aorta and lies between the aorta and probe. The main pulmonary artery is seen to the side of the aorta. The left pulmonary artery is not visible.

Ascending aorta A short segment of the ascending aorta can usually be seen to assess dilatation, dissection, and atheroma.

Superior vena cava The superior vena cava is seen in cross-section close to the aorta and right pulmonary artery.

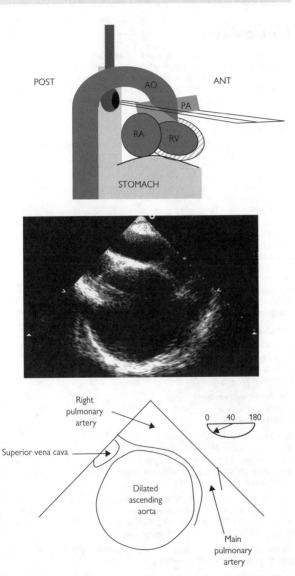

Fig. 4.18 View of the pulmonary artery. Note reverberation artefact at 10'o'clock in the ascending aorta.

Aortic views

The final views are usually the aortic views. They can be important for monitoring dissection or studying atheroma. They can also be used to assess aortic flow in aortic regurgitation. The only limitation is that transoesophageal echocardiography cannot see the distal ascending aorta and proximal part of the aortic arch as the air-filled left bronchus obscures the view.

Finding the view

- The ascending aorta is seen in the pulmonary artery view. Obtain the short axis aortic view at 50° and then withdraw the probe slowly to scan up the aorta as far as images are maintained.
- For descending aorta and aortic arch start from the 4-chamber view with a sector angle of 0° and turn the probe slowly so that it starts to face posteriorly.
- It is usually best to turn the probe anticlockwise until the circular aorta is seen.
- Decrease the depth so that the aorta fills the screen and you usually also need to reduce the gain slightly.
- The probe may then be withdrawn slowly to scan up the aorta. As the aorta curls around the oesophagus some slight turning will be required as the probe is withdrawn.
- The optimal view is a cross-section through the aorta. A long axis view can also be useful and is achieved by changing the sector angle to 90°.

What do you see?

Use this view to assess
- Aortic dissection or dilatation.
- Atheroma and thrombus.
- Aortic flow, e.g. in aortic regurgitation.

Use this view to measure
- Aortic size.
- Aortic flow.

Key features of view
Descending aorta There is good depiction of the aortic walls and their layers as well as thickening and gross atherosclerosis. If measurements are made, annotate images with the depth of the probe so that serial measures are possible.

Aortic arch At the top of the descending aorta the aortic cross-section will disappear and the vessel opens out into the arch. The origin of the left subclavian artery may be seen. By changing the sector angle to 90° at this point a cross-section can be maintained.

Ascending aorta A short segment of the ascending aorta can usually be seen to assess dilatation, dissection, and atheroma.

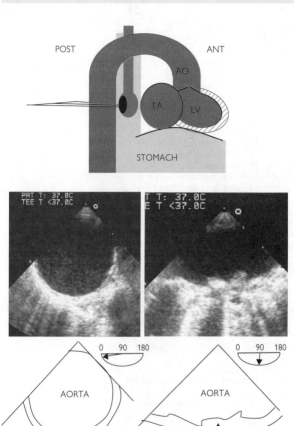

Fig. 4.19 Aortic short (on left) and long (on right) axis views.

Transoesophageal: anatomy and pathology

Mitral valve

Transoesophageal echocardiography is one of the most important tools for the assessment of mitral valve disease and allows superb visualization of the mitral valve. The modality is particularly good for systematic reviews of the different valve segments. Mitral valve anatomy is described on p. 104. Briefly, there are two leaflets, each with three segments (or scallops)—a large anterior and a crescent-shaped posterior leaflet. Assessment of stenosis and regurgitation follows the same criteria as for transthoracic imaging (pp 106 and 110) but there can be more detailed study of the pathology underlying regurgitation or stenosis.

Normal findings

Views

- The mitral valve is sliced through in virtually all the oesophageal views and the 'screen wiper' principle allows rotation through the valve in multiple planes. The oesophageal views also allow alignment of Doppler and colour flow across the valve. The minimum views are oesophageal views at around 0°, 135°, and 80°.
- The transgastric views provide additional information in both the short axis 0° (pulled back slightly) and the long axis 90° view for the subvalvular apparatus.

Normal findings

- 4-chamber 0° view—this classically includes A2, A1, and P1 segments of the valve (however, there is a tendency to cut more through A2 and P2 if the left ventricular outflow tract is seen and the papillary muscles are not evident).
- Long axis 135° view—equivalent to the apical 3-chamber view, this gives a good stable view of A2 and P2.
- 2-chamber 75° view—stable 'commissural' view to see P1 and P3 either side of A2 (Fig 5.1 top right). Rotation of the probe allows you to swing more towards the anterior or posterior leaflet. Slight adjustment of sector angle will bring in the left atrial appendage and localize A1/P1 next to the appendage (Fig 5.1 bottom left).
- Transgastric short axis view or 'fish mouth' view has the A3/P3 segments nearest the probe. The 90° view can be used to look at the papillary muscles and chordae.

Identifying mitral valve leaflets and segments

There are rigorous descriptions of which leaflets are seen in which view. Initially, standard views allow good orientation but, as you become more familiar, you can play with these by slight adjustments of the probe to cut through the 3D structure at any point. There are two tips to identify the segments and leaflets.

- The anterior leaflet is nearest the septum/left ventricular outflow tract and usually appears larger than the posterior leaflet.
- The segments are numbered so that A1 and P1 are nearest the left atrial appendage.

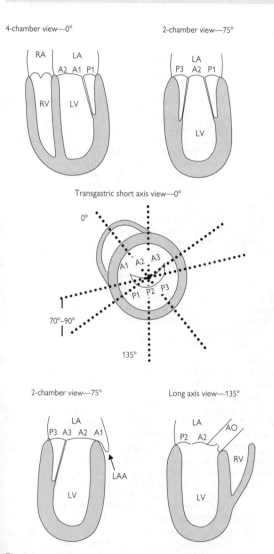

Fig. 5.1 Key views to assess mitral valve. In the 2-chamber view display of the mitral valve can be varied. A classic commisural 2-chamber view is demonstrated in the top right figure and a view adjusted to focus on the anterior leaflet is shown in the bottom left figure.

Mitral regurgitation

Transoesophageal echocardiography should be used to assess mitral regurgitation:
- when transthoracic echocardiography is inconclusive or technically difficult;
- to define the underlying mechanism for planning mitral valve surgery.

Transoesophageal echocardiography is particularly useful to visualize where the regurgitant jet passes through the valve. Higher transducer frequencies and multiple views result in more reliable measurements of both vena contracta and flow convergence. However, the different transducer frequency, pulse repetition frequency, and gain also mean they appear larger on transoesophageal images than transthoracic images.

Assessment

Appearance
- Start in the 4-chamber 0° view and map the regurgitation with colour flow. Scan through the valve at different angles to establish the shape, direction, and pattern of the jet. Comment on:
  - where the regurgitation passes through the valve, e.g. perforation, failure of coaption, prolapse of a leaflet scallop;
  - direction of eccentric jets (anterior or posterior).
  - how far back the jet extends (involving pulmonary veins?);
  - if there are several jets comment on each.
- Use transgastric long axis 90° view to look at subvalvular apparatus. Comment on: papillary muscle and chordae with reference to shortening and rupture.
- Report associated features, e.g. atrial size, ventricular size and function.

Grading severity
Assess severity on vena contracta, flow convergence, pulmonary venous flow, and valve structure. Colour jet area can also be used.

Colour Doppler jet area Difficult to assess with transoesophageal echocardiography because sector width often does not include the whole of the atrium. Proportional jet area is therefore difficult to judge. 4-chamber 0° and long axis 135° views may give the best impression.

Vena contracta Transoesophageal echocardiography provides excellent views and resolution for measurement of colour flow through the valve.
- In oesophageal views choose the plane that cuts though the jet.
- Zoom in on the colour flow through the mitral valve and record a loop. Identify the image with maximal flow through the valve.
- The vena contracta is the narrowest region of the regurgitant jet (usually as it passes through the valve). Report the diameter.

Flow convergence (PISA) Transoesophageal echocardiography is ideal for measurement of flow convergence zone and PISA (proximal isovelocity surface area; p. 118).

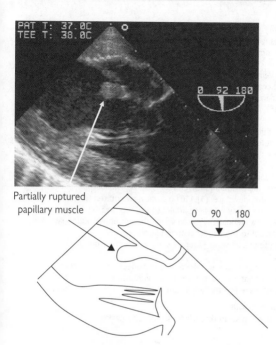

Partially ruptured
papillary muscle

Fig. 5.2 Transgastric long axis view demonstrates subvalvular apparatus. In this example there is a partial papillary muscle rupture.

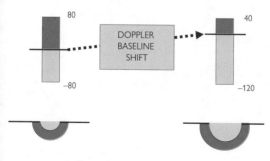

Flow convergence zone becomes
larger and more clearly defined

Fig. 5.3 Flow convergence radius is more clearly defined with Doppler baseline shift.

Pulmonary venous flow

Transoesophageal echocardiography provides a unique opportunity to visualize directly all four pulmonary veins and measure pulmonary vein flow. The contralateral pulmonary vein to an eccentric jet (i.e. left pulmonary veins for an anteriorly directed jet and vice versa) should be used to avoid changes in flow due to washing of the jet into the vein.

- In 4-chamber 0° view rotate to the left to identify the left-sided veins (p. 408). Advance or withdraw the probe to bring them into view. The left upper pulmonary vein usually points towards the probe and left lower pulmonary vein is perpendicular. To help with identification place colour flow by the edge of the atrium and look for the jets of the veins draining into the atrium. Slight changes in the plane angle can optimize the view. Right-sided veins are identified in the same way but with rotation to the right. Again the right upper pulmonary vein points towards the probe and lower vein is perpendicular.
- Alternative views are: (1) 110° bicaval view rotated to the left—right upper pulmonary vein lies parallel to the septum; (2) 2-chamber 75° (left atrial appendage) view, in which the left upper pulmonary vein lies parallel to the left atrial appendage.
- Place the pulsed wave Doppler sample volume around 1cm into the chosen vein.
- Look at the systolic and diastolic components of the spectral trace and comment if the systolic wave is blunted or reversed relative to the diastolic wave (normally the same direction, with systolic dominant).

Supportive measures

These can be measured as for transthoracic imaging (p. 116).

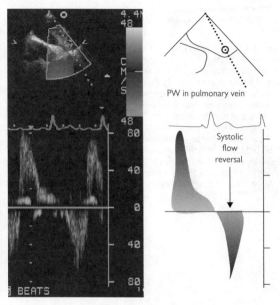

PW in pulmonary vein

Systolic flow reversal

Fig. 5.4 Pulmonary venous flow with an example of abnormal systolic flow reversal.

Carpentier (functional) classification of mitral valve disease

The Carpentier classification (types 1 to 3) is sometimes used to report the functional basis for mitral regurgitation. This categorizes cause according to leaflet motion. It is relevant to different surgical approaches.

• Normal leaflet motion (type 1).
  • Annular dilatation causes regurgitation due to failed coaption.
  • Leaflet perforation (e.g. from endocarditis).
• Excessive leaflet motion (type 2).
  • Prolapse of leaflet edge beyond the plane of the annulus.
  • Mitral valve prolapse, rupture/dysfunction of the papillary muscle.
• Restricted leaflet motion (type 3).
  • Leaflet edge remains below the plane of the annulus during systole. Usually secondary to rheumatic disease, left ventricle dilatation, posterior wall infarction.

Table 5.1 Parameters to assess mitral regurgitation

	SPECIFIC SIGNS OF SEVERITY	
	MILD	**SEVERE**
Vena contracta	<0.3cm	>0.7cm
Jet (Nyquist, 50–60cm/sec)	<4cm^2 or <20% LA; small & central	>40% LA; large & central or wall impinging & swirling
PISA r (Nyquist, 40cm/sec)	None/minimal	
	(<0.4cm)	Large (>1cm)
Pulmonary vein flow	—	Systolic reversal
Valve structure	—	Flail or rupture
	SUPPORTIVE SIGNS OF SEVERITY	
	MILD	**SEVERE**
Pulmonary vein flow	Systolic dominant	
Mitral inflow	A-wave dominant	E-wave dominant (>1.2m/sec)
CW trace	Soft & parabolic	Dense & triangular
LV & LA	Normal size LV if chronic MR	Enlarged LV & LA if no other cause

Report as MODERATE if signs of regurgitation are greater than MILD but there are no signs of SEVERE regurgitation.

Mitral valve prolapse

The clear images of valve leaflets allow identification of the morphology of mitral valve prolapse. Description of mitral valve prolapse is a common indication for transoesophageal echocardiography because of its clinical importance to determine whether a valve can be repaired or will need to be replaced. The commonest prolapse is of the P2 segment of the posterior leaflet. This is amenable to a standard repair procedure.

Assessment of prolapse

- Start by studying the regurgitation. Comment on appearance and severity. Take particular note of the direction of the jet as a guide to the predominant leaflet prolapse. Anteriorly directed suggests posterior leaflet prolapse and vice versa. Centrally-directed suggests bileaflet prolapse. Also comment on changes in left atrial and ventricular size and function.
- Then use the 'screen wiper' principle to scan through the mitral valve at 0°, 135°, 110°, 80°. Ensure each segment has been studied (Fig. 5.6). Comment on which segments prolapse. If the tips of the segment reflect back into the left atrium then report this as 'flail' (important when planning the operation).
- Remember that both leaflets, or more than one segment, may be prolapsing. Report all the abnormalities.
- A transgastric 0° short axis view can be used to confirm the segment prolapse and the long axis 90° view should be used to look at the subvalvular apparatus to identify chordae or papillary muscle rupture.

LONG AXIS VIEW

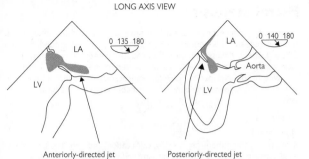

Anteriorly-directed jet   Posteriorly-directed jet

Fig. 5.5 Examples of mitral valve prolapse in 135° long axis views. Left figure shows a posteriorly directed jet due to anterior leaflet prolapse and the right figure shows an anteriorly directed jet.

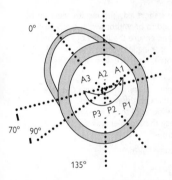

Fig. 5.6 The short axis figure demonstrates which scallops are seen in the 3 key views. The 4-chamber 0° and long axis 135° views are particularly good for studying the central scallops (A2 and P2). The 2-chamber view with sector variation between 70° and 90° can be very useful for looking at the side scallops (A1/P1, A3/P3).

Mitral stenosis

Transoesophageal echocardiography is not routinely used to assess mitral stenosis but stenosis should be commented upon and graded if seen during a study. Assessment may be needed if there are poor transthoracic windows or if the valve is being assessed for percutaneous intervention with balloon valvotomy (p. 366). Transoesophageal echocardiography is also used intraoperatively during percutaneous interventions on the mitral valve.

Assessment

Appearance

Remember to comment on mobility, calcification, and chordae. Comment on associated valvular lesions, left atrium, and right heart.

Grading severity

Grade severity on planimetered area supported by pressure half-time (P1/2) and pressure gradient (p. 108).

Planimetry

- A transgastric 0° view provides a short axis 'fish mouth' view of the mitral valve. The probe may need to be withdrawn and advanced slightly to optimize the image and ensure the *leaflet tips* are being imaged. Identify the maximum opening in diastole and trace along the inner edge of the leaflets. Report the surface area of the orifice.

Pressure half-time and pressure gradient

- In any oesophageal view with good alignment through the valve align the continuous wave Doppler through the mitral valve orifice. For pressure half-time, measure the slope of the E-wave diastolic flow on the spectral trace (p. 108). Trace the Doppler waveform to obtain mean pressure gradient. Remember:

  Mitral valve area = 220/pressure half-time

Table 5.2 Parameters to assess mitral stenosis

Parameter	MILD	MODERATE	SEVERE
MV area (cm^2)	2.2–1.5	1.0–1.5	<1.0
MV P½ time (msec)	100–150	150–220	>220
Mean pressure gradient (mmHg)	<5	Variable	>10
Tricuspid regurgitation velocity (m/sec)	<2.7	Variable	>3
PA pressure (mmHg)	<30	Variable	>50

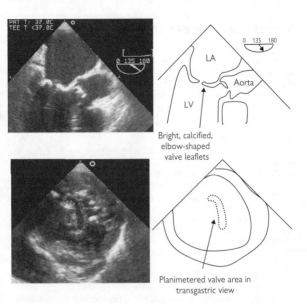

Fig. 5.7 Examples of mitral stenosis in 4-chamber and transgastric views. Note planimetered surface area in short axis view.

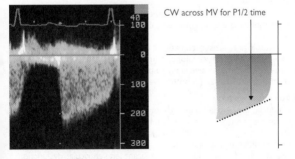

Fig. 5.8 Pressure half-time measured in a long axis view.

Mitral valve pre-operative assessment

Transoesophageal echocardiographic assessment of the mitral valve is essential before surgery. The key surgical decision in the patient with mitral regurgitation is whether the valve is to be repaired or replaced. With mitral stenosis the request for imaging is usually to assess suitability for valvotomy or to determine severity of stenosis and effects on left ventricle and other valves.

What the surgeon wants to know

Mitral regurgitation

The main objectives prior to mitral valve surgery are to define the following.

- Underlying anatomical details of the mitral regurgitation. Include a full assessment (p. 354) and ensure comments on:
  - severity;
  - central or eccentric;
  - if prolapse, which scallops are affected and whether flail elements.
- Size of annuloplasty ring likely to be needed if repaired or size of valve if replaced. Report:
  - mitral annulus size (in both valve axes if possible);
  - leaflet length.
- Presence and location of annulus calcification. There is a risk of annulus leak if in an area of repair.
- If regurgitation secondary to endocarditis, comment on complications of the endocarditis: fistulae from left ventricle to aorta, right ventricle, or left atrium; mitral valve annulus abscess; other valve involvement in endocarditis (typically aortic or tricuspid valve).

Mitral stenosis

- Underlying anatomical details of the mitral stenosis. Include a full assessment and ensure comments on:
  - severity;
  - pathological basis: rheumatic or degenerative.
- Assess suitability for valvuloplasty (p. 366).
- Size of replacement valve likely to be needed. Report:
  - mitral annulus size (in both valve axes if possible).

For all mitral surgery

- Left atrial size. A dilated left atrium (>50mm) provides good surgical exposure of mitral valve directly through a left atrial incision. If the left atrium is normal size or only mildly increased the surgeon may need an alternative surgical approach (e.g. trans-atrial septum).
- Assessment of cardiac function. Significant left ventricular dysfunction caused by mitral regurgitation encourages mitral valve repair rather than replacement if repair results will be predictable and effective.
- Reports of other valve disease, particularly the aortic valve.

Pre-operative versus intraoperative assessment

The severity of mitral regurgitation may be underestimated during intraoperative transoesophageal echocardiography. Preload, afterload, and inotropic state of the heart are reduced during general anaesthesia. Therefore, all patients undergoing valve surgery should have transoesophageal imaging prior to surgery. Assessment of the valve intraoperatively should take into account the pre-operative information and changes in conditions due to the anaesthesia. Volume loading and inotropic agents can sometimes be used to mimic haemodynamics comparable to those without anaesthesia.

Factors that make mitral valve repair unfavourable

- Annular calcification. It is most common in the posterior annulus and can extend into the myocardium and leaflets.
- Marked mitral ring dilatation (>5cm in the 2-chamber view).
- Extensive leaflet disease (3 or more prolapsed or flail segments seen).

Risk of systolic anterior motion of mitral valve post-repair

If repair is planned then it is important to assess, before surgery, the risk of postoperative systolic anterior motion of the anterior leaflet and consequent obstruction of the left ventricular outflow tract. This causes obstruction in ~15% of patients after mitral valve repair. The following findings in the preoperative examination are associated with an increased risk of postoperative systolic anterior motion of the anterior leaflet and should be reported if present.

- Excess mitral leaflet tissue. Particularly elongated anterior leaflet causing an increase in slack leaflet available to obstruct the left ventricular outflow tract.
- Anteriorly displaced papillary muscles.
- Non-dilated left ventricle.
- Narrow mitral–aortic angle.
- More anterior position of the leaflet coaptation point due to relatively large posterior mitral leaflet: Anterior to posterior leaflet ratio <1.
- Distance from the coaptation point to the septum <2.5cm.

In high risk cases the surgical approach may be modified. In patients with an excessive posterior leaflet a sliding leaflet plasty can be carried out after resection of the P2 segment. Another option is the use of a rigid ring to increase the anteroposterior diameter—in particular if the coaptation line is displaced anteriorly after resection of excessive tissue.

Mitral valve balloon valvotomy

Transoesophageal echocardiography is performed routinely to assess suitability for percutaneous valvotomy for treatment of mitral stenosis. Contraindications to intervention that should be reported include:
• left atrial appendage thrombus;
• moderate mitral regurgitation or greater;
• severe aortic or tricuspid valvular disease.

Echocardiographic scoring of mitral valve morphology can be preformed to predict successful outcome. The commonest is the Wilkin's scoring based on 4 features each scored 1–4, giving a minimum score of 4 and maximum of 16. The lower the score the more suitable the valve for balloon valvotomy. A score of >8 suggests poor long-term outcome with percutaneous intervention.

Leaflet mobility
1 Highly mobile with restriction of leaflet tips only.
2 Mid-portion and base of leaflets have reduced mobility.
3 Valve leaflets move forward in diastole mainly at the base.
4 No or minimal forward movement of the leaflets in diastole.

Valvular thickening
1 Leaflets near normal (4–5mm).
2 Mid leaflet thickening, pronounced thickening of the margins.
3 Thickening extends through entire leaflet (5–8mm).
4 Pronounced thickening of all leaflet tissue (8–10mm).

Subvalvular thickening
1 Minimal thickening of chordal structure just below the valve.
2 Thickening of chordae extending up to 1/3 of chordal length.
3 Thickening extending to the distal 1/3 of chordae.
4 Extensive thickening and shortening of all chorda extending down to the papillary muscles.

Valve calcification
1 A single area of increased echo brightness.
2 Scattered areas of brightness confined to the leaflet margins.
3 Brightness extending into the mid-portion of the leaflets.
4 Extensive brightness through most of the leaflet tissue.

Mitral valve repair

Post-operative assessment

Assessment of mitral valve repair should be based on the following.

Residual regurgitation

Despite competent valve at surgical inspection and leak test by the surgeon there may still be significant valvular regurgitation in the beating, volume-loaded heart. This may be due to ischaemic wall dysfunction or systolic anterior motion of the mitral valve. Use standard parameters to assess severity, location, and likely underlying mechanism.

- Moderate to severe residual regurgitation usually requires surgical revision or conversion to valve replacement.
- Para-annulus leak can occur after repair if there was a large posterior leaflet resection. Even mild degrees of para-annulus leak usually require further surgical revision to avoid post-operative haemolysis.

New stenosis

After repair of the mitral valve the repaired leaflet usually appears thickened, shortened, and almost immobile. Use continuous wave Doppler to assess transmitral pressure gradient and pressure half-time. However, pressure-half-time method may be inaccurate immediately post-operatively (the method assumes that the left atrial and ventricular compliance do not affect the pressure decline, but up to 72 hours after surgery compliance is altered). Interpret orifice area taking into account heart rate and stroke volume. Stenosis is often due to under-sized annuloplasty.

Systolic anterior leaflet motion/left ventricular outflow obstruction

Systolic anterior leaflet motion/left ventricular outflow obstruction can be due to the mitral valve repair but also can be caused by haemodynamic factors. Inotropic agents, vasodilators, and low volume states provoke systolic anterior leaflet motion/left ventricular outflow obstruction in susceptible patients and have to be discontinued before considering re-intervention. In some patients beta-blockers may be useful. To demonstrate systolic anterior motion of the mitral leaflet use the aortic long-axis 135° view. 2D can demonstrate abnormal valve movement. However, Doppler measurements have to be performed in gastric views, which may be difficult in theatre.

- Consider whether effects can be reduced by changes in cardiac physiology (improved left ventricular cavity size and diastolic filling): increase left ventricular filling; stop/reduce positive inotropic drugs; commence β-blockade; pace the ventricle. Monitor effectiveness of medical treatments with repeat echocardiography. If medical management fails surgical revision of repair or valve replacement may be indicated.

Left ventricle function

Hypo- or akinesis of the lateral and inferoposterior wall can be due to circumflex artery injury if sutures are too deep into the mitral ring.

Aortic valve

Aortic valve function can be impaired by deep suture placement in the anterior annulus.

Mitral valve replacement

Post-operative assessment

Mechanical valve dysfunction is more likely with: over-sized prosthesis; small left ventricular cavity; double valve replacement; abnormal mechanical prosthesis orientation. Bioprosthesis dysfunction may be due to distorted annulus due to over-sizing or suture looping of cusps. The key features to assess immediately after replacement are the following.

Valve prosthesis regurgitation

Use colour flow to look for normal prosthesis wash jets (closing jets) and differentiate from paravalvular regurgitation. If present consider severity.

- For biological valves mild central jet is normal. Small degrees of para-prosthetic regurgitation (mechanical and biological valves) immediately after surgery often improve with protamine administration. If moderate to severe central regurgitation and restricted prosthetic cusp opening/ closing, surgical intervention is normally indicated.

Valve prosthesis opening

Use 2D imaging to look for symmetrical, synchronized opening and closing of prosthesis leaflets. Look for functional stenosis (measure prosthesis mean gradient and effective orifice area). If abnormal opening consider:

- relation between prosthetic valve and subvalvular apparatus. With mechanical bileaflet prostheses, opening and closing may be reduced because the leaflets impinge on the subvalvular apparatus (posterior leaflet may be preserved in valve replacement);
- left ventricular filling. If not adequately filled re-evaluate when filled and contracting. If still dysfunctional surgical intervention is advisable.

Left ventricular outflow tract obstruction

Assess valve movement with 2D imaging and colour flow mapping in the outflow tract. Pulsed wave Doppler in the outflow tract may be possible in transgastric view. Obstruction may be due to septal hypertrophy combined with a high profile prosthesis intruding into the outflow tract.

Cardiac function

After mitral surgery use 2D imaging to re-assess global and regional left and right ventricular function. With acute correction of regurgitation left ventricular ejection fraction can be expected to drop (e.g. from 60–70% to 40%) due to sudden reduction in left ventricle stroke volume, without proportional reduction in left ventricle cavity size, combined with a variable degree of underlying impaired contractile function. Mitral valve replacement for mitral regurgitation has more adverse physiological effects on left ventricular function than repair.

- If left ventricular filling is adequate but cavity is dilated and global ejection fraction is <30%, consider inotropic support and monitor response with echocardiography until stable haemodynamics.
- If there is a new lateral or inferoposterior wall motion abnormality consider whether the circumflex artery could have been damaged.
- Always consider other general causes for acute severe deterioration in global cardiac dysfunction after cardiopulmonary bypass.

Bileaflet valve (long axis view)—Mitral position

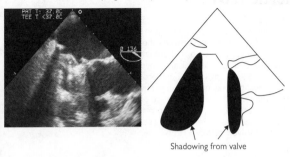

Shadowing from valve

Bileaflet valve (2 chamber view)—Mitral position

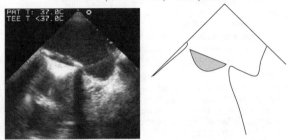

Fig. 5.9 Examples of mechanical mitral valve prostheses in long axis and 2-chamber views. Two views of a St Jude bileaflet mechanical valve protheses at different angles. Long axis (top figure) cuts through both leaflets and 2-chamber (bottom figure) cuts across one of the leaflets.

Aortic valve

Very good views of the aortic valve can be obtained with transoesophageal echocardiography because there is only the left atrium, which is a clear fluid-filled window, between the valve and the probe. Aortic valve anatomy is described on p. 122 but essentially comprises three cusps and associated sinuses of Valsalva, named after the coronary arteries that derive from them (right, left, non-coronary).

Transoesophageal echocardiography is indicated to study the aortic valve when transthoracic images are of insufficient quality or when better spatial resolution is needed to provide complete assessment of valve pathology, e.g. vegetations, aortic root abscesses, aortic valve area, and prosthetic valve function.

Normal findings

Views

- The best views to see the aortic valve are the 50° short axis view and 135° long axis view. These can be supported by the 5-chamber 0° left ventricular outflow view.
- Additional information is obtained from transgastric views, which provide better alignment for Doppler. The aortic valve can be studied with a transgastric long axis 110° view and a deep transgastric 0° view.

Aortic valve

- *5-chamber 0° left ventricular outflow view.* This provides a limited first view of the left ventricular outflow and with colour flow can be used to judge whether there is any aortic regurgitation
- *Short axis 50° view.* This is the first clear view and is similar to the transthoracic parasternal short axis but upside down. A cross-sectional view of the cusps is seen (left on the right, non-coronary on the left, and right nearest the right ventricle). To optimize the image try slight rotation or movement of the probe up and down. Get all three cusps in view, of equal size. Withdraw the probe further to bring the coronary arteries, sinotubular junction, and then the ascending aorta into view. Advance the probe to see the left ventricular outflow tract. Colour flow mapping allows positioning of aortic regurgitant jets. This view also allows the stenotic valve area to be measured.
- *Long axis 135° view.* This view is similar to the transthoracic parasternal long axis. Right and non-coronary cusps are seen (non-coronary nearest the probe and right nearest the right ventricle). Use the view to measure aortic root, sinotubular junction, and valve annulus.
- *Transgastric 110° long axis view.* This view allows the outflow tract to be aligned with Doppler. The aortic cusps are sometimes seen in the far field but it can be difficult to get a clear image. Colour flow can help to pick out the outflow tract.
- *Deep transgastric view.* This is an alternative to align the Doppler with the outflow tract and valve. It provides an equivalent view to the transthoracic apical 5-chamber but is difficult to obtain. If there are good transthoracic windows it will not add more information.

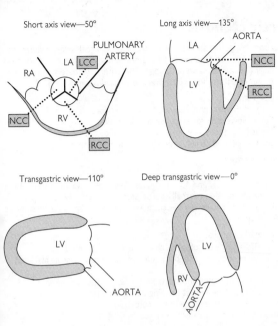

Fig. 5.10 Key views to assess the aortic valve. NCC, Non-coronary cusp; RCC, right coronary cusp; LCC, left coronary cusp.

Aortic stenosis

Evaluation of aortic stenosis with transoesophageal echocardiography follows the same routine as for transthoracic but with more emphasis on 2D imaging to assess valve pathology. The criteria to determine severity are the same as those for transthoracic echocardiography (p. 124).

Assessment

Bear in mind the potential causes of aortic stenosis.
- In all the views look for evidence of calcification.
- In the 50° short axis view look at number of cusps.
- Look at associated structures—aortic root dilatation, etc.

Grading severity

2D imaging

In 50° short axis view and 135° long axis view look at valve motion. If the valve appears to open normally aortic stenosis is unlikely to be present. In the 135° long axis view, if the cusps separate by >12mm aortic stenosis is mild or better.

Planimetered valve orifice
- In 50° short axis view obtain a clear image of all cusp edges.
- Move the probe back and forth until the cusp tips in systole are seen in plane.
- Zoom on to the valve and store a loop. Scroll through the loop and try and identify the largest opening during systole.
- Trace along the inner edge of the cusps.
- Report the surface area of the orifice.

Problems with planimetered measures

Shadowing from heavy calcification can make it difficult to get an accurate area or it may be difficult to the get the open tips in systole in plane with the probe.

Doppler assessment

Both the velocity across the valve and the continuity equation require aortic valve vti (or peak flow), left ventricular outflow tract vti (or peak flow), and left ventricular outflow tract dimension. It is often easier and more accurate to do this with transthoracic echocardiography but can also be done during a transoesophageal examination.
- Use a transgastric 110° long axis or deep transgastric view to line up the continuous wave Doppler with the aortic valve and aorta.
- Acquire a spectral recording and trace the aortic vti.
- In the same view acquire a pulsed wave Doppler in the left ventricular outflow tract and trace the vti.
- Measure the left ventricular outflow tract diameter in the 135° long axis view.
- Report the peak velocity or use the standard continuity equation:

valve area = LVOT area × LVOT vti/aortic vti

Table 5.3 Parameters to assess severity of aortic stenosis

	MILD	MODERATE	SEVERE
Peak velocity (m/sec)	2.0–3.0	3.0–4.0	>4.0
Peak gradient (mmHg)	<35	35–65	>65
Mean gradient (mmHg)	<20	20–40	>40
Valve area (cm²)	2.0–1.5	1.0–1.5	<1.0

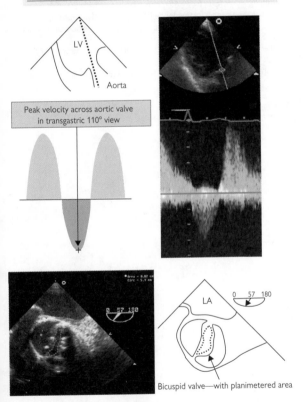

Fig. 5.11 Measurement of aortic stenosis severity from Doppler in a transgastric 110° view (top) and planimetered area in a short axis 50° view (bottom).

Aortic regurgitation

In evaluation of aortic regurgitation with transoesophageal echocardiography there is more emphasis on 2D imaging to assess cause. Doppler criteria to determine severity are as for transthoracic (p. 134).

Assessment

Bear in mind potential causes of regurgitation and study both valve and aortic root (p. 133).

2D imaging

- In all the views look for evidence of abnormal valve motion.
- In the 50° short axis view look at the valve and position of regurgitation. Study the sinuses and aortic root.
- In the 135° long axis view look at the aortic root dimension and check for dissection.
- Comment on the location and direction of jet.

Table 5.4 Parameters to determine severity of aortic regurgitation

	SPECIFIC SIGNS OF SEVERITY	
	MILD	SEVERE
Vena contracta	<0.3cm	>0.6cm
Jet (Nyquist, 50–60cm/sec)	Central, <25% of LVOT	Central, >65% of LVOT
Descending aorta	No or brief early diastolic flow reversal	
	SUPPORTIVE SIGNS OF SEVERITY	
	MILD	SEVERE
Pressure half-time	>500msec	<200msec
Descending aorta	—	Holodiastolic flow reversal
Left ventricle (only for chronic lesions)	Normal LV	Moderate or greater LV enlargement (no other cause)

Report as MODERATE if signs of regurgitation are greater than MILD but there are no features of SEVERE regurgitation.

Grading severity

Colour flow Doppler

- Aortic regurgitation can first be identified in the 5-chamber 0° view although this will not give you an idea of severity.
- The 50° short axis view with colour flow provides an impression of where the regurgitation is and the area of the jet relative to the left ventricular outflow tract.
- The 135° long axis view with colour flow provides the most information to assess severity. This view can be used to assess vena contracta and jet width relative to left ventricular outflow tract.

Aortic flow reversal

- In the 90° long axis aortic view pulsed wave Doppler with some correction for angle will allow assessment of aortic flow in diastole. Some diastolic flow reversal is normal. Holodiastolic flow reversal is associated with severe aortic regurgitation.

Continuous wave Doppler

- For continuous wave assessment of aortic regurgitation a transgastric 110° long axis view or deep transgastric view is required to align the Doppler signal.
- Look at density of signal, deceleration slope, and peak velocity. However, these are less accurate with transoesophageal echocardiography because of technical limitations in alignment.

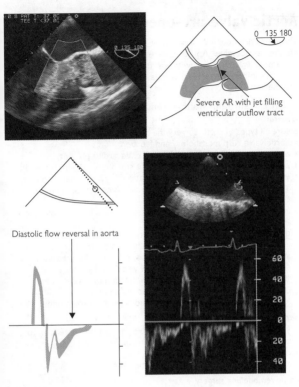

Fig. 5.12 Abnormal aortic flow reversal (bottom) and broad vena contracta filling outflow tract (top) consistent with severe regurgitation.

Aortic valve pre-operative assessment

Thorough pre-operative assessment allows careful planning of surgery on the aortic valve. Aortic valve replacement is the most frequently performed valve surgery with an increasingly elderly population. Pre-operative information should include data on the valve, the left ventricle, and the aorta.

What the surgeon wants to know

General

Before all types of aortic surgery the basic information needed is:
- aortic valve cusp morphology and function;
- aortic root size (look for abscesses if endocarditis present);
- aortic annulus size (to judge prosthesis size if replacement planned);
- evidence of sinotubular junction dilatation (if >25% bigger than aortic annulus then aortic homograft or stentless bioprosthesis may be contraindicated);
- ascending aortic dimension and geometry (ascending aorta dilatation >45mm may require replacement).
- descending aorta size and flow velocity.
- anatomy and dynamics of left ventricular outflow tract (in surgery for stenosis check for a sub-aortic stenosis to account for gradient);
- coronary ostia size, location, and flow velocity (check for ostial stenoses and coronary sinus calcification that might complicate coronary reimplantation in aortic root replacement);
- left ventricular cavity size, function, and degree of hypertrophy.

Bicuspid valves

In young patient with bicuspid aortic valve pay particular attention to:
- concomitant abnormalities in left ventricular outflow tract;
- coronary anatomy;
- aortic root, arch, and descending aortic structure.

Aortic remodelling surgery

In aortic root remodelling check native valve can be preserved. Look at:
- aortic cusp morphology and mobility;
- aortic sinus geometry.

Aortic valve replacement

Post-operative assessment

Assessment of an aortic valve replacement should be based on the following.

- *Valve prosthesis opening*. With 2D imaging (and if appropriate M-mode) look at valve opening and closing. Assess velocity across the aortic valve with continuous wave Doppler from a transgastric view. Expect a mean gradient of <15mmHg.
- *Valve prosthesis regurgitation*. Check for regurgitation with colour flow. There may be small closing jets or some mild paraprosthetic regurgitation early after surgery before protamine is given. If regurgitation is seen, determine severity and location (trans or para-prosthetic). If bio-prosthetic valve consider whether due to annulus distortion. Para-valvular regurgitation is more likely with a calcified aortic annulus, infected aortic valve, or redo aortic valve surgery

Endocarditis

If surgery was for endocarditis ensure any abscesses or fistulae that were present have been treated.

Cardiac function

For all surgery, determine global and regional cardiac function using standard techniques (p. 164). Expect an ejection fraction of >40% if normal before surgery. If significant impairment consider causes as for mitral valve surgery (p. 370) and in particular consider whether there has been damage to coronary artery ostia.

Coronary arteries

Check for proximal coronary obstruction or occlusion. In short axis views assess proximal coronary lumen size and flow velocity. Acute coronary obstruction can be due to acute thrombus, emboli, prosthesis malposition and/or oversizing, or abnormal coronary anatomy in congenital aortic valve disease.

Other

- Monitor for left ventricle outflow tract obstruction and systolic anterior motion of mitral valve (see mitral valve surgery, p. 368).
- If there has been septal myomectomy check for a ventricular septal defect.

Ball and cage valve—aortic position

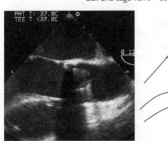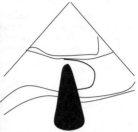

Single disc valve—aortic position

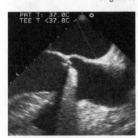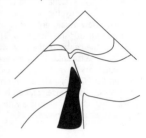

Stented bioprosthesis

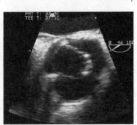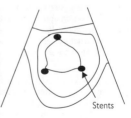

Stents

Fig. 5.13 Examples of prosthetic valves in the aortic position. Top figure is a long axis view of a ball-and-cage valve and the middle figure of a single disc valve. The bottom figure is a short axis view of a stented bioprosthesis.

Tricuspid valve

The tricuspid valve is often included in a transoesophageal study but, unless the indication is a study of endocarditis, is not the primary focus. Generally, the right heart is more difficult to study with transoesophageal echocardiography because it lies furthest from the probe.

Normal findings
Views
- The best views are: 4-chamber 0°; bicaval 110°; short axis 80° (right ventricular inflow/outflow); and right ventricular transgastric 90°.

Findings
- *4-chamber 0° view.* The tricuspid valve lies on the left and the probe may need to be advanced slightly to optimize the image.
- *Bicaval 110° view.* Usually used to study the atrial septum. If the probe is advanced slightly, the tricuspid valve often comes into view in the far field. This view usually gives good alignment for Doppler studies.
- *Right ventricle 80° short axis view.* The aortic valve appears in cross-section in the centre of the view with the right ventricle wrapped around in the far field. This view gives a good image of both tricuspid and pulmonary valves with tricuspid valve on the left.
- *Transgastric 90° long axis view.* From a standard long axis view of the left ventricle, clockwise rotation of the probe to the right can some-times bring the right ventricle with the tricuspid valve and subvalvular apparatus clearly into view.

Tricuspid regurgitation and stenosis

Assessment of regurgitation
Assess regurgitation on appearance and severity according to the standard transthoracic guidelines (p. 144). Vena contracta, PISA, continuous wave tracing, valve structure, and right heart size are usually possible with transoesophageal echocardiography, whereas jet area and hepatic vein flow are not.

Assessment of stenosis
Usually assessment is better by transthoracic echocardiography. Assess stenosis on appearance (leaflet thickening or restriction) and severity according to the transvalvular gradient. Remember: severe tricuspid stenosis is usually associated with a gradient of 3–10mmHg.

Table 5.5 Parameters to assess severity of tricuspid regurgitation

	MILD	SEVERE
Jet (Nyquist, 50–60cm/sec)	<5cm^2	>10cm^2
Vena contracta	—	>0.7cm
PISA r (Nyquist 40cm/sec)	<0.5cm	>1cm
Hepatic vein flow	Normal	Systolic reversal
Valve structure	Normal	Abnormal
CW trace	Soft & parabolic	Dense & triangular
RV/RA/IVC	Normal size	Usually dilated

Report as MODERATE if signs of regurgitation are greater than MILD but
there are no features of SEVERE regurgitation.

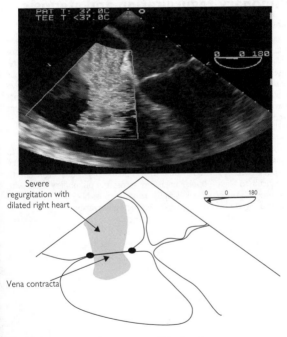

Fig. 5.14 Severe tricuspid regurgitation in 4-chamber view.

Pulmonary valve

Transoesophageal imaging may have limited views of the pulmonary valve. The only views in transoesophageal echocardiography that allow Doppler alignment through the valve are a modified transgastric view of the right heart and a view back from the aortic arch level.

Normal findings

Views and findings

The most useful views are based on the short axis 50–80° (right ventricular inflow/outflow) view. This is a short axis view through the aortic valve in which the pulmonary valve is seen lying behind and slightly to the right of the aortic valve. The image may be optimized by changing the angle slightly from between 50° and 90° until the leaflets of the pulmonary valve are seen opening and closing.

Pulmonary regurgitation and stenosis

Assessment of regurgitation

Colour flow mapping of the pulmonary valve identifies small regurgitant jets in most people—usually to one edge near the aortic valve. If there appears to be more regurgitation than normal, comment on size, site, and severity. Grade severity as *mild*, *moderate*, or *severe* based on colour flow mapping criteria (p. 158). It may also be possible to use pulsed wave Doppler in the pulmonary artery to look for holodiastolic flow reversal consistent with severe pulmonary regurgitation. Remember to comment on the right heart.

Assessment of stenosis

Pulmonary stenosis is usually valvular and congenital (e.g. related to rubella, Noonan's, or tetralogy of Fallot). Comment on valve appearance and appearance of related structures (i.e. pulmonary artery, right heart). It is difficult to align Doppler measures across the pulmonary valve with transoesophageal echocardiography may be possible. The degree of opening using 2D may be used as an estimate of severity.

Table 5.6 Parameters to assess pulmonary regurgitation

	MILD	SEVERE
Jet size on CFM	<10mm long	Large with wide origin
CW density & shape	Soft & slow	Dense & steep
Pulmonary valve	Normal	Abnormal
Pulmonary artery flow	Increased	Greatly increased compared to systemic circulation
Right ventricle size	Normal	Dilated

If features suggest more than MILD regurgitation but no features of SEVERE, grade as MODERATE.

Table 5.7 Parameters to determine severity of pulmonary stenosis

	MILD	MODERATE	SEVERE
Peak gradient (mmHg)	10–25	25–40	>40
Valve area (cm^2)	>1.0	0.5–1.0	<0.5

Left ventricle

Transthoracic echocardiography usually provides sufficient information to assess the left ventricle and should be the echocardiographic modality of choice. With transoesophageal echocardiography the left ventricle is in the far field and it can be difficult to obtain unforeshortened views. Transgastric imaging allows accurate measures from stable short axis views. Nevertheless, during a transoesophageal study assessment should be made of the left ventricle, even if limited, to gain an impression of left ventricle size and function and help interpretation of other findings.

Anatomy is described on p. 162. Briefly, the left ventricle is a muscular cavity with a septum dividing it from the right ventricle. The ventricle has anterior, inferior, lateral, and inferolateral (or posterior) walls.

Indications for transoesophageal imaging

Transoesophageal echocardiography is indicated when transthoracic windows are poor, in particular situations such as intensive care unit or cardiac recovery, or when intraoperative evaluation of cardiac function is needed during cardiac surgery.

Normal findings

Views

The key views to assess the left ventricle are the 4-chamber 0°, long axis 135°, 2-chamber 75°, and transgastric 0° short axis view.

Findings

- *4-chamber 0° view.* Equivalent to the the apical 4-chamber but usually with marked foreshortening of the left ventricle. The septum is on the left and lateral wall on the right. To realign the plane through the apex try probe retroflexion until the apex comes into view. The probe may lose contact with oesophagus on retroflexion.
- *Long axis 135° view.* Equivalent to the parasternal long axis, it is often easier to align through the apex with gentle rotation. The septum (anterior portion) is seen by the left ventricular outflow and the posterior (inferolateral) wall is on the left.
- *2-chamber 75° view:* Equivalent to an apical 2-chamber view. The inferior wall is on the left and anterior wall on the right. This is the preferred oesophageal view for measuring left ventricular size.
- *Transgastric short axis 0° view.* The best view to confidently assess left ventricular function and obtain systolic and diastolic measures of cavity size and wall thickness. Equivalent to a parasternal short axis view. Advancing and withdrawing the probe may make it possible to scan through the left ventricle in cross-section from apex to mitral valve. This is a mirror image of a parasternal short axis, i.e. inferior wall lies nearest the probe and anterior in the far field. Septum is still on the left and lateral wall on the right.

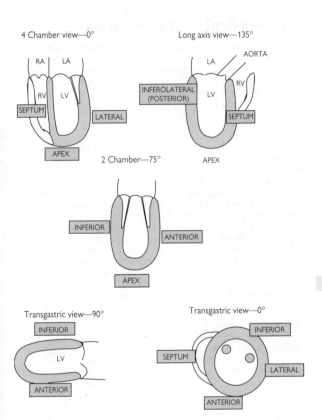

Fig. 5.15 Key views to assess the left ventricle.

Left ventricular size and mass

Report quantitative measures of size (p. 166) if measurements are possible and include a general summary: *normal*, *mild*, *moderate*, or *severe* dilatation; *normal*, *mild*, *moderate*, or *severe* hypertrophy. Both linear and volumetric measures are possible with transoesophageal echocardiography. Start with an overview of the ventricle in all views to gather an impression of appearance, size, and function.

Linear measures

2D imaging

- Optimize a transgastric 0° view at the mid-papillary level and record a loop.
- Identify the end-diastolic frame (widest ventricle). Measure from the inferior wall endocardial border to the anterior wall endocardial border in a line at right angles to each wall. Measurement should be at the junction of the basal and middle thirds of the ventricle. Report the *left ventricular end-diastolic diameter*. Scroll through to identify the end-systolic frame (smallest ventricle) and use the same technique to measure the *left ventricular end-systolic diameter*.
- M-mode, although not usually done, is technically possible in this view.
- The 2-chamber 75° view gives another window to measure left ventricular diameters from anterior to inferior walls (Fig. 5.16).
- Left ventricular hypertrophy can be assessed with measures of wall thickness from the transgastric 2D images at end-diastole in the septum and posterior wall.

Volumetric measures

Simpson's method Simpson's method of discs (p. 168) can be used if the oeso-phageal views allow planes to be set up through the apex. It relies on a good 4-chamber 0° view that is not foreshortened.

- In the 4-chamber 0° view optimize an image of the left ventricle, with clear endocardial border and enough depth to include the apex.
- Record a loop. Trace around the border in diastolic and systolic frames to obtain *left ventricular end diastolic* and *end systolic volumes*.
- Measure left ventricular length from apex to middle of mitral valve in the same view to obtain *left ventricular long axis*.
- For biplane measures repeat the process using an optimized 2-chamber 75° view.

Area–length equation This method (p. 170) can be used based on a transgastric 0° short axis mid-papillary level view and 2-chamber view.

Mass

All the equations and models from transthoracic echocardiography (p. 174) can be applied. Use the transgastric 0° view in place of parasternal short axis. For measurements based on apical 4- and 2-chamber views use the respective 4-chamber 0° and 2-chamber 75° views. Transoesophageal evaluation is reasonably accurate, but tends to report slightly higher left ventricular mass.

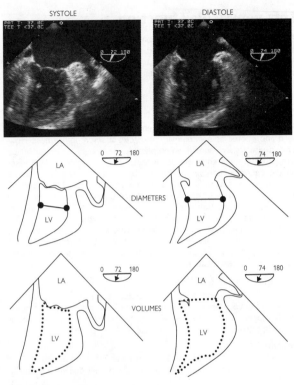

Fig. 5.16 Measures of left ventricular size in 2-chamber view.

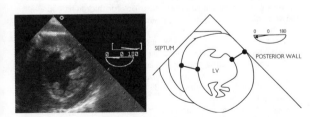

Fig. 5.17 Measures of wall thickness in transgastric view.

Left ventricular function

Assessment of left ventricular function with transoesophageal echocardiography is often needed in the context of intensive care or intraoperatively. Assessment has clinical importance and should be as comprehensive as possible. Minimal requirements are: left ventricular size and shape; systolic function including regional differences. Diastolic function assessment from transmitral and pulmonary vein flow is possible.

Global systolic function

As with transthoracic imaging an eyeball assessment of function is often used and quoted as *normal, mild, moderate, or severe impairment*. However, a visual gauge should, when possible, be backed up by quantification. Use the same equations as for transthoracic imaging (p. 188) based on the equivalent measures. The transoesophageal views for measurement of left ventricular diameters are the 4-chamber 0°, 2-chamber 75°, and transgastric views. Left ventricular diameters in transgastric views are measured from anterior wall to inferior wall in a line perpendicular to the long axis of the ventricle, at the junction of the basal and middle thirds of the long axis. Left ventricular volumes are traced as for transthoracic imaging—with care to avoid using foreshortened images. Doppler-based measures, e.g. dP/dT (p. 192), can be used from the oesophageal views of mitral regurgitation.

Regional systolic function

The usual requirement for regional assessment is to determine wall movement in coronary artery territories. The standard 16-segment model can be applied to transoesophageal images and technically wall motion scores are possible although not normally quoted (p.194).

Wall motion

- Use 4-chamber 0°, long axis 135°, 2-chamber 75°, and transgastric 0° views. Avoid foreshortening. Endocardial border definition is usually very good.
- Look at the segments and decide whether normal, hypokinetic (excursion <5mm), akinetic (excursion <2mm), or dyskinetic (endocardium moves out in systole). If you are unsure look for thickening >50% between diastole and systole. If present report as normal.
- Remember, most commonly:
  - left anterior descending artery supplies: mid and apical septum and lateral wall in 4-chamber 0° view; anterior wall and apex in 2-chamber 75° view, and septum and apex in long axis 135° view;
  - left circumflex artery supplies: basal and mid-segments of posterior (inferolateral) wall in long axis 135° view and lateral wall in 4-chamber 0° view;
  - right coronary artery supplies: inferior wall in 2-chamber 75° view and basal septum in 4-chamber 0° view;
  - transgastric short axis view has right coronary territory nearest the probe, left anterior descending territory in the far field, left circumflex territory supplying the lateral wall (on the right).

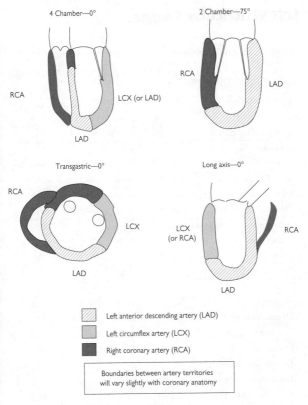

Fig. 5.18 Coronary supply to left and right ventricles.

Left ventricular ranges

Table 5.8 Ranges for measurements of LV size and mass in WOMEN[1]

	NORMAL	MILD	MODERATE	SEVERE
LV dimension				
LV d diameter, cm	3.9–5.3	5.4–5.7	5.8–6.1	>6.1
LV d diameter/BSA, cm/m^2	2.4–3.2	3.3–3.4	3.5–3.7	>3.7
LV d diam/height, cm/m	2.5–3.2	3.3–3.4	3.5–3.6	>3.7
LV volume				
LV d vol, mL	56–104	105–117	118–130	>130
LV d vol/BSA, mL/m^2	**35–75**	**76–86**	**87–96**	**>96**
LV s vol, mL	19–49	50–59	60–69	>69
LV s vol/BSA, mL/m^2	**12–30**	**31–36**	**37–42**	**>42**
Linear method: fractional shortening				
Endocardial, %	27–45	22–26	17–21	<17
Mid-wall, %	15–23	13–14	11–12	<11
2D method: Ejection fraction, %	>54	45–54	30–44	<30
Linear method				
LV mass, g	67–162	163–186	187–210	>210
LV mass/BSA, g/m^2	**43–95**	**96–108**	**109–121**	**>121**
LV mass/height, g/m	41–99	100–115	116–128	>128
LV mass/height^2, g/m^2	18–44	45–51	52–58	>58
Relative wall thickness, cm	0.22–0.42	0.43–0.47	0.48–0.52	>0.52
Septal thickness, cm	**0.6–0.9**	**1.0–1.2**	**1.3–1.5**	**>1.5**
Posterior wall thickness, cm	**0.6–0.9**	**1.0–1.2**	**1.3–1.5**	**>1.5**
2D method				
LV mass, g	66–150	151–171	172–182	>182
LV mass/BSA, g/m^2	**44–88**	**89–100**	**101–112**	**>112**

BSA, Body surface area; d, diastolic; s, systolic.
Bold rows identify best validated measures.

Table 5.9 Ranges for measurements of LV size and mass in MEN[1]

	NORMAL	MILD	MODERATE	SEVERE
LV dimension				
LV d diameter, cm	4.2–5.9	6.0–6.3	6.4–6.8	>6.8
LV d diameter/BSA, cm/m²	2.2–3.1	3.2–3.4	3.5–3.6	>3.6
LV d diam/height, cm/m	2.4–3.3	3.4–3.5	3.6–3.7	>3.7
LV volume				
LV d vol, mL	67–155	156–178	179–201	>201
LV d vol/BSA, mL/m²	**35–75**	**76–86**	**87–96**	**>96**
LV s vol, mL	22–58	59–70	71–82	>82
LV s vol/BSA, mL/m²	**12–30**	**31–36**	**37–42**	**>42**
Linear method: fractional shortening				
Endocardial, %	25–43	20–24	15–19	<15
Mid-wall, %	14–22	12–13	10–11	<10
2D method: Ejection fraction, %	>54	45–54	30–44	<30
Linear method				
LV mass, g	88–224	225–258	259–292	>292
LV mass/BSA, g/m²	**49–115**	**116–131**	**132–148**	**>148**
LV mass/height, g/m	52–126	127–144	145–162	>163
LV mass/height², g/m²	20–48	49–55	56–63	>63
Relative wall thickness, cm	0.24–0.42	0.43–0.46	0.47–0.51	>0.51
Septal thickness, cm	**0.6–1.0**	**1.1–1.3**	**1.4–1.6**	**>1.6**
Posterior wall thickness, cm	**0.6–1.0**	**1.1–1.3**	**1.4–1.6**	**>1.6**
2D method				
LV mass, g	96–200	201–227	228–254	>254
LV mass/BSA, g/m²	**50–102**	**103–116**	**117–130**	**>130**

BSA, Body surface area; d, diastolic; s, systolic.
Bold rows identify best validated measures.

1 Adapted from Recommendations for chamber quantification: a report of the American Society of Echocardiography Guidelines and Standards Committee and the Chamber Quantification Writing Group, developed in conjunction with the European Association of Echocardiography. *J Am Soc Echocardiogr* 2005; **18**: 1440–63.

Right ventricle

The right ventricle is more difficult to see with transoesophageal echocardiography than transthoracic imaging because it lies distant to the probe. However, with an appropriate combination of views it is possible to make a reasonable assessment of right ventricular size and function. Briefly, the anatomy consists of a free wall and the interventricular septum. The cavity is crescent-shaped and wrapped around the left ventricle. Inflow is through the tricuspid valve and outflow through the pulmonary valve.

Normal findings

Views

- The key views are: 4-chamber 0° view and short axis 50–80° view (right ventricular inflow/outflow view). These can be supplemented by transgastric 90° long axis view with the probe rotated clockwise away from the left ventricle.

Findings

- *4-chamber 0° view.* Rotation to the right focuses on the right atrium with the right ventricle furthest from the probe. The right ventricular free wall and septum can be seen. This view permits some assessment of size although the right ventricle is often foreshortened.
- *Short axis 50-80° view.* This is also known as the right ventricular inflow/outflow view and allows assessment of the more basal areas of the right ventricular free wall, as well as, the tricuspid and pulmonary valves.
- *Transgastric 0° view.* This permits a short axis view through the left ventricle. The right ventricle will be seen wrapping around the left ventricle (equivalent to a parasternal short axis). This view can be used to look for septal motion to assess right ventricular overload.
- *Transgastric 90° view (right ventricle).* Rotating the probe away from the standard left ventricular view may demonstrate the right ventricle. The tricuspid subvalvular apparatus is visible.

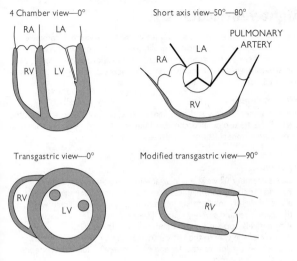

4 Chamber view—0°

Short axis view–50°—80°

Transgastric view—0°

Modified transgastric view—90°

Fig. 5.19 Key views to assess the right ventricle.

Right ventricular size

The complex shape of the right ventricle makes assessment complex and it may be difficult to support a qualitative impression with quantitative measures. Assessment is similar to that for transthoracic imaging (p. 212). Use several views and comment on wall thickness, cavity size, and outflow tract size.

Wall thickness

Use 4-chamber 0° view and comment on thickness of the free wall at the level of the tricuspid valve chordae tendinae. Do not include epicardial fat or coarse trabeculations in the measurement.

Cavity size

Qualitative

- Use 4-chamber 0° view and look at mid-cavity diameter. Right ventricular size is *normal* if less than 2/3 left ventricular size, *mildly dilated* if slightly smaller than left ventricle, *moderately dilated* when the same size, and *severely dilated* if larger than the left ventricle.
- Alternatively, look at the apex and report as *mildly dilated* if greater than 2/3 of the way to the left ventricular apex, *moderately dilated* if it reaches the left ventricular apex, and *severely dilated* if it extends past the left ventricle.

Quantitative

- Use the 4-chamber 0° view optimized to avoid foreshortening. Measure *right ventricular length*, *tricuspid annulus diameter*, and *mid-cavity diameter*.
- Use right ventricular inflow/outflow 80° view to measure *right ventricular outflow diameter, pulmonary valve diameter, and pulmonary artery diameter*. See Table 5.10, p. 402.

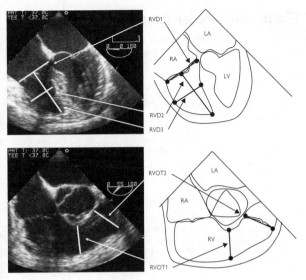

Fig. 5.20 Measures of right ventricular size. These are equivalent to the transthoracic measures (p. 213). RVD1, Tricuspid annulus diameter; RVD2, mid-cavity diameter; RVD3, right ventricle length; RVOT1, diameter of basal part of right ventricle; RVOT2, diameter of outflow tract at pulmonary valve. A further measure can be made of pulmonary artery diameter.

Right ventricular function

The right ventricle contracts in both the long and short axis. The long axis assessment of the free wall is the easiest way to gauge right ventricular function.

Assessment

- Use a 4-chamber 0° view.
- Make a qualitative judgement of global function as normal or impaired impairment based on whether there is less than the accepted 15–20mm movement of the tricuspid annulus towards the apex.
- If you want to quantify the global assessment, measure right ventricular length in diastole and systole and calculate fractional shortening:

$$\frac{\text{RV diastolic length} - \text{RV systolic length}}{\text{RV length in diastole}}$$

  Normal is >35% fractional shortening.

- For regional assessment look at the basal, mid-, and apical segments of the free wall in the same 4-chamber view and report them as hypokinetic, akinetic, or dyskinetic. As with the left ventricle you should be able to see right free wall thickening to corroborate a statement of normal or hypokinetic motion.

Right ventricular ranges

Table 5.10 Parameters to assess right ventricular size and function

	NORMAL	MILD	MODERATE	SEVERE
RV dimensions (apical 4-chamber)				
Basal RV diameter, cm	2.0–2.8	2.9–3.3	3.4–3.8	>3.8
Mid RV diameter, cm	2.7–3.3	3.4–3.7	3.8–4.1	>4.1
Base–apex length, cm	7.1–7.9	8.0–8.5	8.6–9.1	>9.1
RVOT diameter (parasternal short axis)				
Mid-ventricle, cm	2.5–2.9	3.0–3.2	3.3–3.5	>3.5
Pulmonary valve level, cm	1.7–2.3	2.4–2.7	2.8–3.1	>3.1
PA diameter (parasternal short axis)				
Pulmonary artery, cm	1.5–2.1	2.2–2.5	2.6–2.9	>2.9
RV area and fractional area change (apical 4-chamber)				
RV diastolic area, cm^2	11–28	29–32	33–37	>37
RV systolic area, cm^2	7.5–16	17–19	20–22	>22
Fractional area change, %	32–60	25–31	18–24	<18

In relation to Fig. 5.20 apical 4-chamber view: basal RV = RVD1; mid RV = RVD2; base–apex = RVD3.

In relation to Fig. 5.20 parasternal short axis view: aortic valve to free wall = RVOT1; level of pulmonary valve = RVOT2; pulmonary artery = PA1.

Left atrium

The transoesophageal probe lies directly behind the left atrium and provides excellent views of inflow from all pulmonary veins, outflow across the mitral valve, left atrial appendage, and atrial septum. Any left atrial masses are therefore seen much better with transoesophageal than transthoracic imaging.

Normal findings

Views

- The key views are: 4-chamber 0° view, 2-chamber 75° view, long axis 135° view, and bicaval 110° view.
- Further views are needed to look at the pulmonary veins (p. 408).

Findings

- *4-chamber 0° view.* The left atrium lies directly in front of the probe and may allow measurements of left atrial size.
- *Long axis 135° view.* Again the left atrium lies in front of the probe and can be measured.
- *2-chamber 75° view.* With slight adjustments this is perfect for assessment of the left atrial appendage.
- *Bicaval 110° view.* The standard view for assessment of the septum.

Left atrial size

Left atrial size is difficult to assess with transoesophageal echocardiography because the imaging sector does not normally include the whole of the atrium. Volumes are therefore unreliable particularly if the atrium is dilated. Linear measures are possible but may miss longitudinal changes.

Assessment

- Give a qualitative judgement of size based on size relative to the left ventricle. If the left atrium entirely fits into the 4-chamber 0° view it is likely to be small. If it appears similar in size to the left ventricle it is probably severely dilated. There may be supportive qualitative changes of dilatation, such as spontaneous contrast to suggest slow blood movement in a large cavity.
- Use quantitative measures of area in the 4-chamber 0° view if the boundaries of the left atrium can be seen. Trace around the border to estimate left atrial size and use equations as for transthoracic imaging (p. 224).
- Simple linear measures are usually sufficient in the long axis 135° or short axis 50° views. Measure the distance between the probe and the left atrial wall by the aortic valve. Remember that quantitative measures are likely to be unreliable and should be interpreted taking into account other echocardiographic findings and qualitative assessment of atrial size.

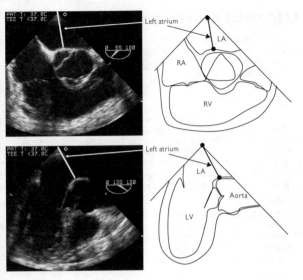

Fig. 5.21 Positions to make linear measures of atrial size.

Left atrial appendage

The left atrial appendage is the most common site for left atrial thrombi in at-risk patients, e.g. those with atrial fibrillation, and is therefore of great clinical relevance, for instance when planning cardioversion or looking for source of emboli.

Normal findings

Views
- The key view is the 2-chamber view.
- However, the left atrial appendage can have a variable shape so modifications of the view may be needed in patients being assessed for cardiac source of emboli, if the left atrium is enlarged, or if atrial fibrillation is found. Once the left atrial appendage is spotted in the 2-chamber view, adjust the scan angle and move the probe up and down to scan through the whole appendage.

Findings
- *2-chamber view.* The left atrial appendage lies on the right, curving around the edge of the mitral valve. Parallel to the appendage and nearer the probe is the left upper pulmonary vein. The appendage and vein are separated by a bright ridge of tissue known as the warfarin or coumadin ridge. This can accumulate fat and may appear bulbous.

Assessment

Assess the appendage as follows.
- Identify the appendage (in some people it can be absent or have been removed/tied/stapled during cardiac surgery).
- Scan through at different planes to identify shape, orientation, and number of lobes (usually 1 lobe but bilobed appendages occur in around 10%). Retroverted appendages (pointing towards the probe) can occur. Inverted appendages are a rare complication of surgery and appear as a mobile mass in the left atrium below the pulmonary vein.
- Look for evidence of thombus or rarely tumours. Differentiate abnormal masses (e.g. thrombus) from pectinate muscles normally present in the appendage. Thrombus is normally associated with low flow. If it is not clear whether there is a mass, colour flow mapping can demonstrate flow down to the apex, or left-sided ultrasound contrast can opacify the appendage (a mass will remain dark).
- Measure filling and emptying velocities. Place pulsed wave Doppler cursor 1cm into the appendage and record a trace. Normal velocities are >40cm/sec. Low velocities are associated with atrial fibrillation or atrial stunning and should make you suspicious that there may be a clot. Less than 20cm/sec indicates a higher risk of clots. Atrial flutter is associated with regular velocities, occurring at a faster rate than the ventricular rate. Look for spontaneous contrast in the atrium or 'smoking' out of the appendage if velocities appear low.

Spontaneous contrast

In the left atrium appears 'smoke-like'. It is classified as *mild* or *severe* (based on qualitative assessment of quantity) and may be seen in both appendage and atrium. Usually spontaneous contrast indicates increased risk of thrombosis. It is due to sludging of the red blood cells when intracardiac velocities decrease. A dilated left atrium and atrial fibrillation increase spontaneous contrast. Anticoagulation does not affect spontaneous contrast. The higher the transducer frequency the better the spontaneous contrast is displayed.

Differentiating pectinate muscle from thrombus

Pectinate muscle
- Strand-like
- Can span the appendage
- Adherent
- Not mobile

Thrombus
- Generally rounded
- May fill the appendage
- Adherent or pedunculated
- Can be mobile
- Often associated spontaneous contrast

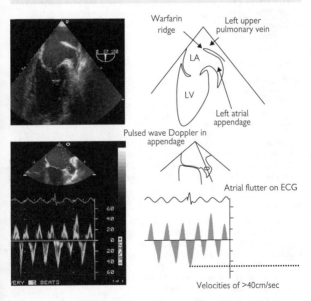

Fig. 5.22 2-chamber view (top) demonstrates prominent left atrial appendage, warfarin ridge, and pulmonary vein. Pulsed wave trace (bottom) demonstrates velocities in appendage consistent with atrial flutter.

Pulmonary veins

Normal anatomy

There are normally four pulmonary veins that drain blood from the pulmonary circulation to the left atrium. Two on the left (lower and upper) and two on the right (lower and upper). They all lie at the back of the atrium. Variations in anatomy include only one pulmonary vein on one side, usually because the upper and lower veins have joined proximally, or significant differences in the size of each vein.

Normal findings

Views

The transoesophageal probe lies behind the atria between the four pulmonary veins. To see all four pulmonary veins modifications of standard views are required. The key views are the 4-chamber 0° view, 2-chamber 75° view, and bicaval 110° view.

Findings

- *4-chamber 0° view.* Start from the 4-chamber view and rotate to right or left; then advance or withdraw the probe to bring each vein into view. The upper pulmonary veins on both sides point towards the probe and are best aligned for Doppler measures. The lower pulmonary veins lie perpendicular to the probe.

How to optimize pulmonary vein views

- *4-chamber 0° view* If the veins are not obvious, colour flow mapping placed in the near field on the left or right can highlight the inflow.
- If the veins are seen but not clearly aligned, rotation of probe angle between 0° and 90° may help to improve the view.

- *2-chamber 75° view.* In this view the the left upper pulmonary vein lies parallel to the appendage, nearer the probe.
- *Bicaval 110° view.* By rotating the bicaval view the right upper pulmonary vein can be brought into view as it drains into the left atrium parallel to the septum.

Assessment

Pulmonary veins are often needed for flow assessment relevant to left atrial pressure, particularly in mitral regurgitation (p. 356). Their anatomy may also be relevant to procedures that use the pulmonary veins as landmarks, such as ablation for atrial fibrillation.

- Comment on whether:
  - all 4 are seen or whether there are more or less than 4;
  - they are in standard locations;
  - there is any discrepancy in size.
- Report pulmonary vein flow patterns.

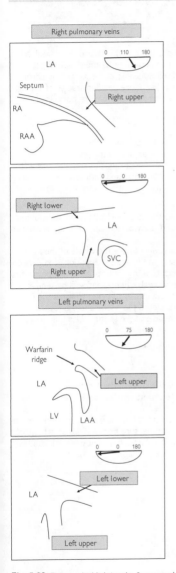

Fig. 5.23 Diagram highlighting the 3 sectors that can be used to identify all 4 pulmonary veins.

Right atrium

There are good views of the right atrium with transoesophageal echocardiography because of its relative proximity to the probe. Right atrial inflows from both superior and inferior vena cavae as well as coronary sinus are also straightforward to image. More detailed studies of the right atrial appendage, Eustachian valve, and atrial septum are possible.

Normal findings

Views

- Key views are 4-chamber 0° view and bicaval 110° view.
- A transgastric view is possible with rotation of the probe from a standard transgastric 90° long axis view of the left ventricle. This will normally bring into view the right ventricle and with some withdrawal of the probe may allow views of the right atrium and tricuspid valve.

Findings

- *4-chamber 0° view.* Equivalent to the apical 4-chamber, rotation of the probe to the right allows focused study of right atrium and a qualitative assessment of size.
- *Bicaval 110° view.* This is the best view to see the whole of the right atrium with inferior cava draining on the left and superior vena cava on the right. The right atrial appendage is invariably present just below the superior vena cava. The Eustachian valve (if present) will be seen at the ostium of the inferior superior cava usually directed towards the fossa ovalis. The atrial septum lies parallel to the probe and the fossa ovalis is usually seen as a 'dip' in the middle of the septum. Use this view to assess the atrial septum.

Right atrial size

- Assess right atrial size qualitatively based on the 4-chamber 0° view. Judge size relative to the left atrium and right ventricle. Normally the two atria are roughly the same size.
- The simplest quantitative assessment is the linear measure of the *minor axis* in a 4-chamber 0° view (linear measure from middle of right atrial lateral wall to mid atrial septum). Volumes have not been validated but can be attempted as for transthoracic imaging (p. 228).

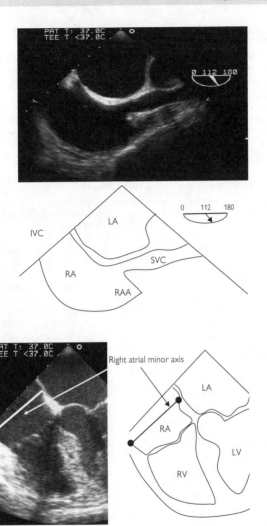

Fig. 5.24 A bicaval view (top) provides excellent depiction of the right atrium. Thrombus, pacing wires, and lines can be seen in the atrium. The 4-chamber view (bottom) can be used for limited measures of the right atrium.

Right atrial features

The following usually do not represent pathological findings, but may be mistaken for abnormalities.

Eustachian valve Best seen in the bicaval 110° view. The Eustachian valve is a membranous structure originating from the junction of the inferior vena cava and right atrium. It represents a remnant from fetal circulation where placental oxygenated blood coming from the inferior vena cava has to be diverted through the foramen secundum into the left heart. Thus the blood flow coming from the inferior vena cava hits the the fossa ovalis. This has implications for contrast application via injections into the arm veins: there is usually a wash-out of contrast close to the fossa, which may impair contrast passage. Size can be highly variable. Rarely, thrombosis or endocarditis can be attached to the valve

Chiari network The Eustachian valve may appear to cross the atrium and have net-like perforations. This is a Chiari network. The Eustachian valve forms from the remnents of one of the valves of the sinus venosus. If the valve does not regress completely, a Chiari network forms instead. Echocardiographically a network of small strands may be seen—sometimes with a broad base, which can be attached to different parts of the right atrium.

Thebesian valve Like the Eustachian valve this does not represent a real valve. It is a muscle and/or fibrous band at the orifice of the coronary sinus in the right atrium. It can be seen in views displaying the orifice of the coronary sinus.

Christa terminalis Separates the smooth part of the right atrium from the pectinated muscle of the right atrium. In the bicaval view the *christa terminalis* is displayed as a ridge at the junction of the right atrium and superior vena cava. When pulling back from a 4-chamber view the christa terminalis can be seen as a bright protrusion of the lateral atrial wall. Further pulling back shows how this structure continues into the superior vena cava.

Coronary sinus

To see the coronary sinus use a 4-chamber 0° view. Advance the probe slightly and retroflex slightly to look below the mitral valve. The coronary sinus should appear across the image draining to the right atrium.

The sinus can enlarge if there is anomalous drainage of a persistent left superior vena cava. Anomalous drainage can be demonstrated by injecting agitated saline into a *left-sided* arm vein. Because the left-sided vena cava drains into the coronary sinus the contrast comes through the coronary sinus into the right atrium.

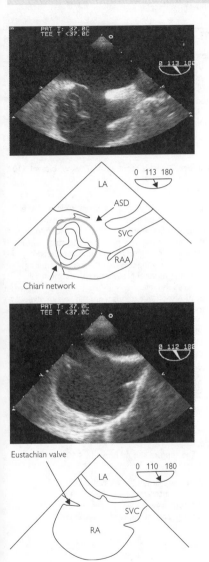

Fig. 5.25 Example of Chiari network (top) and Eustachian valve (bottom) in bicaval views.

Atrial septum

The atrial septum divides the left and right atria and embryologically has two distinct elements, the primum and secundum septum, which fuse after birth. Abnormal development or closure of the septum is fundamental to the emergence of septal defects. Transoesophageal echocardiography is uniquely suited to study the septum because it can be viewed through the left atrium in several planes. These views are suitable for colour flow and continuous wave Doppler, as well as contrast studies.

Normal findings

Views

The key views are 4-chamber 0° view, short axis 50° view, bicaval 110° view.

Findings

- *4-chamber 0° view.* In the 4-chamber view the septum is close to the probe and rotation to the left can be used for an initial assessment. Atrial septal defects are usually first evident in this view and colour flow mapping can identify left to right flow patterns. The atrial septum normally bows slightly towards the right atrium but in ventilated patients there is a mild systolic bowing towards the left both during inspiration and expiration. If right atrial pressure exceeds left atrial pressure it will bows towards the left.
- *Short axis 50° view.* Here the septum extends from the aortic valve ring, in a line at 10 o'clock. This view can be used for stable contrast studies.
- *Bicaval 110° view.* The standard view to study the septum as it lies parallel to the probe. The fossa ovalis is usually easily seen as a depression. This view should be used for colour flow and contrast studies.

Assessment

Assess the septum in all views using 2D. Look for:
- lipomatous hypertrophy (bright thickening of the septum that spares the fossa ovalis);
- septal defects or an appearance of layers in the septum suggestive of a patent foramen ovale;
- atrial septal aneurysms. The septum should move by >10mm towards right or left atrium.

Then use colour flow over the septum in the bicaval view.
- A septal defect will be seen as interatrial flow. Also, screen for patent foramen ovale—a small colour flow jet may be seen in the fossa ovalis into the atrium during a short part of the cardiac cycle.

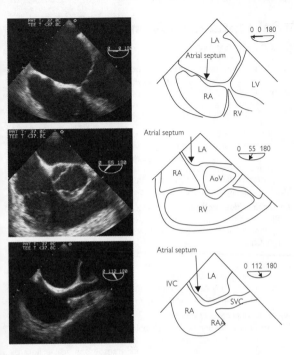

Fig. 5.26 Key views to assess the atrial septum. 4-chamber 0° view (top), short axis 50° view (middle), bicaval 110° view (bottom).

Atrial septal defects and patent foramen ovale

Requests for transoesophageal echocardiography in people with suspected atrial septal defects and patent foramen ovale are usually because:
• there is a high suspicion from transthoracic imaging of a defect;
• the patient is being evaluated for intervention;
• the study is to look for an embolic source.

Assessment

As for transthoracic imaging (p. 232) initial assessment should be with 2D imaging to look for obvious defects, followed by colour flow mapping. If a septal defect is seen, Doppler can be used to quantify the shunt size. Finally, agitated saline contrast injections should always be used if the septal defect or foramen ovale has not clearly been seen.

2D and colour flow mapping

Use all 3 views but in particular the bicaval view. Look for gaps and then overlay the colour flow to look for flow (most likely to be left to right). Comment on:
• defect position including proximity to aortic valve and likely classification (primum or secundum);
• defect size in several directions;
• direction and timing of flow from colour flow mapping;
• associated cardiac defects (particularly relevant for primum defects).

Doppler quantification of shunt

See transthoracic imaging (p. 232). Doppler quantification is not normally needed for patent foramen ovale. Shunt quantification using measurement of Qp and Qs is often limited with transoesophageal echocardiography because alignment of the Doppler beam to flow through the pulmonary valve is difficult. However, measurement of the diameter of the pulmonary artery or right ventricle outflow tract and of the left ventricle outflow tract is more reliable than on transthoracic images. Pulmonary and aortic vti can be determined separately with transthoracic imaging.

Agitated saline contrast versus colour flow mapping

In patent foramen ovale or septal defects the left-to-right shunt can be detected by colour flow mapping. In most patients a right-to-left shunt is present when right atrial pressure increases, for instance, during Valsalva manoeuvre. However, it may be difficult to display these right-to-left shunts with colour Doppler. In these cases contrast echocardiography is indicated. Contrast echocardiography is also needed, when colour flow mapping does not reveal a shunt, since contrast echocardiography appears to be more sensitive.

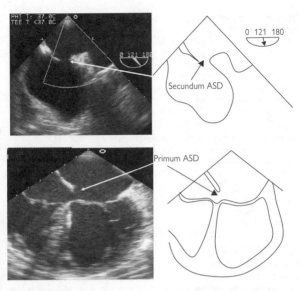

Fig. 5.27 Examples of atrial septal abnormalities. Top figure shows a bicaval view of a secundum defect, note bulky septum due to septal lipomatous hypertrophy. Bottom figure demonstrates a primum defect in a 4-chamber view.

Secundum atrial septal defect—device closure

Transoesophageal echocardiography is indicated to guide transcatheter closure of secundum defects. The key features to record before the procedure to plan closure are:
- size in different scan planes (many ASDs are not circular!);
- presence of multiple defects;
- presence of interatrial septal aneurysm;
- size of rim of normal tissue between defect and adjacent structures for device to fit over. In particular look at rim close to aortic valve;
- other cardiac abnormalities.

During the procedure monitor and advise on:
- guidewire position while crossing the defect;
- defect size for device sizing;
- positioning of closure device during deployment;
- residual shunt after closure.

After the procedure and during follow up look for:
- device position;
- residual shunts;
- clots or other abnormalities on the device.

Primum atrial septal defects

Primum atrial septal defects are usually well displayed with transthoracic echocardiography. During a transoesophageal study the beginning of the defect will be seen at the hingepoints of the mitral and tricuspid valves, which arise from the same level. A 4-chamber 0° view is usually ideal. Transoesophageal echocardiography is useful for a comprehensive assessment of the pathology, which often includes defects of the proximal interventricular septum and mitral and tricuspid valve insufficiency (including cleft anterior mitral leaflet).

Sinus venosus defects

Sinus venosus defects are very difficult to display using transthoracic 2D echocardiography.

Superior sinus venosus defects are best displayed in a modified bicaval view with the probe slightly rotated to the right. There will often be communication between the pulmonary vein and the superior vena cava opposite to the sinus venosus defect. The abnormal drainage of the right upper pulmonary vein can also be displayed in a 0° view pulled back from the standard 4-chamber image to show a short axis view of the superior vena cava and ascending aorta.

Inferior sinus venosus defects are less common and may be associated with abnormal drainage of the right lower pulmonary vein.

Coronary sinus defects are between the coronary sinus and the left atrium. Coronary sinus views are needed to display the shunt, which may be difficult to see.

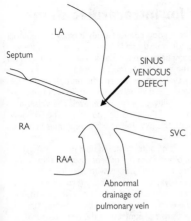

Fig. 5.28 Schematic demonstrating position of a sinus venous defect in a bicaval view.

Contrast study for intracardiac shunts

The three elements to ensure a good contrast study looking for an atrial shunt are identical to those for transthoracic imaging. The sedation with transoesophageal imaging complicates the Valsalva manoeuvre but does not make it impossible and the manoeuvre must be used.

1 **A stable image.** The bicaval 110° view aligns the septum across the image and therefore provides good views of contrast flow. An alternative view is the short axis 50° view at aortic valve level. The Valsalva manoeuvre causes movement of the heart up and down. The 50° view tends to be more stable with this movement as the septum is in line with the image plane.

2 **Good quality contrast.** The contrast should be 8mL of saline, 1mL of air, and (ideally) 1mL of blood from the patient mixed in two connected syringes until 'frothy'. Use syringes with Luer locks to avoid them bursting off the 3-way tap. Inject rapidly through a venflon inserted into the right antecubital vein (if the patient is lying on their left side this arm will not be compressed and will be uppermost). This will ensure the fastest transit of contrast to the heart (ensure the blood pressure cuff does not inflate on this arm during the procedure). Good contrast should completely and rapidly opacify the right atrium. Sometimes rapid flow from the inferior vena cava causes mixing and partitioning of contrasted and uncontrasted blood in the right atrium. As the inferior vena cava directs blood at the foramen ovale the mixing tends to keep contrast away from the septum. If this persists despite fast boluses then an alternative is to inject contrast via a femoral vein.

3 **A good Valsalva.** If further studies are needed after rest injections always do the study with a Valsalva. The critical time is when the patient relaxes, when right-sided pressures transiently elevate relative to left. The patient takes a breath and bears down hard. Inject the contrast and when it fills the right atrium tell them to relax. If there is a shunt a few bubbles appear in the left atrium and left ventricle within 5 beats of the patient relaxing. If bubbles appear later this suggests a pulmonary arteriovenous malformation. This procedure is entirely feasible during transoesophageal imaging with a compliant patient. To improve compliance lighter sedation can be used and/or the shunt study can be near the end of the examination (as sedation becomes lighter). Assistance can be given by asking the patient to press against a hand placed on the stomach.

Image acquisition

Set the system to capture 10 cardiac cycles and start acquisition on contrast injection. Look back through the loop searching for bubbles. Repeat the study with more contrast until you are happy all three elements of the study are perfect.

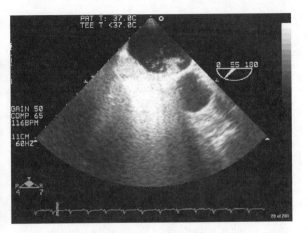

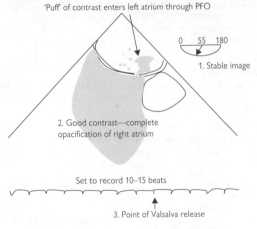

'Puff' of contrast enters left atrium through PFO

0   55   180

1. Stable image

2. Good contrast—complete
opacification of right atrium

Set to record 10–15 beats

3. Point of Valsalva release

Fig. 5.29 The 3 key elements of an agitated saline contrast study. 1. Stable image;
2. Good contrast; 3. Good Valsalva.

Ventricular septum

The ventricular septum can be difficult to see entirely with transoesophageal imaging and therefore it is not indicated for assessment of the septum. However, it is normal to assess the septum routinely during a study and comment if abnormalities are identified incidentally. Transoesophageal echocardiography provides reasonable views of the proximal septum and can be efficient for membranous septal defects. More apical defects, as often occur post-ischaemia, are difficult to see.

Normal findings

Views

The key views are the 4-chamber 0° view and the long axis 135° view. These can be supplemented by the short axis 50° view to look at septum around the aortic valve. The transgastric short axis 0° view can also be useful.

Findings

- *4-chamber 0° view.* The septum lies between the left and right ventricles. With an unforeshortened view it may be possible to see to the apex but the views are not aligned for colour flow mapping. The view gives good depiction of the proximal septum. Withdrawal to the 5-chamber view allows imaging of the septum below the aortic valve.
- *Short axis 50° view.* With a slight advance of the probe the membranous and outlet septum just below the aortic valve can be seen.
- *Long axis 135° view.* This also demonstrates the septum close to the aortic valve.
- *Transgastric view.* This gives equivalent information to the parasternal short axis view and provides information on the muscular (trabecular) septum in the mid-ventricle.

Assessment

Assess the septum in all views with 2D and then overlay colour flow to look for defects. If there is evidence of hypertrophy, particularly in the outflow tract, then colour flow can also be used to look for sub-aortic valve flow acceleration.

- If comments on the septum are required then report septal thickness (this can be measured from transgastric views) and comment on any irregular thickening of the septum.
- To identify a ventricular septal defect first look in 2D for evidence of a 'gap'; then use colour flow to identify definite flow across the septum. If there is a gap measure the size in two different directions/planes. Finally, if Doppler alignment is possible consider calculation of a shunt. However, if a septal defect is sufficient to cause major shunts these can often be seen most easily with transthoracic imaging.

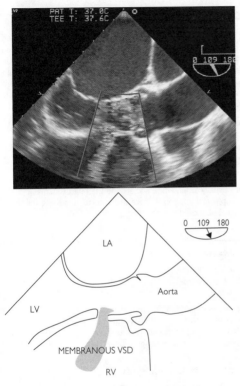

Fig. 5.30 Example of a large perimembranous ventricular septal defect seen in a long axis 135° view. A left to right shunt is demonstrated with colour flow mapping.

Pericardium

Transthoracic echocardiography usually gives all the information needed to assess the pericardium. However, the pericardium should be assessed routinely during transoesophageal studies. Transoesophageal echocardiography can be useful in peri-operative cardiac patients to assess localized collections or because of poor post-operative windows. Assessment of the pericardium should follow the same routine as with transthoracic imaging (p. 242).

Normal findings

Views

Part of the pericardium can be seen (and should be assessed) in all views.

Findings

Pericardial surfaces

The surfaces are usually a thin white line around the heart (normal 1–2mm thick). Transoesophageal imaging is more accurate for assessing thickness than transthoracic but should not be relied upon.

Pericardial space

The space, if it contains fluid, is a black, lucent area associated with the pericardial surfaces.

Transverse and oblique sinuses

Transoesophageal echocardiography is good for studying the transverse and oblique sinuses.

Transverse sinus lies between left atrium and aorta/pulmonary trunk.
- Use atrioventricular short axis 50° view and then long axis 135° view.
- Fluid or haematoma in the sinus appears as space—shaped like a crescent or triangle—between ascending aorta and left atrium (Fig. 5.31).

Problems with the transverse sinus

To differentiate the space from the left atrium or left atrial appendage (roof lies in transverse sinus) use colour flow Doppler. There will be no flow in the sinus. Beware: because of the position of the sinus it can be mistaken for abscess or cyst or—if containing fat—an atrial mass.

Oblique sinus lies between the pulmonary veins on back of left atrium.
- Use 4-chamber 0° view.
- Fluid or haematoma in sinus appears as a space between left atrium and the probe tip in the oesophagus.

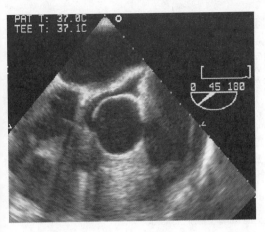

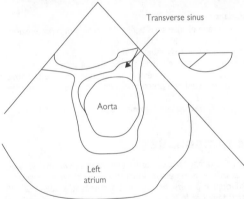

Fig. 5.31 Oesophageal, 50° view just above aortic valve. Fluid in transverse sinus is seen as echolucent area between aorta and left atrium.

Pericardial effusion

Assessment

Global effusions

- Use all views. Seen well in 4-chamber 0° view or transgastric short axis view.
- Report depth in several different sites and report where the measurements were made.
- Gauge global effusion on same parameters as transthoracic imaging (<0.5cm, minimal; 0.5–1cm, mild; 1–2cm, moderate; >2cm, large).
- Comment on appearance (fibrin strands, masses, haematoma).

Differentiate between pleural and pericardial fluid by using descending aorta and left atrium (as for transthoracic imaging). In 4-chamber view rotate probe to focus on the space between the left heart and descending aorta. Pericardial fluid will pass between aorta and left heart (sometimes widening the gap), whereas pleural fluid will extend to the lateral side of the aorta.

Localized effusions

- Common sites are in *oblique sinus* behind left atrium or a *posterolateral collection* against right atrium or right ventricle.
- Both can be seen in the 4-chamber 0° view.
- Space between probe and left atrium is the *oblique sinus* collection.
- Rotate probe to focus on right heart. Look at right ventricle and atrium for evidence of localized compression or collapse from a *posterolateral* effusion.
- Use long axis 135° view to check *transverse sinus*.

Cardiac tamponade

Features of cardiac tamponade can usually be assessed with transthoracic imaging. If assessment is required during transoesophageal imaging use the 2D and Doppler parameters as for transthoracic studies (p. 240). Remember that tamponade is a clinical diagnosis (hypotension, tachycardia, etc.) and echocardiography will only provide supportive evidence.

Problems in ventilated post-surgery/ITU patients

- There will not be the normal respiratory variation in Doppler indices of mitral and tricuspid inflow and these should not be used. Rely on 2D features.
- Look for right or left ventricular or atrial collapse.
- Look for localized collection compressing left or right ventricle or atria reducing chamber function.
- With *oblique sinus* collection look at pulmonary vein flow. Local compression will reduce flow velocity in vein.

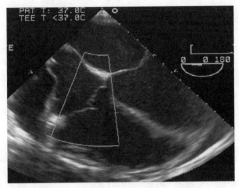

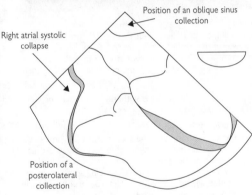

Fig. 5.32 4-chamber 0° view showing global pericardial effusion with exaggerated right atrial collapse during atrial systole. Annotation demonstrates where an oblique sinus and posterolateral collection would be seen in this view.

Aorta

The close proximity of the oesophagus to the aorta makes transoesophageal imaging ideal for assessment of the ascending and descending thoracic aorta. Parts of the aortic arch including the origin of the brachiocephalic vessels can also be visualized. The views allow diagnosis and assessment of aortic dissection and severity of aortic atheroma. The portability of transoesophageal imaging also permits assessment of traumatic aortic transsection.

Normal findings

Views

The key aortic views are the 50° short axis aortic valve view at aortic valve level and, withdrawn slightly, the 135° long axis view and dedicated descending aorta and aortic arch views. Deep transgastric and 110° long axis transgastric views can be used for alignment of Doppler in the ascending aorta.

Proximal ascending aorta

Proximal ascending aorta is best seen in the 50° short axis view with slight withdrawal of the probe to scan up the aorta. The 135° long axis view also allows measures of aortic root size. Transgastric views sometimes allow Doppler alignment through the proximal ascending aorta.

Aortic arch

Seen as the last views as the probe is withdrawn in the aortic views and can be seen in long and short axis.

Descending thoracic aorta

- The descending thoracic aorta can be seen in short (0°) and long axis (90°) with the dedicated posteriorly-directed aortic views. Advancing and withdrawing the probe allows scanning of the entire length of the aorta. This view can help demonstrate descending aortic aneurysm and atheroma. Rotation will differentiate artefact from true abnormality, particularly when dissection suspected.
- Aortic views can also demonstrate the aortic isthmus, and the ostium, and proximal part, of the left subclavian artery. This landmark is used to describe extent of dissection or help assess placement of intra-aortic balloon pumps.

Emergency evaluation of the aorta

In an emergency where aortic dissection is a major indication proceed immediately to the 135° long axis view. This view shows the aortic annulus, aortic valve, and proximal ascending aorta with sinuses of Valsalva and right and non-coronary leaflets of the aortic valve. A proximal aortic dissection flap or excessive dilatation of the sinus of Valsalva is therefore readily diagnosed. Pericardial fluid and aortic regurgitation can also be detected.

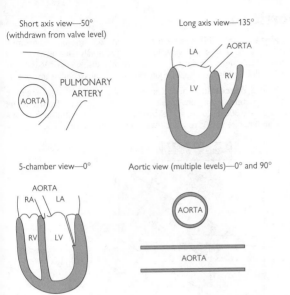

Fig. 5.33 Key views to assess the aorta.

Aortic size

Proximal aorta Make measurements in 2D imaging from mid-oesophageal 135° long axis view in systole (with valve leaflet tips open to their maximum). Standard measures are annulus, sinus of Valsalva at aortic leaflet tip level, sinotubular junction, proximal ascending aorta.

Arch and descending aorta In aortic short axis 0° view measure aortic diameter at different levels. Record the distance from incisors (40cm, 35cm, 30cm, 25cm) for each measure. When withdrawn to the aortic arch rotate to 90° to get a cross-section and measure diameter.

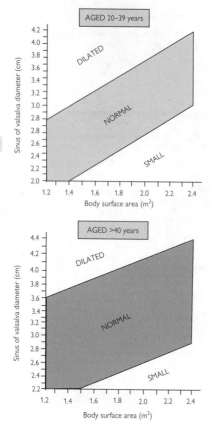

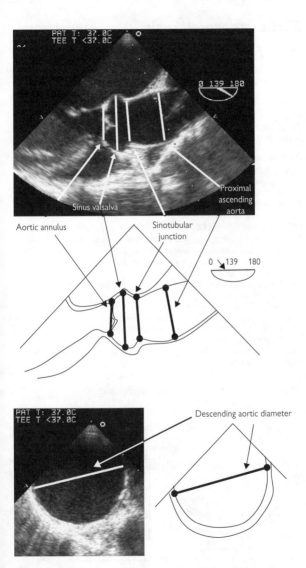

Fig. 5.34 Standard measures of aortic root and proximal aorta in long axis 135° view and of descending aorta diameter from short axis aortic views.

Aortic atherosclerosis

Aortic atherosclerosis is easily seen with transoesophageal echocardiography. Assessment is important when hunting for embolic source or before surgery for impression of likely coronary atherosclerotic disease. Risk of embolic events increases incrementally with extent of atheroma and is dramatically higher once plaque extends beyond 4mm. Severity is strongly associated with risk factors for atheroma and incidence and severity of carotid and coronary disease. Site of atherosclerosis is not always correlated with stroke localization and presence of atherosclerosis may simply be a marker of generalized atherosclerosis.

Assessment

Atherosclerosis is seen as wall thickening, irregular plaque, or as ulcerated, thrombotic, mobile plaque. Significant atherosclerosis increases the risk for dissection and aneurysm formation.

- In aortic views scan up the descending aorta and aortic arch. Also assess proximal ascending aorta.
- Measure wall thickness at several sites and in particular at any position where there are irregularities. Aortic thickness is *intima-media thickness*. The wall is seen as a two white lines separated by a black space. Intima media thickness is the thickness of the inner white and black bands added together.
- Grade atherosclerosis within the different sections of the aorta as *mild, moderate,* or *severe.*
  - Normal, wall thickness <2mm.
  - Mild atherosclerosis, wall thickness 2–4mm.
  - Moderate atherosclerosis, wall thickness >4mm.
  - Severe atherosclerosis, irregular protruding plaque.
- Comment on specific lesions, such as thrombus or ulcerated plaques, and comment on location and depth.

Measurement of aortic intima media thickness

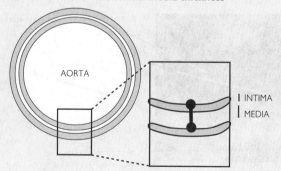

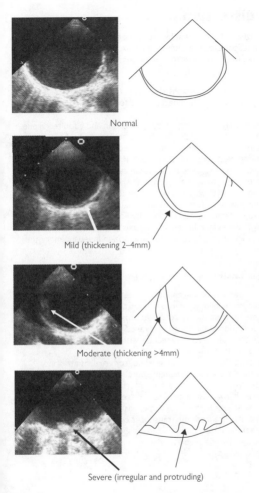

Normal

Mild (thickening 2–4mm)

Moderate (thickening >4mm)

Severe (irregular and protruding)

Fig. 5.35 Grades of atheroma within the aorta.

Aortic dissection

Transoesophageal echocardiography allows diagnosis and serial monitoring of aortic dissection. Diagnostic utility with experienced operator is good and comparable to that of other modalities (sensitivity and specificity >97%).

Diagnosis

- Transthoracic echocardiography should routinely be performed first as this may be diagnostic and negate need for transoesophageal echocardiography.
- For transoesophageal imaging adequate sedation and good technique are essential. Excessive retching can cause acute blood pressure rise, which could extend dissection and cause acute haemodynamic deterioration. Therefore, if concerns, particularly if haemodynamic instability, consider performing study in theatre with cardiac surgeon available.
- Use all aortic views to scan all of aorta in short and long axes. In short axis, look for an enlarged aorta with a line across lumen dividing *true* and *false* lumens. True lumen is usually smaller. Colour flow mapping can be used to demonstrate high velocity flow in the true lumen and no, or slow, flow in false lumen. In long axis views *dissection flap* may be seen as a linear mobile structure with motion independent of the aortic wall.

Limitations—false negative and false positive findings

- The distal ascending aorta cannot be assessed by transoesophageal echocardiography due to interposition of trachea and left bronchus. Thus pathology in about 5cm of length may be missed. However, isolated dissection in this location is rare. False negative studies can occur due to localized root dissection with pericardial haematoma but no false lumen.
- Linear artefacts have to be distinguished from real intimal flaps. Reverberation is the most frequent source of these artefacts. Strong backscatter from various tissue–fluid interfaces such as the anterior aortic valve or Swan–Ganz catheters in the pulmonary artery can cause linear echoes in the aortic lumen. They are typically found at double the distance from the transducer compared to the source of the reverberation. Also mirror artefacts showing a reduplication of the aortic lumen are possible. A real intimal flap should be visible in at least two planes.

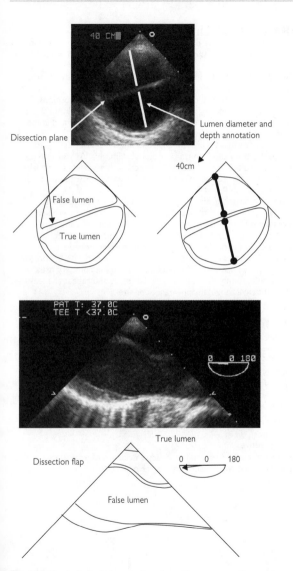

Fig. 5.36 Short axis (top) view of a dissection with measures or false and true lumen, Long axis view (bottom) of aorta demonstrating dissection flap.

Assessment

If an aortic dissection is diagnosed or the study is for serial monitoring of a known dissection the objectives of the investigation should be as follows.

- Perform all standard aortic measures and measure diameter of true and false lumens at different levels.
- Try and identify start and end of dissection and record positions. This allows serial monitoring of size and length of dissection. In the ascending aorta dissections tend be along the greater curvature and in the descending aorta may spiral around the true lumen.
- Multiple tears may be present and sometimes it is not possible to locate the entry site with transoesophageal imaging. As you scan up aorta use colour flow to identify connections between true and false lumens (will be seen as colour flow jets). If seen, measure positions and direction of flow.
- Comment on and quantify aortic regurgitation. Aortic valve insufficiency can occur due to dilatation of the aortic root, impaired cusp movement by ring haematoma, impaired cusp support, and cusp prolapse or prolapse of the dissecting flap into outflow tract.
- Comment on pericardial fluid and evidence of tamponade.
- Assess global and regional left ventricular function in case of coronary artery involvement. 10% of dissections involve the coronary ostia.
- When monitoring dissection, review last study and repeat all measures. Highlight any changes in appearances or size.

Surgery for aortic dissection

Pre-operative

If performing echocardiography before type A dissection surgery:

- check diagnosis and differentiate between acute dissection, leaking aneurysm, or intramural haematoma. Type and timing of surgery will vary significantly;
- look at aortic valve cusps and aortic root. If normal cusps and aortic annulus and sinotubular junction normal size, then, even if regurgitation, interposition ascending aortic graft replacement, rather than total aortic root replacement, can be considered.

Post-operative

Ensure successful repair and no residual evidence of dissection. If native valve was preserved, ensure normal valve function.

Differentiating true from false lumen

	True lumen	False lumen
Diameter	True < false	False > true
Pulsation	Systolic expansion	Systolic compression
Blood flow	Systolic, antegrade	Reduced
Spontaneous contrast	Rare	Frequent
Thrombus	Rare	Frequent, depending on flow communication
Localization	Inner, anterior contour	Outer, posterior contour

Differentiating intimal flap from artefact

	Intimal flap	Artefact
Borders	Definite	Indistinct
Movement	Rapid, oscillatory	Parallel to strong reflector proximal to artefact
Extension	Within aorta	Beyond aortic wall
Colour Doppler	Different colour communicating jets	Homogeneous colour on both sides

Intramural haematoma

There is debate as to whether aortic intramural haematoma is a discrete pathological entity or precursor of aortic dissection. Haematoma tends to occur in older patients with hypertension.

Diagnosis and assessment

- Intramural haematoma is seen as a generalized thickening of the media without obvious disruption of the intima and no flow communication.
- Wall thickness >7mm suggests haematoma (normal <4mm).
- Can affect any area of aorta. Intramural haematoma in ascending aorta is usually managed similarly to type A dissection.

Differential diagnosis of haematoma is atherosclerotic disease with a penetrating aortic ulcer. Penetrating ulcer is always associated with heavy atheroma and predominantly affects descending aorta; intima is irregular with thickening above the intima. Atherosclerosis is also suggested by inward displacement of any intimal calcification with homogeneous mottled thickening of wall either side of the displacement.

Aortic transection or traumatic aortic disruption

Usually occurs at aortic isthmus following acceleration/deceleration injury (e.g. restrained passenger or driver in road traffic accident). Usually other traumatic injuries.

To differentiate from dissection:

- Transection is disruption of media rather than intima, resulting in relatively thick flap, usually very mobile, and perpendicular to aortic wall (aortic dissection is intimal, with thin flap parallel to wall)
- Not usually thrombus in false lumen but may be mediastinal haematoma.
- Usually asymmetric aortic shape. >4mm difference in anteroposterior and lateral aortic dimensions (dimensions similar with dissection).
- Colour flow mapping reveals similar velocities on both sides of any flap, with turbulence around the point of disruption (turbulence unusual in dissection and usually slower velocities in false lumen).

Aortic coarctation

Usually diagnosed from transthoracic assessment of Doppler flow in suprasternal view. Accurate transoesophageal imaging can be difficult but images are best obtained by examining the descending aorta at 0° in multiple sections to identify the isthmus. At level of isthmus, rotate to a 90° longitudinal view to identify the origin of the left subclavian artery. Look for irregularity of aortic lumen. Morphology of aortic coarctation is often complex and further imaging is usually necessary.

Assessment

- Measure size of aorta proximal, distal, and at the coarctation. For follow up, post-repair, compare with previous studies to look for repair dilatation or persistent gradient.
- Pulsed wave Doppler in long axis aortic views can be used to look for flow acceleration across a coarctation.

Sinus of Valsalva aneurysm

A rare, congenital abnormality (<1:1000 patients). Acquired aneurysms are even rarer and are predominantly due to endocarditis, trauma, syphilis, or tuberculosis. Often an incidental finding. When symptomatic, rupture causes chest pain and breathlessness or, with smaller ruptures, more insidious onset congestive cardiac failure.

Assessment

- Use the 135° long axis view (>95% originate from either right or non-coronary cusps, both visualized). Aneurysm usually has a wind-sock appearance blowing in either right atrium or right ventricle.
- Colour flow mapping will show an aortic to cardiac chamber shunt. Continuous wave Doppler assessment confirms continuous flow.
- Use a 50° aortic short axis view with slight probe withdrawal to level of coronary sinus to identify coronary arteries and exclude coronary artery fistula as an important differential diagnosis.
- Haemodynamic effect of a ruptured coronary sinus is best assessed from size of atria and left ventricle, reflecting extent of volume overload.

Thoracic aortic aneurysm

Thoracic aortic aneurysm is usually suspected on chest X-ray or transthoracic echocardiography. Confirmation can be by CT, magnetic resonance imaging, or transoesophageal echocardiography. CT and magnetic resonance imaging have the advantage of showing the true extent of the aneurysm and clear identification of the origin of the head and neck vessels, while transoesophageal echocardiography more accurately delineates flow patterns within the aneurysm, the presence of thrombus, involvement of the aortic valve and the presence of atherosclerotic debris.

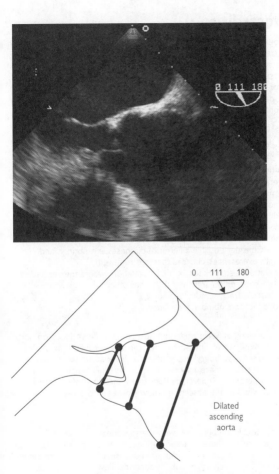

Fig. 5.37 Measurements of a dilated ascending aorta. From left to right: aortic annulus, sinotubular junction, and proximal ascending aorta.

Endocarditis

Transoesophageal echocardiography has better sensitivity and specificity than transthoracic echocardiography for identifying vegetations. The higher spatial and temporal resolution can identify smaller vegetations with rapid movement. Image quality is also better to identify complications of endocarditis: aortic root; fistulae; and valve dysfunction such as leaflet perforation. Remember a normal echocardiogram, including transoesophageal echocardiography, never excludes endocarditis.

Assessment

Use a full systematic examination (p. 282) with focus on both left and right-sided valves. Report on the following.

Vegetations

- Vegetations tend to appear as masses on valves (rarely septum and chamber walls). Focus on each valve (aortic, mitral, tricuspid, and pulmonary valve) and vary position slightly while watching for 'flicking' objects attached to valve. Record loops and scroll through frame-by-frame to pick out any abnormal mobile elements.
- If one is seen, move probe position and see if you can see it in multiple planes. Consider possible differential diagnoses, e.g. fibrin strand (Lambl's excrescence), chordae (perhaps ruptured).
- If vegetation, also look for 'seeded' vegetations where the vegetation (or its associated regurgitant jet) touches other valves or walls (e.g. outflow tract, septum, and aorta).
- Report: location, number, size, functional effect.

Abscess

Look particularly at valve rings (but also study leaflets); focus on aortic root and mitral valve. The aortic root can be seen particularly well so look for thickening, 'boggy' appearances or frank abscesses. If after valve surgery, remember there may be some normal inflammation associated with the operation. Report position, size, functional effects (compression), and whether the abscess has now opened into a cavity (if so, say which).

Fistulae

These can usually be best seen with transoesophageal echocardiography. Suspect a fistula if there is a known abscess, a new murmur has been heard, or there has been a sudden haemodynamic change in the patient. Use colour flow mapping to look for abnormal flow and cavity jets. Fistulae can be between any adjacent cavities where there has been infection, e.g. around valves, aorta to right heart.

Valve dysfunction

If there is a vegetation give details of functional effect on valve. Even if you have not seen a vegetation look for suspicious valve dysfunction in a systematic manner and report.

Pericardial effusion See p. 426.

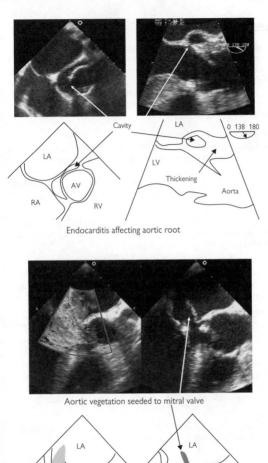

Endocarditis affecting aortic root

Aortic vegetation seeded to mitral valve

Fig. 5.38 Examples of aortic root abscess (top). Bottom figure shows aortic regurgitant jet (left figure) associated with aortic vegetation and seeded mitral valve vegetations (right figure).

Masses

Masses are usually much clearer on transoesophageal echocardiography than transthoracic echocardiography and therefore transoesophageal echocardiography is indicated for definition of masses. Abnormal masses are vegetations or very rarely thrombi or tumours (see pp 284–7).

Report position, size, and functional effects. Comment on any suspicions as to the nature of the mass but remember that echocardiography is unlikely to give the definitive diagnosis.

Differential diagnosis of masses

Like transthoracic echocardiography, transoesophageal imaging does not provide a specific tissue pattern of the tumours (the exception being lipomas). Therefore it is not possible to differentiate masses (tumours, thrombi, and vegetations) according to their structure on echocardiography. However, there are associated features that help to make a diagnosis.

Myxomas

Myxomas are the most frequent cardiac tumours and usually originate from the fossa ovalis of the interatrial septum. They also may be found in other chambers.

Fibroelastoma

Fibroelastoma are mobile tumours on the upstream side of the aortic valve (rarely mitral valve). In comparison to vegetations there are usually no other valvular lesions.

Lipomatous interatrial hypertrophy, lipoma in the tricuspid ring

These lipomatous changes have a characteristic high density appearance but do not result in acoustic shadowing like calcification.

Thrombi

Thrombi are usually associated with reduction in blood flow (atrial fibrillation, dilated heart chambers, altered or artificial valves, or atheroma)

Exceptions to this principle are thrombi associated with coagulopathy and left ventricular non-compaction or on aortic atherosclerosis.

Vegetations

Vegetations are associated with other clinical signs of endocarditis (e.g. raised inflammatory markers, positive blood cultures).

Transoesophageal imaging for tumours

If the study is for benign or malignant tumours, and there is suspicion of an extracardiac tumour, consider whether there might be oesophageal involvement. If this is possible then consider an endoscopy or other imaging before performing transoesophageal imaging.

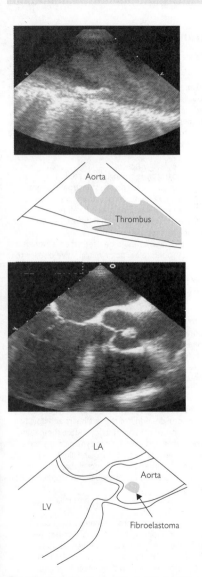

Fig. 5.39 Examples of aortic thrombus (top) and fibroelastoma (bottom).

Cardiopulmonary bypass and coronary artery surgery

If cardiopulmonary bypass is used for coronary artery surgery in a patient with normal left ventricular function and no significant valve disease, it remains a matter of debate whether intraoperative transoesophageal echocardiography is used routinely. However, a comprehensive study performed before establishing cardiopulmonary bypass, provides a comparison for post-operative studies. Transoesophageal imaging can also be useful during *de-airing* and *weaning off bypass*.

Indications

- Transoesophageal echocardiography is strongly indicated in coronary artery surgery complicated by: severe cardiac dysfunction; significant ischaemic mitral regurgitation; large left ventricular aneurysm; mural thrombus; left ventricular remodelling (Dor procedure); recent myocardial infarction; ischaemic ventricular septal defect; requirement for left ventricular assist device support post-surgery.
- Transoesophageal echocardiography should be used when a patient pre-operatively has mild to moderate aortic or mitral valve disease to determine whether valve surgery is also required. Post-operative echocardiography is required to assess cardiac function and valve performance whether the valve was operated on or not.

De-airing

During cardiopulmonary bypass air can be trapped in pulmonary veins, the left ventricular apex, or left atrial appendage. This air is mobilized by the surgeon before coming off bypass and enters the left ventricle and aorta. As it is expelled it resembles agitated saline (as might happen if there was a massive right-to-left shunt during contrast echocardiography). Remaining air can be scanned for after de-airing.

Coming off bypass

Start monitoring with transoesophageal imaging soon after the aortic cross-clamp is removed. Monitor de-airing of the left heart and aorta and then watch to ensure restoration of cardiac function. After the patient is weaned off bypass, ensure stable systemic haemodynamics (i.e. systolic blood pressure >100mmHg, adequate left ventricular filling) then assess effectiveness of surgery. For all surgery, determine global and regional cardiac function using standard techniques. If global cardiac dysfunction develops consider the following.

- Was there satisfactory myocardial preservation, in particular with concomitant coronary artery disease?
- Was there a large amount of air emboli into a coronary (particularly the right as this is uppermost in the supine patient)? Usually causes severe right, and some left, ventricular failure with significant tricuspid and mitral regurgitation. Further cardiopulmonary bypass may be required to wash out air emboli. Monitor recovery with echocardiography.
- Is there insufficient flow in the bypass grafts (kinking, sutures, etc.) causing regional wall motion abnormality?

Failure to wean off bypass

A possible urgent call for transoesophageal echocardiography is to evaluate a patient who has failed to come off bypass following surgery. Ensure you are familiar with what surgery is being performed and what the pre-operative investigations and transoesophageal findings were, i.e. valve disease, left ventricular function, and degree of coronary disease. Although there could be many causes look for:

- massive mitral or aortic regurgitation due to prosthesis failure;
- acute right ventricular failure due to air emboli (the right coronary artery is particularly prone to air emboli because of its proximal position and therefore 'upper' position in the supine patient);
- left ventricular failure due to intraoperative myocardial infarction. This could be due to concomitant coronary disease without sufficient coronary protection or surgical injury (to a coronary ostia in aortic surgery or the circumflex coronary artery in mitral surgery). Check regional wall motion abnormalities as a guide to which artery may be affected. Look at coronary ostia lumen size and flow in short axis views.

Off-pump coronary artery bypass

Transoesophageal monitoring may be useful in off-pump coronary artery bypass graft surgery to monitor cardiac function and potential mitral regurgitation. Beware of the following aspects of off-pump surgery.

• Imaging of left ventricular wall motion is limited by the stabilizer apparatus, which tethers the adjacent myocardium.
• During right coronary artery and circumflex grafting major displacement of the heart does not allow reliable imaging.
• Distortion of the heart can also cause transient mitral regurgitation or increase in right atrial pressure and a shunt via a patent forman ovale.
• It is best to restart imaging after completion of anastomoses and release of the stabilizer.
• For a short period after the anastomosis regional wall motion abnormalities are seen, representing stunned myocardium. If wall motion abnormalities are persistent, graft patency should be checked.

Ischaemic mitral regurgitation

Ischaemic mitral regurgitation is regurgitation due to incompetent mitral valve systolic coaption with normal valve leaflet structure, in the presence of ischaemic heart disease. Commonly due to tethered valve leaflets after basal posterior myocardial infarction, combined with mild to moderate mitral annulus dilatation. Less frequently due to papillary muscle dysfunction or detachment.

• It may be present before surgery. In this case imaging has to assess the severity to decide on the need for mitral valve repair or replacement. To plan surgery (approach, mitral valve ring size, etc.) measure leaflet tethering distance (distance between posterior papillary muscle and mitral valve posterior annulus) and mitral valve annulus diameter.
• Ischaemic regurgitation may also evolve during coronary bypass surgery due to insufficient grafting to the right coronary artery or diffuse myocardial ischaemia. Ischaemic mitral regurgitation is dynamic so tends to be less severe during surgery because of the reduced left ventricular afterload and the general anaesthetic. Moderate to severe regurgitation on intraoperative echocardiography requires surgical intervention.

Aneurysm repair

Before and during ventricular aneurysm resection or apex remodelling (Dor procedure) echocardiography should focus on:

• presence, mobility, and distribution of mural thrombus;
• involvement of mitral valve apparatus and papillary muscle;
• mitral regurgitation caused by surgery;
• amount and function of residual myocardium.

Haemodynamic instability

On the Intensive Care Unit and during intraoperative monitoring transoesophageal echocardiography provides a quick and reliable way to investigate the cause of haemodynamic instability. *Haemodynamic instability* usually means *unexplained hypotension* in some cases associated with *unexplained hypoxaemia*. Transoesophageal echocardiography provides information on both intrinsic cardiac causes (e.g. ventricular function, valvular function) and extra-cardiac factors (e.g. left ventricular preload and afterload). Assessment should take into account the clinical history and follow a standard routine to try and exclude common causes.

Hypotension due to hypovolaemia

Hypovolaemia causes reduced left ventricular preload/filling. A simple measure of preload/filling is the *left ventricular end-diastolic area* in the short-axis transgastric view. This view can be used for monitoring during surgery. It is useful if a baseline area is known (e.g. pre-operative or at start of surgery) in order to judge change from normal filling.

- Hypovolaemia causes a reduced end-diastolic left ventricular volume and, with preserved left ventricular function, an even greater reduction in end-systolic volume. This results in a very high fractional area change.
- If hypovolaemia is diagnosed response to fluid therapy should be monitored. Optimal filling of the left ventricle is achieved when further volume supplements do not result in further increase in end-diastolic left ventricular area. Further volume then merely causes increase in left ventricular end-diastolic pressure.

Hypotension due to reduced peripheral resistance

Reduced peripheral resistance (e.g. due to sepsis) results in much higher stroke volumes. End-diastolic volume therefore remains normal but the end-systolic volume is reduced. This again leads to an increased fractional area change.

Hypotension due to ischaemia

If there is clinical suspicion of myocardial ischaemia it is useful to compare any new findings to the pre-operative assessment of cardiac function. Look for the following.

- Left ventricular systolic global and regional function.
- Right ventricular systolic dysfunction. Right ventricular dysfunction is often associated with right ventricular dilatation, tricuspid regurgitation, and paradoxical septal movement, and a decrease in left ventricular chamber size can sometimes occur.
- True or pseudo aneurysm and/or right ventricular rupture in those known to have had an infarct.
- Ischaemic ventricular septal defect or papillary muscle rupture.

Table 5.11 Conditions causing hypotension. Severe aortic stenosis can also be associated with hypotension and is identified from changes to the aortic valve and transvalvular gradient. Aortic dissection can cause hypotension due to associated pericardial effusions and tamponade, hypovolaemia, or aortic regurgitation

Condition Associated findings	End-diastolic volume*	End-systolic volume*	Ejection fraction[†]	Cardiac output
Decreased preload Hypovolaemia	↓	↓↓	↑	↓
Decreased afterload Vasodilation/sepsis	↔	↓↓	↑↑	↑
LV dysfunction Global/regional wall motion, rupture	↑	↑↑	↓↓	↓
RV dysfunction Dilated right heart, thrombus in pulmonary artery	↓	↓	(↓)	↓
Tamponade Effusion	↓	↓	↓	↓

* Left ventricular end-diastolic and end-systolic areas in the short axis transgastric views may be used as markers of left ventricular volume.
† Fractional area change can be substituted for ejection fraction.

Unexplained hypoxaemia

Hypoxaemia suggests inadequate lung perfusion. Cardiac causes can include right ventricular dysfunction, pulmonary embolism, or right-to-left shunts. Investigations should also look for primary lung pathology (e.g. pneumonia with associated sepsis).

Pulmonary embolism

Pulmonary embolism is not easy to diagnose (and cannot be excluded) because large emboli are needed to induce haemodynamic changes or to be visualized. Helpful features to suggest pulmonary embolism include the following.

Indirect signs

- Dilated right atrium. Dilated and diffusely hypokinetic right ventricle. Dilated pulmonary artery. (An increased right ventricular wall thickness suggests a more chronic problem, e.g. pulmonary hypertension).
- An increase in tricuspid regurgitation because of raised pulmonary artery pressure. Judge pressure from the tricuspid regurgitation. (However, cardiac shock can lead to a normal gradient.)

Direct signs

- Thrombus in the inferior or superior vena cava, or pulmonary artery.
- There are two types of thrombi. Type A are highly mobile and vermiform. They derive from deep veins and can become trapped in a Chiari network, tricuspid valve chordae, or right ventricle trabeculae. Type B originate from chamber walls, leads, or prostheses.
- To see the pulmonary artery withdraw the probe slightly from an aortic 50° view and angulate the probe forward. The right pulmonary artery can be seen wrapping around the aorta. The left pulmonary artery is obscured by the bronchus (see p. 346).

Patent foramen ovale

In suspected pulmonary embolism always assess the interatrial septum. High right atrial pressure opens the foramen and can cause significant right-to-left shunting. With successful treatment of the embolism the shunt reduces and then disappears. Paradoxical embolism is possible and sometimes thrombi can be trapped in the septum.

Right-to-left shunt

Right-to-left shunts can be intracardiac or intrapulmonary. Base initial survey on colour flow mapping of the atrial and ventricular septa. If no shunt is displayed by colour flow mapping use agitated saline contrast, injected through a central line.

- If an *intracardiac shunt*, contrast will pass from right to left atrium, or from right to left ventricle immediately after arrival in the right atrium.
- If an *intrapulmonary shunt*, contrast will appear in the left atrium via the pulmonary veins at least five beats after the right atrium.
- If there is a known pre-existing left-to-right shunt this may be turned into a right-to-left shunt by the surgery, ventilation, or a pulmonary embolism. Positive end-expiratory pressure ventilation may open a patent foramen ovale in the presence of severe pulmonary embolism.

Mechanical cardiac support

Intra-aortic balloon pump

Transoesophageal echocardiography can be used to identify contraindications to a balloon pump and ensure the balloon is correctly placed in the thoracic descending aorta, distal to the subclavian artery.

Complicating factors

Possible contraindications include: descending aortic aneurysm; moderate to severe aortic regurgitation; severe atheroma.

Placement

To localize the balloon tip start with an aortic arch view. Try and locate the left subclavian artery origin; then advance the probe until the tip of the balloon pump comes into view. It should be several centimetres below the left subclavian artery. The tip appears as a bright mark in the centre of the aorta, with associated artefacts. If the probe is advanced further the balloon may be seen deflating and inflating in the aorta.

Left ventricular assist devices

Left ventricular assist devices take blood from a cannula placed in the left atrium or left ventricle, pass it though an extracorporeal pump, and then pass the blood back into the circulation via a tube inserted into the thoracic aorta. Transoesophageal echocardiography can help in placement, assessment of device function, and device weaning.

Complicating factors

Before placement, imaging should be used to identify possible contraindications and complications.

- Aortic regurgitation may deteriorate after device placement because of increased backflow into a relatively decompressed left ventricle. In moderate aortic regurgitation valvular surgery has to be considered prior to device placement.
- Thrombi within the ventricular cavities may be mobilized by assist device tubes and should be excluded.
- Aortic atheroma may be dislodged during cannula insertion.
- Right ventricular dysfunction should be assessed in case right ventricular assistance is required.
- Patent foramen ovale should be identified. Significant right-to-left shunting can be found after left ventricular assist device placement. The device significantly offloads the left heart and drops left atrial pressure, whereas the right atrium remains at a relatively high pressure.

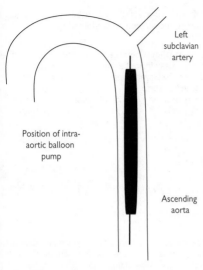

Fig. 5.40 Position of intra-aortic balloon pump in aorta. The top of the balloon can be imaged in aortic views.

Placement

During placement of a left ventricular assist device use transoesophageal echocardiography to report to the surgeon on the following.

Cannulae

- Position of the atrial cannula (should be in centre of atrium). It should not lie against a wall and be away from the subvalvular apparatus.
- Flow in the cannulae (can be displayed using colour flow mapping).
- Flow pattern in the descending aorta.
- De-airing of the system by observing clearing of bubbles through the ascending or descending aorta.

Changes to valves and septum

- Patent foramen ovale, which may have been missed pre-placement.
- Presence of tricuspid regurgitation.
- Competence of the aortic valve.

Changes to chamber function

- Whether adequate left ventricular offload is achieved.
- Left atrial filling status and size.
- Right ventricular volume status and contraction.

During use

After placement, transoesophageal echocardiography should monitor for bleeding and pericardial effusion. This is common during the first 24 hours of support and can cause cardiac tamponade.

Weaning

On removal, transoesophageal echocardiography should be used to judge weaning off left ventricular assist support. The emphasis should be on watching the effect of reducing support on left ventricular function. The left ventricle should gradually improve and take over haemodynamic function.

- Monitor response of the left ventricle to resumed volume loading at both regional and global levels.
- Look at mitral valve competence and systemic haemodynamics.
- Check that improvement in left ventricular is sustained with minimal support rather than just a short-lived improvement of left ventricular contraction.

Pleural space and lungs

As the probe is rotated posteriorly during the study the lungs and pleura may come into view. It is difficult to give accurate information about lung pathology because they are full of air, which does not allow good ultrasound views. Pleural effusions are easily recognized as crescent or 'tiger claw' -shaped areas of fluid. The principle to determine whether it is a right or left effusion is to look at the way the 'tiger claw' points. If it points to the right it is a right-sided effusion and if to the left, a left-sided effusion (Fig. 5.41).

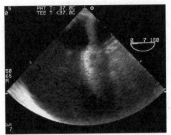

Right-sided effusion

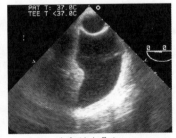

Left-sided effusion

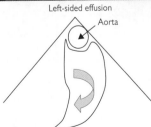

Fig. 5.41 Pleural effusions.

Pacing wires and other implants

As well as prosthetic valves a series of other artifical devices will be seen during transoesophageal studies. Right-sided implants include pacing and defibrillator wires in the right atrium and ventricle, and central lines in the superior vena cava and right atrium.

Increasingly, percutaneous closure devices are being implanted. Most commonly these are seen across the atrial septum but they can also be positioned in the ventricular septum or beside prosthetic valves to close paraprosthetic leaks. Left atrial appendage occluder devices are also implanted in some centres. Make sure you check the notes before and during the procedure if there is an unusual feature identified.

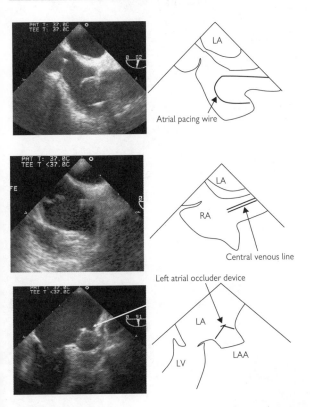

Fig. 5.42 Example of an atrial pacing wire (top) and central venous catheter (middle) in bicaval views. A left atrial occluder device (bottom) is seen in a 2-chamber view.

Stress echocardiography

Introduction

Stress echocardiography has become a valuable method for cardiovascular stress testing. It plays a crucial role in the initial detection of coronary artery disease, in determining prognosis, and in therapeutic decision-making. The major use of stress echocardiography is to assess myocardial ischaemia or viability in patients with coronary artery disease. Stress echocardiography can also be applied to evaluation of valvular disease and cardiomyopathies.

Stress echocardiography or nuclear myocardial perfusion scanning?

The two techniques have similar sensitivity and specificity so choice of test often depends on local availability and expertise. The indications for stress echocardiography widely overlap with the indications for myocardial scintigraphy.

There are clinical situations where myocardial scintigraphy is relatively contraindicated (left bundle branch block, bifascicular block, and ventricular paced rhythms). In these situations dynamic exercise leads to perfusion abnormalities of the septum and adjacent walls in the absence of obstructive coronary disease. If there is local expertise, stress echocardiography is an option.

For assessment of viability/hibernation stress echocardiography and myocardial perfusion imaging are joined by magnetic resonance imaging and positron emission tomography. All are potential methods and currently there is no consensus as to whether one of these methods is superior. The decision depends on local availability and expertise.

Pre-test probability

In patients referred for stress echocardiography the likelihood of having coronary artery disease can usually be estimated from their symptoms and history. This *pre-test probability* is useful because the gain by performing a stress test depends on the pre-test probability. Based on the accuracy of stress echocardiography to detect coronary artery disease it is also possible to calculate the probability of coronary artery disease with a negative or positive result of stress echocardiography (*post-test probability*).

If there is a *high* pre-test probability, >70% (see Table 6.1) (e.g. typical angina and risk factors) the risk of a cardiac event remains high even if there is a negative test. In patients with a *low* pre-test probability, <30% (e.g. young patients with atypical chest pain) a positive test does not necessarily indicate disease. Therefore, when used for diagnosis, stress echocardiography (like nuclear perfusion imaging) is ideal for patients with *intermediate* pre-test probability (e.g. women with atypical chest pain and some risk factors). In this group of patients a negative test predicts a low risk of further cardiac events, whereas a positive test indicates a high risk and warrants further invasive diagnostics.

Although stress echocardiography in patients with high pre-test probability is of limited *diagnostic value*, it is still of *clinical value*. In patients with known coronary artery disease stress echocardiography can help to define the location and extent of ischaemia.

Table 6.1 Combined Diamond–Forrester and CASS data of pre-test likelihood of coronary artery disease in symptomatic patients. (Modified from Committee on the Management of Patients with chronic stable angina. ACC/AHA 2002 guideline update for the management of patients with chronic stable angina. *J Am Coll Cardiol* 2003;**41**(1);159–68.)

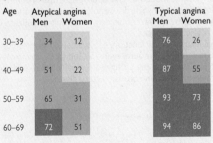

Age	Atypical angina		Typical angina	
	Men	Women	Men	Women
30–39	34	12	76	26
40–49	51	22	87	55
50–59	65	31	93	73
60–69	72	51	94	86

Values represents % with coronary artery disease on angiography

■ >70%   ■ 30–70%   ▨ <30%

Detection of ischaemia

Principle

The rationale for the diagnosis of myocardial ischaemia with stress echo-cardiography is a relative reduction in myocardial blood flow on stress sufficient to cause a decrease in myocardial contraction. The ischaemic changes in left ventricle wall motion appear earlier than ECG changes and angina (the *ischaemic cascade*). During stress, in a normal subject, coronary and myocardial blood flow increase 3- to 4-fold to comply with the increased oxygen demand of the myocardium. This can occur because myocardial arteriolar resistance reduces. If there is a significant stenosis of an epicardial coronary artery, the resistance of the arteriolar vessels is already reduced at rest. This is known as *autoregulation* and allows preservation of coronary blood flow at rest, and at low levels of stress, in the territory supplied by the stenosed artery. Therefore, at rest severe occlusions do not result in wall motion abnormalities. However, with stress and increased oxygen demand the blood flow cannot be further increased and the corresponding myocardial segment cannot contract as well as myocardial segments supplied by patent arteries. The more severe the epicardial stenosis, the smaller the possible increase in coronary blood flow and the earlier wall motion abnormalities occur.

Limitations

- Coronary atherosclerosis can only be detected when epicardial stenosis exceeds 50%.
- There has to be a significant increase in oxygen demand to disclose regional wall motion abnormalities—in particular for moderate stenoses. This is only possible by reaching or exceeding target heart rates as in exercise ECG stress testing.
- Even severe stenosis may be missed if there is a well developed collateral circulation.
- Worsening of wall motion or an inappropriate loss of contractility in comparison to other myocardial segments is the hallmark of stress echocardiography. However, this may be difficult to visualize if resting function is already reduced.
- Abnormal microvascular function, e.g. in arterial hypertension or diabetes, may reduce the autoregulation and cause abnormal responses to stress. However, the changes are usually diffuse and not segmental as observed in coronary artery disease.

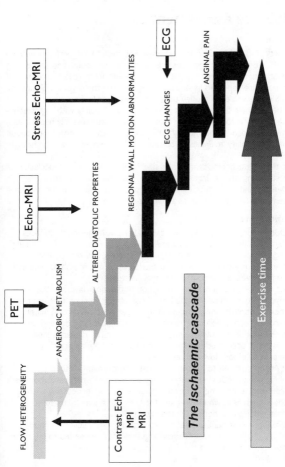

Fig. 6.1 The ischaemic cascade.

Viability assessment

Principle

Viability studies based on left ventricle wall motion are performed when akinetic (or severely hypokinetic) segments are found and there is a question as to whether the patient will benefit from revascularization. If segments are reported as *viable* this implies that the myocardial function is still preserved even though their blood supply is limited.

The rationale for the diagnosis of *myocardial viability* with stress echocardiography is to demonstrate that the akinetic (or severely hypokinetic) segments improve contractility when exposed to low doses of dobutamine. This ability to increase contractility is referred to as a *contractile reserve*.

If there is a haemodynamically significant stenosis or an occlusion of the supplying artery, higher dosages of dobutamine may then result in ischaemia and the contractility decreases. This improvement and then deterioration is referred to as a *biphasic response*.

Limitations

- Dobutamine increases oxygen demand and at higher doses induces ischaemia in hibernating myocardium (biphasic response). This usually requires doses exceeding 20mcg/kg/min. However, very severe stenoses may cause ischaemia at the lowest doses of dobutamine and no improvement of contractility may be seen.
- Contractility depends on preservation of the inner layers of the myocardium. Therefore, the lack of contractile reserve does not mean there is no viable myocardium in the outer layers. Although major recovery of function after revascularization appears to depend on preserved contractility, segments with irreversibly damaged inner layers but preserved outer myocardial layers still may benefit from improved blood flow and remodelling.
- It may be difficult to differentiate passive movement (tethering, i.e. being pulled with a normally moving segment) of a myocardial segment from active movement due to contraction. Image processing analysis tools, such as strain imaging and tissue tracking, may be useful to differentiate but there is limited experience.
- Viability assessment using stress echocardiography relies on good image quality. Contrast echocardiography may be needed to improve border delineation.

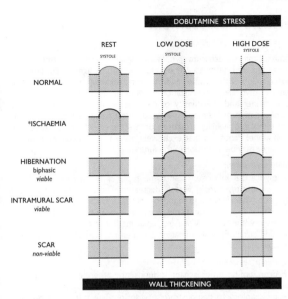

Fig. 6.2 Changes in wall thickening with dobutamine stress. *Decline in wall thickening with ischaemia can be variable in degree and timing.

Table 6.2 Causes of akinetic left ventricle segments

Scar (non-viable)
- Irreversible loss of myocardium.
- Often reduced diastolic wall thickness <0.6cm.

Stunning (viable)
- Transiently reduced contractility after ischaemia.
- Usually spontaneous recovery (e.g. transient coronary occlusion in infarction with early recanalization, or poststress in severe stenosis).
- Stunning usually diagnosed by follow-up studies that demonstrate recovery in function.
- If complete occlusion during infarction this can take 4–6 weeks

Hibernation (viable)
- Permanently reduced contractility.
- Permanent coronary occlusion or high grade stenosis with insufficient collateral blood flow: 'too little to live, too much to die'.
- Transient recovery with low dose dobutamine.
- Worsening with high dose 'biphasic response'.

Intramural scar (viable)
- As for hibernation but does not worsen with high dose dobutamine.

Perfusion assessment

Principle

Myocardial contrast echocardiography (perfusion imaging) describes echo-cardiography with intravascular ultrasound contrast agents. These result in opacification of the cavities and the intramyocardial blood vessels. The amount of myocardial opacification depends on the settings of the ultra-sound scanner and the density of the myocardial microvessels (where most of the myocardial blood is located). Most guidelines for assessment of ischaemia and viability are based on assessment of left ventricle wall motion alone. Protocols that exclusively make the diagnosis from perfusion images may be an option in the future.

Viability assessment

After myocardial infarction scar tissue replaces the myocytes and the density of intramyocardial vessels decreases. Therefore the myocardial opacification decreases and 'dark' or 'black' areas are seen within the myocardium. Typically scar tissue does not opacify because the amount of contrast within the few vessels remaining is not enough to cause an ultrasound signal. Perfusion imaging can then be used at rest to identify non-viable scar.

Ischaemia assessment

As myocardium becomes ischaemic during stress there is an early relative reduction in perfusion in the ischaemic area. This principle is used in nuclear cardiology to demonstrate a perfusion defect. It is also possible for ultrasound contrast agents to demonstrate this reduction in perfusion during a stress study. Segments that have normal perfusion at rest will start to have reduced perfusion and take on an appearance similar to scar.

Limitations

- There is limited experience using contrast echocardiography for viability studies. Contrast echocardiography may be used only in addition to dobutamine stress echocardiography.
- Scar tissue sometimes can cause a very echogenic tissue signal. This makes it very difficult to assess changes in myocardial opacification after contrast injection.
- Artefacts caused by inadequate machine settings and contrast dosage can cause false-positive and false-negative findings.

Pre-operative assessment

In patients undergoing major vascular surgery a dobutamine stress echocardiogram allows determination of the peri-operative risk for cardiovascular complications. This is particularly useful if patients have three or more of the following characteristics: age >70yrs; current angina; prior myocardial infarction; congestive heart failure; prior cerebrovascular event; diabetes mellitus; or renal failure.

The main method to protect patients with known coronary artery disease peri-operatively is to prescribe effective beta-blockade. The risk of peri-operative cardiac complications has been assessed in clinical trials and is related to the number of wall segments that become ischaemic on dobutamine stress echocardiography. Patients without new wall motion abnormalities have a low risk (<5%). Patients with 1–4 segments showing new wall motion abnormalities have a slightly higher peri-operative risk but can be protected with beta-blockers. If >4 segments exhibit new wall motion abnormalities during stress, there is a high risk (>30%) of cardiac complications peri-operatively. This risk cannot be reduced by beta-blockers and there is therefore a potential theoretical benefit from revascularization (although currently unproven to reduce risk).

Table 6.3 Odds ratios for risk of cardiovascular complications peri-operatively relative to a low risk patient on beta-blocker. Risk is assessed from a risk score based on age and other disease (score 1 for each factor present: age >70 years; current angina; prior myocardial infarction; congestive heart failure; prior cerebrovascular event; diabetes mellitus; or renal failure) combined with presence of new wall motion abnormalities on stress echocardiography. Note benefit of beta-blockers in those with one to two risk factors and for those who have more risk factors but less than four ischaemic segments on stress*

Risk score	Wall motion abnormality	Beta-blocker	
		No	Yes
0	—†	1.2	0
1–2	—†	3.0	0.9
≥ 3	None	5.8	2.0
≥ 3	1–4 segments	33.0	2.8
≥ 3	>4 segments	33.0	36.0

† In patients with two or less risk factors pre-operative risk assessment using stress echocardiography is not absolutely necessary, particularly if patients are already on beta-blockers.

* Data from Boersma, E, Poldermans, D, *et al.* Echocardiographic cardiac risk evaluation applying stress echocardiography. Predictors of cardiac events after major vascular surgery: role of clinical characteristics, dobutamine echocardiography, and beta-blocker therapy. *JAMA* 2001;**285**(14);1865–73.

Indications

The main indication for stress echocardiography is in assessment of coronary artery disease patients. ECG stress testing is the most frequently used initial stress test to evaluate patients with suspected coronary artery disease. Stress echocardiography is used in addition to stress ECG or as the initial diagnostic tool. However, stress echocardiography has been applied to several other pathologies. The key indications are to aid management of patients with the following.

Suspected coronary artery disease

- As part of an investigational strategy for the diagnosis of patients in whom stress ECG was inconclusive.
- For people for whom treadmill exercise is difficult or impossible because of poor mobility or inability to perform dynamic exercise.
- For people for whom stress ECG poses particular problems of poor sensitivity or difficulties in interpretation, including women, patients with cardiac conduction defects (for instance, left bundle branch block and resting ST segment abnormalities), and diabetes.
- For people with a low or intermediate likelihood of coronary artery disease and future cardiac events. Likelihood of coronary artery disease depends on clinical assessment of risk factors including age, gender, ethnic group, family history, associated co-morbidities, clinical presentation, physical examination, and results from other investigations (e.g. blood cholesterol levels or resting ECG).

Known coronary artery disease

- To determine the likelihood of future coronary events, for instance after myocardial infarction or risk assessment for proposed non-cardiac surgery (p. 472).
- To assess myocardial viability and hibernation, particularly with reference to planned myocardial revascularization.
- To guide strategies of myocardial revascularization by determining the haemodynamic significance of known coronary lesions.
- To assess the adequacy of percutaneous and surgical revascularization.

Valvular heart disease

- Aortic stenosis with a low gradient and poor left ventricle function (p. 130).
- Aortic stenosis with a high gradient in asymptomatic patients.
- Mitral stenosis with discrepancy between haemodynamic and clinical findings (e.g. dyspnoea despite low gradient at rest, asymptomatic patient with high grade stenosis).
- Mitral regurgitation (organic, severe) in asymptomatic patients.
- To establish evidence of inducible ischaemic mitral regurgitation.
- To evaluate aortic regurgitation (severe) in asymptomatic patients.

Hypertrophic cardiomyopathy or sub-aortic muscular obstruction

- Assessment for dynamic gradient.

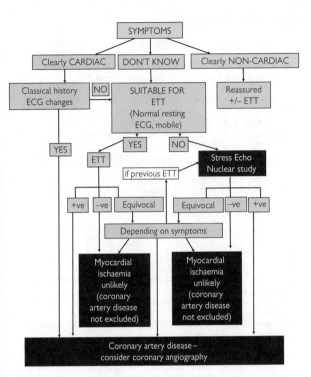

Fig. 6.3 An approach to investigate a patient with suspected coronary artery disease. Adapted from Gershlick, AH *et al*. Role of non-invasive imaging in the management of coronary artery disease. *Heart* 2007: 93(4); 423–31.

Contraindications

Absolute contraindications for all stress modalities

- Non-ST-segment elevation acute coronary syndrome. Once stabilized, exercise stress can be considered 24–72h after chest pain, in low or intermediate risk patients. High dose dobutamine should not be performed within the first week after a myocardial infarction.
- ST segment elevation myocardial infarction within the previous 4 days.
- Left ventricular failure with symptoms at rest.
- Recent history of life-threatening arrhythmias.
- Severe dynamic or fixed left ventricular outflow tract obstruction (aortic stenosis and obstructive hypertrophic cardiomyopathy).
- Severe systemic hypertension (systolic blood pressure >220mmHg and/or diastolic blood pressure >120mmHg).
- Recent pulmonary embolism or infarction.
- Thrombophlebitis or active deep vein thrombosis.
- Known hypokalaemia (particularly for dobutamine stress).
- Active endocarditis, myocarditis, or pericarditis.
- Left main coronary artery stenosis that is likely to be haemo-dynamically significant.

Absolute contraindications for vasodilator stress

- Suspected or known severe bronchospasm.
- Second and third degree atrioventricular block in the absence of a functioning pacemaker.
- Sick sinus syndrome in the absence of a functioning pacemaker.
- Hypotension (systolic blood pressure <90mmHg).
- Xanthines taken in the last 12 hours, or dipyridamole use in the last 24 hours.

Relative contraindications to vasodilator stress

- Bradycardia of less than 40 beats/min. Initial dynamic exercise normally increases the rate sufficiently to start the infusion.
- Recent cerebral ischaemia or infarction.

Contraindications to contrast imaging

- See p. 500.

Equipment and personnel

Equipment

Because analysis of wall motion abnormalities is difficult and not reliable in the presence of poor quality images, every effort has to be made to optimize visualization of the endocardial border and the myocardium.

- The scanner should provide tissue harmonic imaging and a contrast-specific imaging modality in order to be applicable in the majority of patients.
- Use of digital frame grabbers and split or 'quad-screen' displays allows side-by-side comparison of rest and stress images using the same echocardiographic views and is the current standard for performing stress echocardiograms.
- Doppler tissue imaging is optional but may add clinical information. 3D imaging is not widely available but has the potential to generate more detailed information.

Personnel and experience

- Two people are required to record and monitor stress echocardiography—one of them should have substantial experience in the evaluation of patients with ischaemic heart disease and in analysis of wall motion/thickening abnormalities.
- Recordings should be performed by a skilled echocardiographer (technician or physician).
- If a physician is not participating in the study, one should be available in the immediate locality in case of acute problems. One of the personnel present should be qualified in advanced life support.
- Recording and interpretation of stress echocardiograms require extensive experience in echocardiography and should be performed only by technicians and physicians with specific training in the technique. Most recommendations suggest physicians should perform and interpret a minimum of 100 studies under supervision before they can perform stress echocardiography independently. Supervised over-reading of at least 100 stress echocardiograms is required to attain the minimum level of competence for independent interpretation.

Drugs

- Depending on the stress protocol chosen the appropriate drugs (dobutamine, adenosine, dipyridamole, atropine) and agents to reverse their effects should be prepared (aminophyline if dipyridamole used, beta-blockers).
- Standard resuscitation drugs and equipment will need to be available in the room.

Patient preparation

Patients should be provided with information or have a detailed verbal explanation. Informed consent is usually considered appropriate especially for pharmacological stress or with the use of contrast agents.

Sample information sheet

You have been asked to attend for stress echocardiography. A stress echocardiogram is an ultrasound scan of your heart, performed after increasing your heart rate. A stress echocardiogram provides information about the performance of your heart at stress and helps your doctors to identify symptoms you may have on exertion.

Before the procedure? Please continue to take all your medications as usual except for your beta-blocker which should not be taken on the morning of the test. You will be seen by the doctor who will take a medical history and after explaining the procedure will ask you to sign a consent form. If you have any concerns, please do not hesitate to ask, as we would like you to be as relaxed as possible and are happy to answer questions.

What happens during the procedure? The doctor will insert a small tube into your arm (cannula) to infuse the drug (dobutamine) that increases the heart rate. A blood pressure cuff will be placed on your arm. You will be asked to lie on your left side and the ultrasound scan will be performed. Dobutamine will be given via the cannula, which will gradually increase the heart rate. In addition, ultrasound contrast agents may be given to improve image quality. There will be a doctor present, also a technician. The procedure takes 20–30 minutes to examine all areas carefully. When the examination is finished the dobutamine is stopped and the heart rate will come down quickly.

Benefits? The benefits from stress echocardiography are that it can: (1) define the nature of cardiac symptoms; (2) point out the status of the cardiovascular system; (3) decide which further therapeutic and diagnostic procedures you have to undergo following the information derived from this examination.

Risks? Usually the investigation is tolerated well; some patients could have some mild symptoms during the test (mostly palpitations, tremor, light-headed sensation). Serious risks are very rare, less than 0.3% (1 in every 330 patients), and include heart rhythm problems, myocardial infarction, and low blood pressure. Your doctor would not recommend that you have a stress echocardiogram unless she/he felt that the benefits of the procedure outweighed these small risks.

After the procedure? After the procedure you will be asked to stay for another 30 minutes. This is the time needed to completely clear the infused drugs. You will be offered refreshments. The doctor will return and discuss the results of your procedure. Any relevant advice and literature will then be given. Your cannula will be removed and you may go home with your relative/friend. A letter with the results of your procedure will be sent to your GP and any referring doctor.

Safety

A large international study of stress echocardiography[1] reported on 85,997 patients undergoing stress echocardiography. The incidence of life-threatening adverse events in those undergoing stress with exercise was 1:6574, dobutamine 1:557, and dipyridamole 1:1294. There were six deaths (1:14333) related to the procedure (5 with dobutamine, and 1 with dipyridamole). These were mainly due to ventricular arrhythmias. It was pointed out that the subgroup of patients receiving dobutamine may have been at higher risk because of viability studies in those with established coronary disease.

1 Varga, A, Garcia, MA, and Picano, E International stress echo complication registry. Safety of stress echocardiography. *Am J Cardiol* 2006:98(4);541–3.

Performing the study

The image acquisition is structured to make it easy to identify changes from baseline in wall motion and thickening of the left ventricle. The fundamental requirement is high quality 2D echocardiographic recordings with good endocardial border definition in all segments. These basic images need to be acquired confidently and quickly during stress. Additional data can include Doppler tissue profiles (global and regional parameters of function) and direct assessment of myocardial perfusion by myocardial contrast enhancement (depending on local experience).

Views

Multiple views are required to ensure all left ventricular segments are monitored and all three major coronary distributions are assessed. The key four views are: apical 4- and 2-chamber; parasternal short and long axis (or apical long axis). Subcostal or additional short-axis views can be substituted when necessary or when more appropriate for visualization of specific anatomy.

Set up

- Spend time ensuring good patient position (they will be in this position throughout the stress). A clear, stable ECG recording is required.
- Study all four views and spend time optimizing the images.
  - *Machine settings*. Select harmonic imaging and adjust focus zone. Ideally, frame rate should be >25 frames/sec (if heart rate >140 then frame rates >30 frames/sec may be better).
  - *Probe position*. Be very careful not to foreshorten apical views. The patient may need to do held inspiration or expiration for clear, stable, unforeshortened images.
  - *Contrast*. Decide whether there is good endocardial border definition in each view and whether images can be acquired confidently and smoothly during the stress in each window. If two or more segments are not seen or the images are difficult use contrast.

Image acquisition

- Record a set of baseline images (use a stress protocol preset if available). Use a standard acquisition order, e.g. parasternal long axis, parasternal short axis, apical 4-chamber, and apical 2-chamber (alternatively the apical views can be recorded first).
- Start the stress (e.g. pharmacological/physical).
- At the preset time-points (depending on stress and clinical response) record a complete set of images. Some machines have a 'compare' mode to ensure your images are in exactly the same position.
- Look for changes in wall motion and thickening during image acquisition so that you interpret the test as you go along.
- Once all the images are acquired, review them off-line, ideally with a second experienced reviewer, to create the final report.

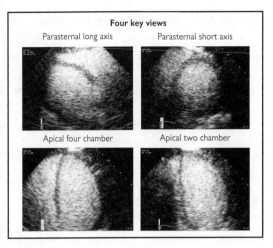

Fig. 6.4 There are four key views. The parasternal long axis and apical 3-chamber provide very similar information.

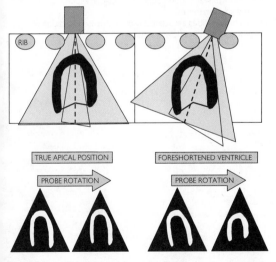

Fig. 6.5 It is vital that all apical views are unforeshortened to avoid missing apical wall motion abnormalities. If the probe is not on the true apex then, even though the apex may be included in the initial plane, probe rotation for the next view will create a foreshortened image.

Monitoring and termination criteria

Monitoring

As with other forms of stress testing, standard ECG and blood pressure monitoring should be performed. This may provide diagnostic and prognostic information during exercise studies. With pharmacological stress ECG monitoring has limited diagnostic value but is needed to trigger loop recording and monitor for arrhythmias. However, if a 12 lead ECG is not performed during pharmacological stress, a 12 lead ECG recorder should be readily available in case of problems.

Termination criteria

Treadmill exercise echocardiography should be terminated at traditional endpoints:
- attainment of target heart rates;
- cardiovascular symptoms;
- significant ECG changes or arrhythmias.

Bicycle exercise and pharmacological stress provide additional echocardiographic endpoints because they allow on-line, continuous visualization of wall motion and thickening. Stress echocardiography with on-line monitoring should be terminated at:
- traditional endpoints (as above);
- the development of wall motion abnormalities corresponding to two or more coronary territories;
- wall motion abnormalities associated with ventricular dilatation and/or global reduction of systolic function.

Maximum age predicted heart rate = 220 – Age of patient

Target heart rate = 85% × Maximum age predicted

e.g. Age = 67
Maximum age predicted = 220 – 67 = 153 bpm
Target heart rate = 0.85 × 153 = 130

Target heart rate according to age

Age	100%	85%
85	135	115
80	140	119
75	145	123
70	150	128
65	155	132
60	160	136
55	165	140
50	170	145
45	175	149
40	180	153
35	185	157
30	190	162
25	195	166
20	200	170

Fig. 6.6 Target heart rates for stress.

Exercise stress protocols

Exercise is the most physiological stressor for assessment of myocardial ischaemia in patients able to exercise.

Stress protocol

- The protocols are the same as for exercise stress ECG testing.
- A Bruce treadmill protocol with 3min stages of graded increases in speed and gradient, or an ergometer with 3min stages of graded cycling resistance at a fixed cycling rate.
- Treadmill exercise should be terminated at traditional endpoints such as attainment of target heart rates, cardiovascular symptoms, and/or significant ECG changes suggestive of ischaemia.
- Supine and upright bicycle exercise appear to have equivalent degrees of accuracy. Supine bicycle ergometry on a special bed, which can be rotated, provides additional echocardiographic endpoints because it allows continuous visualization of wall motion at incremental levels of stress, including peak exercise. Bicycle exercise should be terminated at traditional endpoints and, if a supine bicycle is used, when wall motion abnormalities develop that correspond with two or more coronary territories, or wall motion abnormalities associated with ventricular dilatation and/or global reduction of systolic function.

Image acquisition

Imaging should be performed at:

- baseline;
- post-treadmill exercise (because ischaemia-induced wall motion abnormalities may resolve quickly, post-exercise imaging should be accomplished within 60–90sec of termination of exercise). If the patient is asymptomatic and there are no ECG changes then extending the exercise up to 100% of target heart rate provides more time post-exercise to acquire images;
- if supine bicycle ergometry is used imaging should also be performed during exercise and an intermediate stage can be recorded.

Exercise or dobutamine

For the diagnosis of myocardial ischaemia, there appears to be no difference in the accuracy and prognostic information obtained with dobutamine compared to exercise stress. It is possible that, for milder forms of coronary artery disease, treadmill may be advantageous. Exercise stress echocardiography presents a challenge to obtain good quality images. For patients unable to exercise, dobutamine is indicated. An advantage of dobutamine is that it has a rapid onset and cessation of action, and its effects can be reversed by β-blocker administration. If there is a contraindication to dobutamine then dipyridamole, adenosine, or pacing may be used. For risk assessment prior to non-cardiac surgery the accuracy of dobutamine stress echocardiography is proven. For assessment of myocardial viability use of low and high dose dobutamine seems to be the best stress method for echocardiography.

Bruce exercise protocol

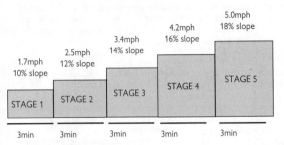

Modified Bruce has 2 extra 3 minute stages at start
(1.7mph/0% slope and 1.7mph/ 5% slope)
then continues as above

Ergometer protocol

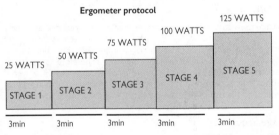

AT CONSTANT PEDAL RATE OF 50 CYCLES PER MINUTE

Fig 6.7 Standard protocols for exercise testing.

Dobutamine stress for ischaemia

Myocardial ischaemia is assessed by graded dobutamine infusion. This increases myocardial oxygen demand in a fashion analogous to staged exercise. Contractility, heart rate, and to a minor degree systolic blood pressure are all increased.

Dobutamine infusion

- Start the infusion at 5 or 10mcg/kg/min dobutamine.
- At 3min intervals increase the infusion to 20, 30, and then 40mcg/kg/min.
- If the rise in heart rate is minimal by 30mcg/kg/min dobutamine, then consider using atropine. Check for contraindications to atropine, in particular glaucoma, before administration.
- Atropine should be used at the minimum effective dose. Administer 0.3mg doses at 60sec intervals until the desired heart rate response is seen. Maximum dose should be 1.2mg. The effect on accuracy is not fully established but appears beneficial.

Dobutamine stress and beta-blockers

In patients with ongoing beta-blocker treatment a reduced sensitivity for reversible ischaemia has been found. This is seen even if target heart rate is reached with additional atropine injections due to the negative inotropic effect of beta-blockers. Therefore stop beta-blockers ideally 48h prior to the test to increase sensitivity. However, if not possible, patients can still be accepted for exercise or dobutamine stress, with the use of atropine, accepting that sensitivity is lower.

Image acquisition

Images should be recorded at:
- baseline;
- intermediate stage (70% of the age-predicted heart rate);
- peak stress (>85% of the age-predicted heart rate);
- recovery.

The minimal images are baseline and peak. More than four stages can be recorded as felt clinically needed.

Termination of test (see p. 484)

Dobutamine stress echocardiography, like bicycle echocardiography, allows on-line monitoring of ventricular function. Termination of the test should occur at both traditional endpoints (target heart rate—85% of maximum age-predicted heart rate—or significant symptoms) and for development of wall motion abnormalities or systolic dysfunction.

Dobutamine ischaemia protocol

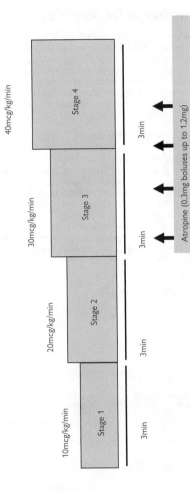

Fig. 6.8 Standard protocol for dobutamine ischaemia stress testing.

Dobutamine stress for viability

The basis for the diagnosis of myocardial viability is contraction of the myocardium either spontaneously or after inotropic stimulation by activating contractile reserve. The principle of low dose dobutamine stress is to assess contractile reserve, i.e. look for evidence of improvement in wall motion abnormalities or clear inotropic response in areas that are thought to have coronary stenoses. The rationale for viability assessment is usually to determine the value of performing revascularization.

Dobutamine infusion

- Start the infusion at 5mcg/kg/min dobutamine.
- Continue the infusion for up to 5min and then increase to 10mcg/kg/min. This can be increased to 20mcg/kg/min.
- A 10% increase in heart rate marks the end of the low-dose protocol.
- After completing the low-dose protocol higher doses of dobutamine (30 and then 40mcg/kg/min for 5min periods) may be given to look for a biphasic response (improved contraction at low dose followed by reduced contraction at peak).
- The presence of a biphasic response indicates inducible myocardial ischaemia and is perhaps the strongest predictor for recovery of myocardial dysfunction following revascularization. It will indicate a viable but jeopardized myocardial region.

Image acquisition

A full set of images should be recorded at:
- baseline;
- low stress (10% increase in heart rate);
- high stress (if performed).

Viable or non-viable?

```
                    LOW DOSE DOBUTAMINE

SCAR or LIMITED VIABILITY          SIGNIFICANT VIABILITY
1. No improved wall motion         1. Improved wall motion in
   or <4 segments improve*            >4 segments improve*
2. Diastolic wall thickness <0.6cm 2. Diastolic wall thickness >0.6cm
3. End-systolic volume >140ml**    3. End-systolic volume <140ml**


                    HIGH DOSE DOBUTAMINE


   INTRAMURAL SCAR                         HIBERNATION
1. No change in wall motion         1. Ischaemic response
                                    2. Worsening wall motion
```

*Improvement in >4 segments is a good predictor for recovery of left ventricle function after coronary revascularization in patients with hibernating myocardium.
** End systolic volume >140ml indicates an advanced stage of remodelling. Revascularization may not result in reverse remodelling.

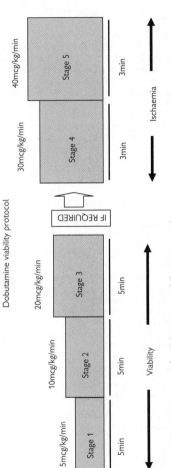

Fig. 6.9 Standard protocol for dobutamine viability stress testing.

Vasodilator stress

Vasodilator stress echocardiography should only be considered when physical stress is not possible and there are contraindications to dobutamine. It is less sensitive for identification of mild to moderate coronary artery disease. Vasodilator stress, however, may become more important as perfusion imaging becomes more widely clinically applicable.

Vasodilators are effective because they induce regional variation in coronary blood flow. Dipyridamole or adenosine cause a 2- or more fold increase in myocardial blood flow in segments supplied by normal coronary arteries, whereas in segments supplied by stenotic arteries flow is unchanged or decreased. If oxygen demand increases with flow changes, regional abnormalities in wall motion and thickening appear.

Because vasodilator stress acts via change in perfusion, theoretically, it should be more suitable for direct assessment of myocardial perfusion using contrast echocardiography.

Dipyridamole protocol for myocardial ischaemia

The protocol for dipyridamole is based on continuous ECG and echocardiographic monitoring during a two-stage infusion.

Infusion

- Check for contraindications to dipyridamole (p. 476).
- Initially infuse 0.56mg/kg of dipyridamole over 4min.
- Monitor for 4min. If there are no adverse effects and no clinical or echocardiographic endpoints occur (significant anginal symptoms, wall motion abnormalities) infuse 0.28mg/kg over 2min.
- As with dobutamine (p. 488), atropine can be used after the second stage to increase heart rate and improve sensitivity.
- Aminophylline (240mg, IV) should be available for immediate use in case of an adverse dipyridamole-related event.

Imaging

Imaging should be performed continuously, and images captured at baseline, end of phase one, end of phase two (if performed), and during recovery. The minimal images are baseline and hyperaemia.

Adenosine protocol for myocardial ischaemia

Adenosine works on a 6min protocol with ECG and echocardiographic monitoring.

Infusion

- Check for contraindication to adenosine (p. 476).
- Infuse at a maximum dose of 140mcg/kg/min over 6 min.
- Stop the infusion if clinical or echocardiographic endpoints are reached (limiting symptoms or wall motion abnormalities).

Imaging

Image continuously. Record at baseline, and during hyperaemia.

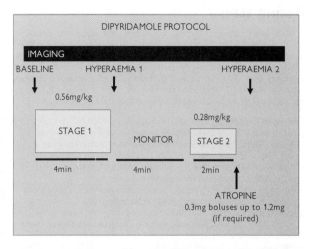

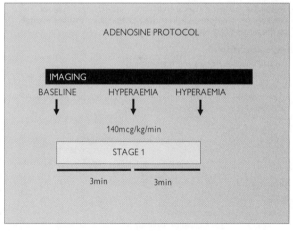

Fig. 6.10 Standard protocols for vasodilator stress testing.

Pacing stress

In most paced patients exercise, dobutamine, and vasodilator protocols are applicable. Pacing stress can be considered when an increase in heart rate cannot be achieved by exercise or dobutamine. Since pacing alone only produces chronotropic stress, it is usually considered to have lower sensitivity than the inotropic and chronotropic stress achieved by pharmacological stress. Dobutamine can be given at the same time as increasing the pacing rate to create both chronotropic and inotropic stress.

Pacing protocol

- Pacing stress should preferably be performed with atrial pacing to ensure natural ventricular contraction and to avoid pacing-induced wall motion abnormalities.
- In patients with permanent pacemakers ensure the assistance of a pacemaker programmer and experienced operator.
- Pacing by temporary intravascular or oesophageal leads is usually not needed for clinically indicated stress echocardiography.
- Record baseline images and then increase pacing rate to an intermediate level (70% of maximum age-predicted heart rate). Finally, increase heart rate to target heart rate and record a further set of images.
- Terminate the test if clinical endpoints occur (changes in blood pressure or symptoms), regional wall motion abnormalities emerge, or the target heart rate is reached.

Image acquisition

- Record baseline images and then monitor.
- During pacing record images if termination criteria are met and/or when heart rate reaches an intermediate level (70% maximum age-predicted heart rate) and when heart rate reaches peak level (85% maximum age-predicted heart rate).

Contrast agents: introduction

Indications for contrast

Since image quality is crucial for reliable stress echocardiography, review all baseline images prior to beginning the stress procedure. If endocardial borders are not visible (or barely visible) in two or more myocardial segments consider using ultrasound contrast agents. Alternatively, the patient can be referred for another imaging test such as myocardial scintigraphy or magnetic resonance imaging.

Principle of action and products

Left-sided contrast agents work because they are highly reflective. They consist of a shell surrounding a gas (air or usually a fluorine-based inert gas). All agents have very favourable safety profiles. SonoVue®, Optison®, and Definity® (Luminity®) are products manufactured for endocardial definition (local licensing and availability should be verified).

Imaging presets and analysis

When ultrasound contrast agents are used, contrast-specific imaging modalities should be employed. There is a range of manufacturer-specific presets. The standard is a real-time, low power mode. The low-power contrast-specific imaging technology provides excellent ventricular opacification. Real time is needed for wall motion analysis. Without low-power modes use harmonic imaging but with a mechanical index of less than 0.6 to minimize bubble destruction and thereby reduce left ventricular swirling.

Perfusion imaging

The ability of contrast echocardiography to supplement wall motion information with information on perfusion can expand the diagnostic value of stress echocardiography. Perfusion is judged from the appearance of contrast within the myocardium. Black represents no perfusion and speckling perfusion. Poor perfusion is usually seen as a black rim around the endocardial border. Perfusion should be graded at rest as normal or abnormal and then compared to perfusion on stress. Furthermore, refilling can be judged by giving an ultrasound flash to destroy the contrast bubbles. The time for the myocardium to refill can then be judged as normal, slow, or complete absence of perfusion.

No contrast

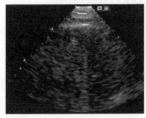

With contrast

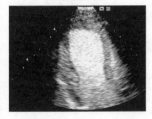

Fig. 6.11 Examples of contrast-specific imaging. Without contrast agent there are only faint signals from myocardial tissue. After contrast injection there is bright opacification of the blood within the left ventricle cavity and excellent delineation of the endocardium. Opacification of the myocardium is not as intense as that of the cavity but provides a good display of left ventricle wall thickness.

Contrast agents: preparation and administration

Contrast agents are licensed 'as transpulmonary echocardiographic contrast agents for use in patients with suspected or established cardiovascular disease to provide opacification of cardiac chambers, and enhance left ventricular endocardial border delineation'. They are indicated when image quality on native imaging is not adequate to provide reliable assessment of resting and inducible wall motion abnormalities.

There are several contrast agents but all consist of a shell usually of an inert substance filled by an inert gas. They can be given as boluses with a flush or some can be given as a constant infusion by a pump. Possible agents include the following.

Optison™ (Amersham)

Structure Composed of an albumin shell containing perflutren gas.

Preparation and storage It comes in a vial that requires reconstitution and manual agitation. It is then drawn up into a 2 or 1mL syringe. A second needle is used to vent the vial (this can be removed if repetitive doses are withdrawn. Normally, the agent is reconstituted directly before injection and the vial agitated before each dose is withdrawn. It should be stored in a refrigerator between 2°C and 8°C.

Dose and administration The recommended dose is 0.5–3.0mL per patient injected into a peripheral vein. However, that dosage derives from studies using fundamental imaging, which should be avoided. For harmonic imaging bolus injections of 0.2–0.4mL are adequate. Total dose should not exceed 8.7mL. The bolus should be followed by a 3–5mL bolus of 0.9% sodium chloride or 5% glucose.

SonoVue® (Bracco International BV)

Structure Composed of a phospholipid shell filled with sulphur hexafluoride (SF_6).

Preparation and storage It is reconstituted with sodium chloride. Normally, the contrast is reconstituted within a few minutes of injection and the vial is agitated before each injection is withdrawn. If given as an infusion it needs to be agitated in a special agitating pump during delivery.

Dose and administration
- *Bolus.* Recommended dose is 2.0mL. However, the dose derives from studies using fundamental imaging, which should be avoided. For harmonic imaging bolus injections of 0.2–0.4mL are adequate. The bolus should be followed by a 3–5mL bolus of 0.9% sodium chloride or 5% glucose. Total dose should not exceed 1.6mL.
- *Infusion.* For Sonovue® a special agitation pump is used. For stress studies two vials should be drawn up into the syringe. The rate of infusion should be initiated at 0.8mL/min, but titrated as necessary to achieve optimal image enhancement (the range is 0.6–1.2mL/min).

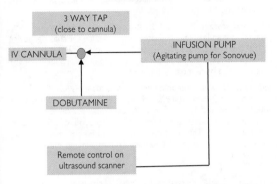

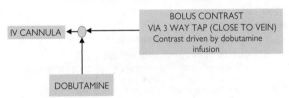

Fig. 6.12 Most contrast agents can be given as a bolus or an infusion. When given with a dobutamine infusion the agent can be given via the same cannula using a 3-way tap. The contrast agent is driven by the dobutamine infusion. No boluses of saline are necessary. There is no risk of dobutamine boluses since the amount of contrast is very low.

Luminity® (Bristol Myers Squib)

Structure Composed of lipid-encapsulated perflutren microspheres. The spheres are between 1 and 10μm in diameter.

Preparation and storage It should be stored in a refrigerator at 2–8°C until activated. It needs to be activated by a mechanical shaking device (Vialmix) and then can be used for up to 12h (although if left standing for more than 5min it requires 10sec of shaking by hand before further use). It can be reactivated once more within 48h.

Dose and administration Recommended bolus dose is 0.1–0.4mL followed by a bolus of 3–5mL of 0.9% sodium chloride or 5% glucose. Total dose should not exceed 1.6mL. For an intravenous infusion it is recommended that 1.3mL of contrast should be added to 50mL of 0.9% sodium chloride or 5% glucose. This mixture should then be infused at a starting rate of 4mL/min and be titrated to achieve optimal image enhancement (not to exceed 10mL/min).

Complications and contraindications to contrast agents

All contrast agents have potential side-effects. They range from headache and flushing with an incidence of around 1% to anaphylactic reactions in <1:1000.

Specific contraindications
- Hypersensitivity to any of the constituents of the contrast agent

Special considerations and precautions with use
- Right-to-left, bidirectional, or transient right-to-left cardiac shunts
- Mechanical ventilation
- Clinically significant pulmonary disease, including diffuse interstitial pulmonary fibrosis and severe chronic obstructive pulmonary disease
- Adult respiratory distress syndrome
- Severe heart failure (NYHA IV)
- Endocarditis
- Acute myocardial infarction with ongoing angina or unstable angina, hearts with prosthetic valves
- Acute states of systemic inflammation or sepsis
- Known states of hyperactive coagulation system
- Recurrent thromboembolism
- Pregnant women

Analysis

Echocardiographic recordings have to be evaluated during image acquisition in order to assess for echocardiographic endpoints. This should be followed by a comprehensive assessment after the stress test with side-by-side comparisons of recordings captured at baseline and stress.

Stress echocardiograms can be analysed on several planes of complexity, which range from a qualitative assessment of segmental wall motion in response to stress to highly detailed schemes for quantitative analysis.

For image interpretation, multiple cine loop display allows up to 4 different stress levels for each imaging plane to be displayed simultaneously.

Standard review

- Start with assessment of image quality. Endocardial border definition can be used as an indicator of image quality. If endocardial border is not seen or is barely visible, wall motion and thickening cannot be reliably assessed in this segment. Grade image quality as *good*, *acceptable*, or *poor* and identify non-diagnostic segments.
- On resting images assess global function by left ventricle ejection fraction using a visual estimate or from measuring end-diastolic or end-systolic volumes in two apical views.
- Compare rest and stress images for the development of global LV dysfunction (left ventricular enlargement and shape changes) and re-measure global function at stress if there appears to be a change.
- Then evaluate segmental wall motion at rest and at each level of stress using a 16- or 17-segment model. Use a 4-step visual score for each segment: 1, *normal*; 2, *hypokinetic*; 3, *akinetic*; 4, *dyskinetic*.
- Calculate a wall motion score at each stage, if required, to facilitate serial comparison. Divide the sum of the points by the number of segments analysed. Normal contraction has a wall motion score of 1; a higher score indicates wall motion abnormalities.
- For assessment of myocardial viability wall thickness is useful. Diastolic wall thickness <5mm at rest indicates non-viability and increases diagnostic confidence in combination with absent contractile response to dobutamine.
- If using contrast during stress echocardiography, it may be useful to assess the myocardial contrast enhancement. With current knowledge the results of perfusion imaging should be used in conjunction with the findings of visual left ventricle wall motion analysis.
- The adequacy of stress should be noted and record kept of the exercise time, symptoms, haemodynamic observations, and ECG changes.

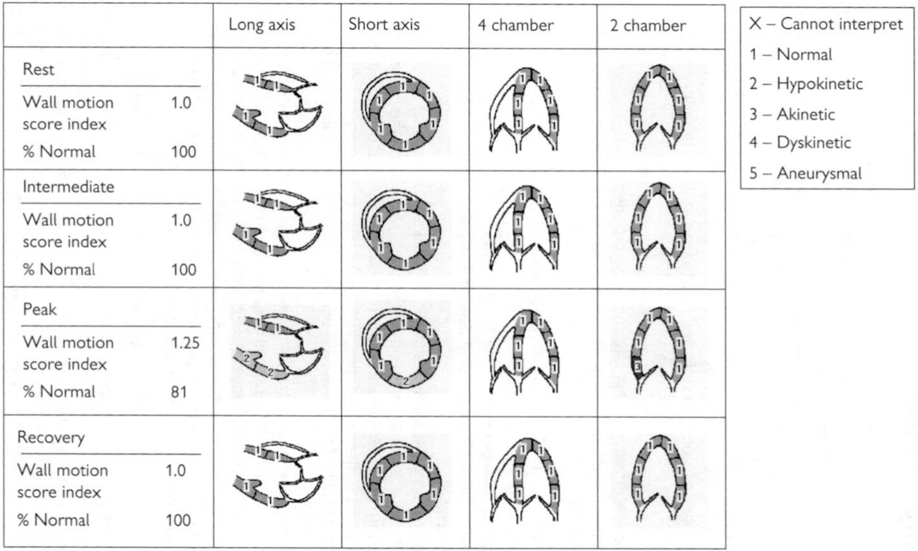

Fig. 6.13 Example of an annotated table to report segmental abnormalities.

Sample report

Section 1. Demographic and other information

All the standard demographic details should be included. Stress echocardiography should also include the following.

- The clinical indication, including relevant clinical history and medications. This provides justification for the study and summarizes clinical information from a number of sources to focus the final conclusion.
- The stress protocol and imaging technique used with justification, including the name and dosage of contrast agents.
- Changes of blood pressure and heart rate should be described briefly. Reporting resting and peak stress blood pressure is usually sufficient.
- For exercise and dobutamine stress echocardiography the age, sex, and specific target heart rate should be included.
- Further measurements or details of ECG changes can be included if relevant.

Section 2. Description of observations and diagnostic statements

- Start with a statement about the completeness of the study and image quality, since diagnostic confidence heavily depends on high quality recordings.
- Next report the baseline analysis. If global and/or regional left ventricular function is abnormal, the segments involved and the degree of abnormality (hypokinetic, akinetic, dyskinetic) should be demonstrated or listed. Schematics of the single views help to illustrate the distribution of wall motion abnormalities. Non-diagnostic segments can be marked.
- Then report each of the stress recordings in the same way describing whether there was a normal response to stress or abnormal response with worsening wall motion. Segments that deteriorate should be listed or marked on the schematic and degree of abnormality noted.
- In viability studies it is important to evaluate whether the akinetic segments show improvement during stress.

Section 3. M-mode, 2D, and Doppler measurements

In stress echocardiography this section will include quantitative measures of left ventricular function (e.g. ejection fraction) at baseline and on stress. There may also be information on left ventricular outflow velocities in patients with suspected stress-induced gradients or changes in mitral valve function. If tissue Doppler imaging or other analysis methods were used these can be documented.

Section 4. Conclusions

The conclusion should comment on any suboptimal aspect of the study (e.g. image quality, target heart rate reached, etc.) and any complications or adverse events. It should then address the clinical question and detail the main abnormalities that occurred during stress, or summarize the response as normal.

Audit and quality control

It is usually accepted that operators should interpret a minimum of 10 stress echocardiograms per month to maintain interpretational skills and sonographers should perform a minimum of 10 stress echocardiograms per month to maintain an appropriate level of skill.

Regular audits are useful to review the quality and accuracy of the stress echocardiograms. The audit should include: the total number of stress echocardiograms performed per month for the time period audited; the number of procedures per sonographer and reads per physician; indications; imaging technology; use of contrast; stress protocols; quality of the studies; termination criteria; results (negative or positive for assessment of ischaemia, viable or non-viable for viability studies); and complications. For those patients undergoing coronary angiography, it would be ideal to have the results of coronary angiography for quality control with routine review of false positive and negative findings.

Future technologies

Echocardiography technology is progressing rapidly and has been developed to ensure assessment of left ventricular wall motion is more objective. Automatic wall tracking software, tissue Doppler imaging, and strain imaging are becoming clinically viable. 3D echocardiography has introduced a further exciting option for stress echocardiography with rapid acquisition of 3D volume datasets and reconstruction of 3D motion.

Chapter 7

Reporting and normal ranges

Reporting

A standard approach to reporting ensures complete studies and improves comprehension for other readers during interpretation or follow up. Below is a suggested structure and on the following pages examples of appropriate descriptions (section 2) (adapted from the British Society of Echocardiography guidelines). The calculations (section 3) will have been collected as part of the minimal dataset (Chapter 2) and can be interpreted based on tables of expected values for different anatomy and pathology (these tables have been replicated in this chapter).

Section 1. Demographic and other information
- Patient's name, date of birth, gender, hospital number.
- Date on which study was performed.
- Location (inpatient, outpatient) and urgency.
- Indications for test.
- Referring physician.
- Sonographer/physician performing and interpreting the study.
- Height, weight, blood pressure (if available).
- Ultrasound machine and data storage.
- Image quality and any suboptimal views (if applicable).

Section 2. Description of observations and diagnostic statements
A brief description of each anatomical feature should be given. The description should summarize findings from all views (comments should be able to be supported from measurements later in report). It is impractical to include all statements if everything is normal and usually it is sufficient just to call them normal in structure and function. However, there should be a protocol or check list to ensure all comments are based on facts (visual and quantitative assessment). For each anatomical detail, when appropriate, there should also be a diagnostic statement such as 'appearances suggestive of rheumatic mitral disease'.

Section 3. M-mode, 2D, and Doppler measurements
This section is based on a minimal dataset that should be included in every report, supplemented with additional measures as required to describe any pathology. Ideally, the report should include normal values for particular measurements.

Section 4. Conclusions
This section is often read first by the referring physicians, who may not be cardiologists. It has to be easily understood and should summarize the whole study. Identify any abnormality, its cause (if identifiable), and any secondary effect. This may involve repeating some of the information from sections 2 and 3. The questions of the referring physicians should be answered. If not possible, then the reasons should be included and alternative methods suggested (e.g. transoesophageal echocardiography or contrast echocardiography). Medical advice should be separated from the report of the study.

Sample report: normal

John Smith   DoB:10:07:1935   Inpatient: Ward A
Height: 182cm   Weight: 74kg   BP: 120/70
Indication: ?LV function
Referring Physician: Dr Smith   Sonographer: John Brown
Interpreting Physician: Dr Jones
Machine: Ultrasound Machine A   Images saved: Server
Image Quality: Good

Descriptions

1. Left ventricle: normal cavity size, normal wall thickness, normal systolic and diastolic function
2. Right ventricle: normal size, normal wall thickness, normal systolic function
3. Ventricular septum: normal
4. Left atrium: normal size
5. Right atrium: normal size
6. Atrial septum: normal
7. Inferior vena cava: normal diameter, normal response during respiration
8. Aortic valve: normal structure and function
9. Mitral valve: normal structure and function
10. Tricuspid valve: normal structure and function
11. Pulmonary valve: normal structure and function
12. Pulmonary artery: normal diameter
13. Pericardium: no thickening, no effusion
14. Aorta: normal diameter of root and ascending aorta

Measurements

1. Left ventricle LVED, 5.0cm; LVES, 3.5cm; FS, 30%; IVS, 1.0cm; LVPW, 0.9cm; normal diastolic LV function
2. Right ventricle RVED, 2.0cm
3. Left atrium LA diameter, 3.2cm
4. Right atrium —
5. Inferior vena cava —
6. Aortic valve peak velocity, 1.2m/sec
7. Mitral valve E:A ratio, 1.1
8. Tricuspid valve TR maximum velocity, 1m/sec
9. Pulmonary valve PW peak velocity, 1m/sec
10. Pulmonary artery Root diameter, 2.6cm
11. Pericardium —
12. Aorta Root diameter, 2.7cm

Conclusions

Normal echocardiogram. Normal left ventricular size. Normal left ventricular systolic and diastolic function.

Dr Jones

Mitral valve

Descriptive terms

Structure
Normal, rheumatic, myxomatous, degenerative.

Annulus
Normal, dilated, calcified (mild/moderate/severe).

Leaflet thickness
• Normal, thickened (mild/moderate/severe).
• Leaflet tips, leaflet body (aMVL/pMVL).

Commissures
Anterolateral fusion, posteromedial fusion.

Calcification
• Focal calcification (aMVL/pMVL), diffuse calcification.
• Commissural calcification (anterolateral/posteromedial).

Cleft
Anterior leaflet, posterior leaflet.

Chordal disease
• Shortening, fusion/thickening, elongation.
• Rupture, calcification.

Papillary muscle
• Rupture, partial rupture (anterolateral/posteromedial).
• Calcification/fibrosis (anterolateral/posteromedial).

Leaflet mobility
• Normal, reduced (mild/moderate/severe).
• Doming, prolapse, bowing.
• Systolic anterior motion (mild/moderate/severe—based on outflow tract gradient).
• Chordal systolic anterior motion.

Prolapse
• Anterior, posterior leaflet (mild/mod/severe/flail).
• A1, A2, A3, P1, P2, P3 (mild/moderate/severe/flail).

Vegetation
• Location (aMVL/pMVL).
• Mobility (non-mobile/mobile), pedunculated.
• Size (small/moderate/large), dimensions.

Abscess
• Location (aorto-mitral/pMVL/annulus).
• Size (small/moderate/large), dimensions.

Mass
Location (aMVL/pMVL), description (see 'Masses', this chapter).

Mitral stenosis

- None, present (mild/moderate/severe).
- Quantitative measurements:
  - peak and mean transmitral velocity/gradient;
  - pressure half-time, mitral valve area.
- Suitable for commissurotomy.

Mitral regurgitation

- None, present (trace, mild, moderate, severe).
- Jet direction:
  - anteriorly, posteriorly, centrally directed;
  - wall-impinging jet, directed down pulmonary veins.
- Diastolic mitral regurgitation (present/absent).
- Quantitative measurements :
  - MR:LA area ratio, regurgitant volume;
  - vena contracta width, EROA.
- Pulmonary venous flow (normal, blunted systolic flow, systolic flow reversal).

Table 7.1 Parameters to determine severity of mitral stenosis

	MILD	MODERATE	SEVERE
MV area (cm^2)	2.2–1.5	1.5–1.0	<1.0
MV P1/2 time (msec)	100–150	150–220	>220
Mean pressure gradient (mmHg)	<5	Variable	>10
TR velocity (m/sec)	<2.7	Variable	>3
PA pressure (mmHg)	<30	Variable	>50

Table 7.2 Parameters to assess severity of mitral regurgitation

	SPECIFIC SIGNS OF SEVERITY	
	MILD	SEVERE
Jet (Nyquist, 50–60cm/sec)	<4cm^2 or <20% LA; small & central	>40% LA; large & central or wall impinging & swirling
Vena contracta	<0.3cm	>0.7cm
PISA r (Nyquist, 40cm/sec)	None/minimal (<0.4cm)	Large (>1cm)
Pulmonary vein flow	—	Systolic reversal
Valve structure	—	Flail or rupture
	SUPPORTIVE SIGNS OF SEVERITY	
	MILD	SEVERE
Pulmonary vein flow	Systolic dominant	
Mitral inflow	A-wave dominant	E-wave dominant (>1.2m/sec)
CW trace	Soft & parabolic	Dense & triangular
LV & LA	Normal size LV if chronic MR	Enlarged LV & LA if no other cause

Report as MODERATE if signs of regurgitation are greater than MILD but there are no signs of SEVERE regurgitation.

Aortic valve

Descriptive terms

Structure
- Normal, degenerative, rheumatic.
- Bicuspid, fused (RCC–LCC, RCC–NCC, NCC–LCC).
- Unicuspid, quadricuspid.

Leaflet thickness
- Focal thickening (RCC/LCC/NCC), diffuse thickening.
- Severity (mild/moderate/severe).

Calcification
- Present (mild/moderate/severe).
- Focal calcification (RCC/LCC/NCC).
- Diffuse calcification.

Leaflet mobility
- Normal, reduced (mild/moderate/severe), doming.

Other
- Leaflet perforation (RCC/LCC/NCC).
- Leaflet prolapse/flail (RCC/LCC/NCC).

Vegetation
- Location (RCC/LCC/NCC).
- Mobility (non-mobile/mobile), pedunculated.
- Size (small/moderate/large) + dimensions.

Abscess
- Location (RCC–annulus/LCC–annulus/NCC–annulus).
- Size (small/moderate/large) + dimensions.

Mass
- Location (RCC/LCC/NCC), description (see 'Masses', this chapter).

Aortic stenosis

- None, present (mild/moderate/severe).
- Quantification:
  - peak and mean transaortic velocity/gradient;
  - aortic valve area.

Aortic regurgitation

- None, present (trace, mild, moderate, severe).

Aortic stenosis

Table 7.3 Parameters to assess severity of aortic stenosis

	MILD	MODERATE	SEVERE
Peak velocity (m/sec)	2.0–3.0	3.0–4.0	>4.0
Peak gradient (mmHg)	<35	35–65	>65
Mean gradient (mmHg)	<20	20–40	>40
Valve area (cm^2)	2.0–1.5	1.0–1.5	<1.0

Aortic regurgitation

Table 7.4 Parameters to determine severity of aortic regurgitation

	SPECIFIC SIGNS OF SEVERITY	
	MILD	SEVERE
Vena contracta	<0.3cm	>0.6cm
Jet (Nyquist, 50–60cm/sec)	Central, <25% of LVOT	Central, >65% of LVOT
Descending aorta	No or brief early diastolic flow reversal	
	SUPPORTIVE SIGNS OF SEVERITY	
	MILD	SEVERE
Pressure half-time	>500msec	<200msec
Descending aorta	—	Holodiastolic flow reversal
Left ventricle (only for chronic lesions)	Normal LV	Moderate or greater LV enlargement (no other cause)

Report as MODERATE if signs of regurgitation are greater than MILD but there are no features of SEVERE regurgitation.

Tricuspid valve

Descriptive terms

Structure
- Normal, rheumatic, myxomatous (redundant).
- Ebstein.

Annulus
- Normal, dilated.
- Calcified.

Leaflet thickness
- Normal, increased.
- Leaflet tips, leaflet body (anterior/posterior/septal).

Calcification
- Focal calcification (anterior/posterior/septal).
- Diffuse calcification.

Papillary muscle
Rupture.

Leaflet mobility
- Normal, reduced (mild/moderate/severe).
- Doming, prolapse, bowing.

Prolapse
- Anterior leaflet (mild/moderate/severe/flail).
- Posterior leaflet (mild/moderate/severe/flail).
- Septal leaflet (mild/moderate/severe/flail).

Vegetation
- Location (anterior/posterior/septal).
- Mobility (non-mobile/mobile), pedunculated.
- Size (small/moderate/large) + dimensions.

Abscess
- Location (anterior-annulus/posterior-annulus/septal).
- Size (small/moderate/large) + dimensions.

Mass
- Location (anterior/posterior/septal).
- Description (see 'Masses', this chapter).

Tricuspid stenosis
- None, present.
- Quantitative measurements:
  - peak and mean transtricuspid gradient;
  - tricuspid valve area.

Tricuspid regurgitation
- None, present (trace, mild, moderate, severe).
- Jet direction: free wall-directed, septal-directed; centrally directed.
- Hepatic vein flow:
  - normal, blunted systolic flow;
  - systolic flow reversal.

Tricuspid stenosis

Table 7.5 Parameters to assess tricupsid stenosis

	MILD	MODERATE	SEVERE
Mean gradient (mmHg)	<4	4–7	>7
Valve area (cm^2)	–	–	<1

Tricuspid regurgitation

Table 7.6 Parameters to assess severity of tricuspid regurgitation

	MILD	SEVERE
Jet (Nyquist, 50–60cm/sec)	<5cm^2	>10cm^2
Vena contracta	—	>0.7cm
PISA r (Nyquist 40cm/sec)	<0.5cm	>1cm
Hepatic vein flow	Normal	Systolic reversal
Valve structure	Normal	Abnormal
CW trace	Soft & parabolic	Dense & triangular
RV/RA/IVC	Normal size	Usually dilated

Report as MODERATE if signs of regurgitation are greater than MILD but there are no features of SEVERE regurgitation.

Right atrial pressure

Table 7.7 Parameters to assess right atrial pressure

	Right atrial pressure (mmHg)		
	5	10	15
Right atrium	Normal	Dilated	Very dilated
TR	Mild	Moderate	Severe
TR velocity (m/sec)	<2.5	2.5–4	>4
IVC	Normal, <1.7cm	Dilated	Dilated; no respiratory variation

Pulmonary valve

Descriptive terms

Structure
- Normal, dysplastic, bicuspid.

Mobility
- Normal, reduced.
- Doming.

Vegetation
- Location.
- Mobility (non-mobile/mobile), pedunculated.
- Size (small/moderate/large) + dimensions.

Mass
Location, description (see 'Masses', this chapter).

Stenosis
- None, present (mild/moderate/severe).
- Location (valvular, infundibular, valvular + infundibular, supravalvular, branch).
- Left or right main pulmonary artery.
- Quantitative measurements: peak and mean transpulmonary gradient.

Regurgitation
None, present (trace, mild, moderate, severe).

Pulmonary pressure
- Normal.
- Elevated systolic pressure (mild/moderate/severe).
- Elevated diastolic pressure (mild/moderate/severe).
- Estimated pulmonary artery.

Pulmonary artery

Descriptive terms

Appearance
Normal, abnormal.

Dilatation
Absent, present (mild/moderate/severe).

Thrombus
Main/right/left pulmonary artery.

Pulmonary artery stenosis
Main/right/left pulmonary artery (mild/moderate/severe).

Patent ductus arteriosus
Absent, present.

Pulmonary regurgitation

Table 7.8 Parameters to assess pulmonary regurgitation

	MILD	SEVERE
Jet size on CFM	<10mm long	Large with wide origin
CW density & shape	Soft & slow	Dense & steep
Pulmonary valve	Normal	Abnormal
Pulmonary artery flow	Increased	Greatly increased compared to systemic circulation
Right ventricle size	Normal	Dilated

If features suggest more than MILD regurgitation but no features of SEVERE, grade as MODERATE.

Pulmonary stenosis

Table 7.9 Parameters to determine severity of pulmonary stenosis

	MILD	MODERATE	SEVERE
Peak gradient (mmHg)	10–25	25–40	>40
Valve area (cm^2)	>1.0	0.5–1.0	<0.5

Left ventricle

Descriptive terms

Cavity size
- Normal, dilated (mild/moderate/severe), decreased.

Wall thickness
- Normal, hypertrophy (mild/moderate/severe).
- Pattern (concentric, eccentric, asymmetric + location).
- Decreased.

Mass
- Normal, mild, moderate, severe increase.

Shape
- Normal, aneurysm, pseudoaneurysm (+ location).

Global systolic function
- Normal, borderline, low normal.
- Decreased (mild, mild to moderate, moderate, moderate to severe, severe).
- Increased (hyperdynamic).
- Estimated ejection fraction.

Regional systolic function
- Normal, hypokinetic, akinetic, dyskinetic, scar.
- Asynchronous, not seen—describe for each segment of the following walls:
  - anterior (basal, mid, apical), antero-septal (basal, mid);
  - infero-septal (basal, mid, apical);
  - inferior wall (basal, mid, apical);
  - posterior (inferolateral) wall (basal, mid, apical);
  - lateral wall (basal, mid, apical).

Diastolic filling
- Normal, abnormal (impaired relaxation, pseudonormal, restrictive);
- Elevated left atrial pressure (E/E' >15, normal <10).

Left ventricular outflow tract
- No obstruction, obstruction (mild/moderate/severe).
- Septal hypertrophy, subaortic membrane.
- Associated with mitral valve systolic anterior motion.

Thrombus
- Absent, present (+ location and description).

Mass
- Absent, present (+ location and description).

Left ventricular size, mass, and function

Table 7.10 Ranges for measurements of LV size and mass

	WOMEN			
	NORMAL	MILD	MODERATE	SEVERE
LV dimension				
LV d diameter, cm	3.9–5.3	5.4–5.7	5.8–6.1	>6.1
LV d diameter/BSA, cm/m²	2.4–3.2	3.3–3.4	3.5–3.7	>3.7
LV volume				
LV d vol, mL	56–104	105–117	118–130	>130
LV d vol/BSA, mL/m²	**35–75**	**76–86**	**87–96**	**>96**
LV s vol, mL	19–49	50–59	60–69	>69
LV s vol/BSA, mL/m²	**12–30**	**31–36**	**37–42**	**>42**
Linear method: fractional shortening				
Endocardial, %	27–45	22–26	17–21	<17
2D method:				
Ejection fraction, %	**>54**	**45–54**	**30–44**	**<30**
Linear method: wall thickness				
Relative wall thickness, cm	0.22–0.42	0.43–0.47	0.48–0.52	>0.52
Septal thickness, cm	**0.6–0.9**	**1.0–1.2**	**1.3–1.5**	**>1.5**
Posterior wall thickness, cm	**0.6–0.9**	**1.0–1.2**	**1.3–1.5**	**>1.5**
2D method				
LV mass, g	66–150	151–171	172–182	>182
LV mass/BSA, g/m²	**44–88**	**89–100**	**101–112**	**>112**

BSA, Body surface area; d, diastolic; s, systolic. Bold rows identify best validated measures.

Table 7.11 Ranges for measurements of LV size and mass

	MEN			
	NORMAL	MILD	MODERATE	SEVERE
LV dimension				
LV d diameter, cm	4.2–5.9	6.0–6.3	6.4–6.8	>6.8
LV d diameter/BSA, cm/m²	2.2–3.1	3.2–3.4	3.5–3.6	>3.6
LV volume				
LV d vol, mL	67–155	156–178	179–201	>201
LV d vol/BSA, mL/m²	**35–75**	**76–86**	**87–96**	**>96**
LV s vol, mL	22–58	59–70	71–82	>82
LV s vol/BSA, mL/m²	**12–30**	**31–36**	**37–42**	**>42**
Linear method: fractional shortening				
Endocardial, %	25–43	20–24	15–19	<15
2D method:				
Ejection fraction, %	**>54**	**45–54**	**30–44**	**<30**
Linear method: wall thickness				
Relative wall thickness, cm	0.24–0.42	0.43–0.46	0.47–0.51	>0.51
Septal thickness, cm	**0.6–1.0**	**1.1–1.3**	**1.4–1.6**	**>1.6**
Posterior wall thickness, cm	**0.6–1.0**	**1.1–1.3**	**1.4–1.6**	**>1.6**
2D method				
LV mass, g	96–200	201–227	228–254	>254
LV mass/BSA, g/m²	**50–102**	**103–116**	**117–130**	**>130**

BSA, body surface area; d, diastolic; s, systolic. Bold rows identify best validated measures.

Right ventricle

Descriptive terms

Cavity size
- Normal, dilated (mild/moderate/severe), decreased.

Wall thickness
- Normal, hypertrophy, decreased.

Global systolic function
- Normal, decreased (mild, moderate, severe).
- Increased (hyperdynamic).

Regional systolic function
- Normal, hypokinetic, akinetic, not seen.
- Describe for free wall/apex/outflow tract.

Thrombus
- Absent, present (+ location and description).

Mass
- Absent, present (+ location and description).

Right ventricular size and function

Table 7.12 Parameters to assess right ventricle size and function

	NORMAL	MILD	MODERATE	SEVERE
RV dimensions (apical 4-chamber)				
Basal RV diameter, cm	2.0–2.8	2.9–3.3	3.4–3.8	>3.8
Mid RV diameter, cm	2.7–3.3	3.4–3.7	3.8–4.1	>4.1
Base–apex length, cm	7.1–7.9	8.0–8.5	8.6–9.1	>9.1
RVOT diameter (parasternal short axis)				
Mid-ventricle, cm	2.5–2.9	3.0–3.2	3.3–3.5	>3.5
Pulmonary valve level, cm	1.7–2.3	2.4–2.7	2.8–3.1	>3.1
PA diameter (parasternal short axis)				
Pulmonary artery, cm	1.5–2.1	2.2–2.5	2.6–2.9	>2.9
RV area and fractional area change (apical 4-chamber)				
RV diastolic area, cm^2	11–28	29–32	33–37	>37
RV systolic area, cm^2	7.5–16	17–19	20–22	>22
Fractional area change, %	32–60	25–31	18–24	<18

In relation to Fig. 5.20 apical 4-chamber view: basal RV = RVD1;
mid RV = RVD2; base–apex = RVD3.
In relation to Fig. 5.20 parasternal short axis view: aortic valve to free
wall = RVOT1; level of pulmonary valve = RVOT2; pulmonary artery = PA1.

Ventricular septum

Descriptive terms

Abnormal septal motion

- Abnormal (paradoxical) motion consistent with right ventricle volume overload.
- Abnormal (paradoxical) motion consistent with post-operative status.
- Abnormal (paradoxical) motion consistent with left bundle branch block.
- Abnormal (paradoxical) motion consistent with right ventricle pacemaker.
- Abnormal (paradoxical) motion due to pre-excitation.
- Flattened in diastole ('D' shaped left ventricle) consistent with right ventricle volume overload.
- Flattened in systole consistent with right ventricle pressure overload.
- Flattened in systole and diastole consistent with right ventricle pressure and volume overload.
- Septal 'bounce; consistent with constrictive physiology.
- Excessive respiratory change consistent with tamponade, constriction, ventilation-related.
- Other (specify).

Ventricular septal defect

- Absent, present.
- Location (peri-membranous, subpulmonary/doubly committed, inlet, muscular, multiple.
- Size (small/moderate/large).
- Shunt (left-to-right/right-to-left/bidirectional).

Left atrium

Descriptive terms

Cavity size
- Normal, dilated (mild/moderate/severe), decreased.

Thrombus
- Absent, present (+ location and description).

Mass
- Absent, present (+ location and description).

Spontaneous contrast
- Absent, present.

Other
- Cor triatriatum, hypoplastic left atrium, consistent with cardiac transplantation.

Right atrium

Descriptive terms

Cavity size
- Normal, dilated (mild/moderate/severe), decreased.

Thrombus
- Absent, present (+ location and description).

Mass
- Absent, present (+ location and description).

Catheter/pacing wire
- Absent, present.

Right atrial pressure
- Septum bowed to left consistent with elevated right atrial pressure.
- Dilated coronary sinus consistent with elevated right atrial pressure or left superior vena cava.
- Persistent left superior vena cava.
- Normal inferior vena cava size/respiratory variation—right atrial pressure normal.
- Normal inferior vena cava size/reduced variation—right atrial pressure mildly increased (10mmHg).
- Dilated inferior vena cava size/reduced variation—right atrial pressure moderately increased (15mmHg).
- Dilated inferior vena cava/absent variation/dilated hepatic veins—right atrial pressure severely increased (20mmHg).

Other
- Prominent Eustachian valve, Chiari network.

Atrial size

Table 7.13 Parameters to assess left and right atria

	WOMEN			
	NORMAL	MILD	MODERATE	SEVERE
Atrial dimension				
LA diameter, cm	2.7–3.8	3.9–4.2	4.3–4.6	>4.6
LA diameter/BSA, cm/m^2	1.5–2.3	2.4–2.6	2.7–2.9	>2.9
RA minor axis, cm	2.9–4.5	4.6–4.9	5.0–5.4	>5.4
RA minor axis/BSA, cm/m^2	1.7–2.5	2.6–2.8	2.9–3.1	>3.1
Atrial area				
LA area, cm^2	<20	20–30	31–40	>40
Atrial volume				
LA vol, mL	22–52	53–62	63–72	>72
LA vol/BSA, mL/m^2	**<29**	**29–33**	**34–39**	**>39**
	MEN			
	NORMAL	MILD	MODERATE	SEVERE
Atrial dimension				
LA diameter, cm	3.0–4.0	4.1–4.6	4.7–5.2	>5.2
LA diameter/BSA, cm/m^2	1.5–2.3	2.4–2.6	2.7–2.9	>2.9
RA minor axis, cm	2.9–4.5	4.6–4.9	5.0–5.4	>5.4
RA minor axis/BSA, cm/m^2	1.7–2.5	2.6–2.8	2.9–3.1	>3.1
Atrial area				
LA area, cm^2	<20	20–30	31–40	>40
Atrial volume				
LA vol, mL	18–58	59–68	69–78	>78
LA vol/BSA, mL/m^2	**<29**	**29–33**	**34–39**	**>39**

BSA, Body surface area. Bold rows identify best validated measures

Atrial septum

Descriptive terms

Atrial septal defect
- Absent, present.
- Location (primum, secundum, sinus venosus).
- Size (dimensions in two planes).
- Shunt (left-to-right, right-to-left, bidirectional).
- Qp/Qs.

Patent foramen ovale
- Absent, present.

Contrast study
- Normal, shunt present (small, <5 bubbles; moderate, 5–20 bubbles; large, >20 bubbles).

Prosthetic valves

Descriptive terms

Type
- Mechanical (tilting disk/bileaflet/ball and cage/other).
- Bioprosthesis (stented xenograft/homograft/stentless).
- Autograft (Ross)/other).
- Manufacturer and size.
- Annuloplasty ring, valve repair.

Sewing ring
Well seated, rocking, dehisced.

Occluder mechanism
- Normal, thickened leaflets (bioprosthesis).
- Normal mobility, restricted mobility, flail.

Abnormal masses
- Strand(s), microcavitations, pannus, thrombus.
- Vegetation (+description), abscess (+description), fistula.

Stenosis
Present, severity (as for native valve).

Regurgitation
- Physiological, prosthetic, para-prosthetic.
- Severity (as for native valve).

Prosthetic valve velocities

Table 7.14 provides a guide to maximal expected velocities for different valve types. Refer to manufacturer guidelines for definitive measures and take into account the clinical scenario. Velocities depend on left ventricle function, volume, and inotropic status. Therefore minimal gradients are not presented. In individual cases the threshold may be exceeded with a functionally normal prosthesis—in particular if there is a hyperdynamic state.

Table 7.14 Maximum prosthetic velocities from normal Doppler data

AORTIC PROSTHETIC VALVES						
Bileaflet valve (e.g. St Jude)						
Size (mm)	19	21	23	25	27	29
Vmax (m/sec)	4.5	3.5	3.5	3.5	3.1	2.5
Tilting disc (e.g. Medtronic Hall, BS)						
Size (mm)	—	21	23	25	27	29
Vmax (m/sec)	—	3.7	3.0	2.4	2.1	2.1
Ball and cage (e.g. Starr–Edwards)						
Vmax (m/sec)	3.6					
Bioprostheses (e.g. Hancock, Carpentier Edwards)						
Size (mm)	19	21	23	25	27	29
Vmax (m/sec)	3.5	3.0	3.0	2.9	2.9	2.5
MITRAL PROSTHETIC VALVES						
Bileaflet valve (e.g. St Jude)						
Size (mm)	19	21	23	25	27	29
Vmax (m/sec)	4.5	3.5	3.5	3.5	3.1	2.5
Tilting disc (e.g. Medtronic Hall, BS)						
Size (mm)	—	21	23	25	27	29
Vmax (m/sec)	—	3.7	3.0	2.4	2.1	2.1
Ball and cage (e.g. Starr–Edwards)						
Vmax (m/sec)	3.6					
Bioprostheses (e.g. Hancock, Carpentier Edwards)						
Size (mm)	19	21	23	25	27	29
Vmax (m/sec)	3.5	3.0	3.0	2.9	2.9	2.5

Pericardium

Descriptive terms

Appearance
Normal, abnormal.

Effusion
- Absent, present.
- Size (small/moderate/large).
- Location:
  - circumferential;
  - localized (near... left ventricle, right ventricle, left atrium, right atrium).
- Appearance/content (clear fluid, fibrinous, focal strands/masses, effusive-constrictive

Thickening/calcification
Absent, present.

Mass
Absent, present.

Haemodynamic effects
- Septal bounce.
- Chamber collapse (absent/present + chamber).
- Increased respiratory variation (absent, present + location).
- Compatible with tamponade or constrictive.

Pericardial fluid

Table 7.15 Assessment of pericardial effusion based on thickness and volume

	TRACE	MILD	MODERATE	SEVERE
Thickness (cm)	<0.5	0.5–1	1–2	>2
Volume (mL)	50–100	100–250	250–500	>500

Aorta

Descriptive terms

Appearance
Normal, abnormal.

Dilatation
- Absent, present (mild/moderate/severe).
- Location and dimensions:
  - dilated atrioventricular annulus;
  - dilated aortic root/sinuses;
  - dilated sinotubular ridge;
  - dilated ascending aorta;
  - dilated transverse aorta;
  - dilated descending thoracic aorta;
  - dilated abdominal aorta.

Aneurysm
- Absent, sinuses of Valsalva (left/right/non-coronary).
- Aortic root, ascending aorta, transverse aorta.
- Descending thoracic aorta, abdominal aorta.
- Dimensions, type (fusiform, saccular).
- Ruptured sinus of Valsalva (to right atrium, right ventricle, left atrium, left ventricle).

Atheroma/thrombus
- Absent, present.
- Location (aortic root, ascending aorta, transverse aorta, descending thoracic aorta, abdominal aorta).
- Appearance (layered/mural, protruding, ulcer).
- Severity (mild/moderate/severe).
- Mobility (immobile/mobile).
- Graft (prosthetic/homograft) + location.

Dissection
- Location, entry point, exit point(s).
- False lumen thrombus (absent/partial/present).
- Stanford type A or B.
- Intramural haematoma and location.
- Transection and location.

Coarctation
- Absent, repaired/residual, present.
- Severity (mild/moderate/severe).
- Measurements (minimum diameter, gradient).

Aortic size

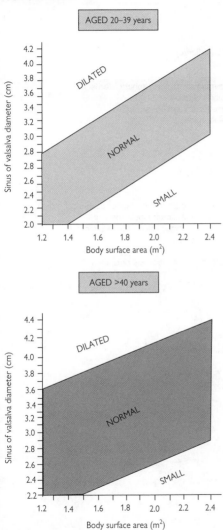

Fig. 7.1 Ranges of normal sinus of Valsalva size according to age.

Masses

Descriptive terms

Thrombus
- Absent, present.
- Size (small/moderate/large).
- Location.
- Description:
  - shape (flat or mural/protruding/spherical/other);
  - surface (regular/irregular);
  - texture (layered/solid/part solid/calcified);
  - mobility (mobile/fixed).
- Dimensions.

Tumour
- Absent, present.
- Size (small/moderate/large).
- Location.
- Description:
  - shape (flat or mural/pedunculated/papillary/spherical/other);
  - surface (regular/irregular/multilobular/other);
  - texture (solid/layered/cystic/calcified/heterogeneous);
  - mobility (mobile/fixed).
- Dimensions.
- Type (suggestive of myxoma, fibroelastoma, etc.).

Endocarditis

Descriptive terms

Vegetation
- Valvular/mural mass consistent with a vegetation.
- Location (atrial or ventricular side of valves, ventricular...).
- Mobility (non-mobile, mobile, pedunculated).
- Size (small, moderate, large).
- Dimensions.

Abscess
- Perivalvular or valvular cavity suggesting abscess.
- Location (annulus, right coronary cusp, etc.).
- Size (small, moderate, large).
- Dimensions.

Fistula
- From... to ...
- Size/haemodynamically relevant.

Severity of valvular lesion See native valves.

Pericardial effusion See pericardial disease.

Index